Atlas of
Skeletal Muscle
Pathology

Current Histopathology

Consultant Editor
Professor G. Austin Gresham, TD, ScD, MD, FRC Path.
Professor of Morbid Anatomy and Histology, University of Cambridge

Volume Nine

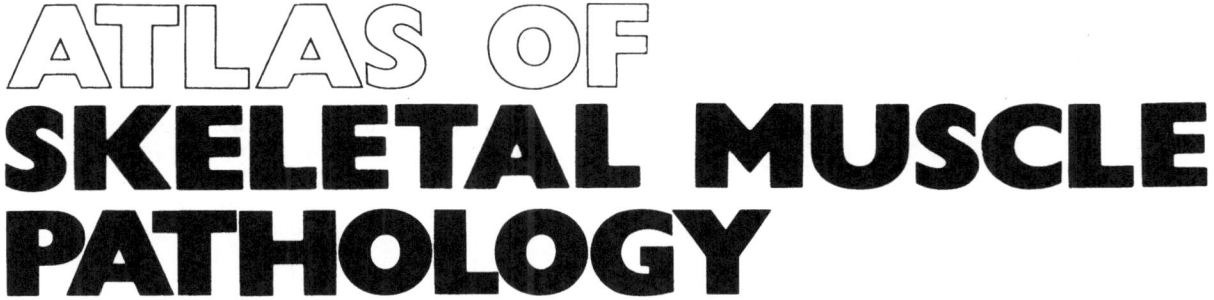

ATLAS OF SKELETAL MUSCLE PATHOLOGY

BY JANICE R. ANDERSON

Consultant Histopathologist
Department of Morbid Anatomy and Histopathology
Addenbrooke's Hospital
Cambridge

Springer-Science+Business Media, B.V.

Published by
MTP Press Limited
Falcon House
Queen Square
Lancaster, England

British Library Cataloguing in Publication Data

Anderson, Janice R.
  Atlas of skeletal muscle pathology.—(Current
histopathology; v. 9)
  1. Muscles—Diseases
  I. Title   II. Series
  616.7′407   RC925.5

ISBN 978-94-010-8653-0   ISBN 978-94-009-4866-2 (eBook)
DOI 10.1007/978-94-009-4866-2

Library of Congress Cataloging in Publication Data

Anderson, Janice R.
  Atlas of skeletal muscle pathology.

  Includes bibliographies and index.
  1. Striated muscle—Biopsy—Atlases. 2. Striated
muscle—Diseases—Diagnosis—Atlases. 3. Histochemistry—Atlases. 4. Diagnosis, Cytologic— Atlases.
I. Title. [DNLM: 1. Muscular Diseases—pathology—
atlases. W1 CU788JBA v.9/WE 17 A5468a]
RC 925.5.A53 1985   616.7′407′58   85–2956

Phototypesetting by Georgia Origination, Liverpool.
Colour origination by Tradescanning Limited,
Stockport.
Printed by Cradley Print PLC, Warley, W. Midlands.

Contents

Current Histopathology Series

Consultant Editor's Note

At the present time books on morbid anatomy and histology can be divided into two broad groups: extensive textbooks often written primarily for students and monographs on research topics.

This takes no account of the fact that the vast majority of pathologists are involved in an essentially practical field of general Diagnostic Pathology providing an important service to their clinical colleagues. Many of these pathologists are expected to cover a broad range of disciplines and even those who remain solely within the field of histopathology usually have single and sole responsibility within the hospital for all this work. They may often have no chance for direct discussion on problem cases with colleagues in the same department. In the field of histopathology, no less than in other medical fields, there have been extensive and recent advances, not only in new histochemical techniques but also in the type of specimen provided by new surgical procedures.

There is a great need for the provision of appropriate information for this group. This need has been defined in the following terms.

(1) It should be aimed at the general clinical pathologist or histopathologist with existing practical training, but should also have value for the trainee pathologist.
(2) It should concentrate on the practical aspects of histopathology taking account of the new techniques which should be within the compass of the worker in a unit with reasonable facilities.
(3) New types of material, e.g. those derived from endoscopic biopsy should be covered fully.
(4) There should be an adequate number of illustrations on each subject to demonstrate the variation in appearance that is encountered.
(5) Colour illustrations should be used wherever they aid recognition.

The present concept stemmed from this definition but it was immediately realized that these aims could only be achieved within the compass of a series, of which this volume is one. Since histopathology is, by its very nature, systemized, the individual volumes deal with one system or where this appears more appropriate with a single organ.

This atlas of muscle pathology is a valuable addition to the *Current Histopathology* series. It reflects the increasing use of new methods in diagnostic work and illustrates the importance of proper sample preparation and full clinicopathological correlation in achieving diagnostic success. Histochemical reactions of muscle are well illustrated here and different enzyme reaction patterns are shown in serial sections. Electron micrographs are included when they assist diagnosis. Careful consultation with clinicians is essential for accurate diagnosis: this information is provided by detailed clinical information accompanying the photomicrographs.

Methods of diagnostic histopathology are frequently changing. New methods are appearing, old ones are being refined and the role of the histopathologist as part of the clinical team is increasingly emphasized. The changing scene is well illustrated by this excellent addition to the series.

G. Austin Gresham
Cambridge

Foreword

With the advent of enzyme histochemistry, which revealed hitherto unseen pathological differences between muscle disorders, muscle biopsy assumed an important diagnostic role. The investigation is easily performed and is being undertaken with increasing frequency. Nevertheless there is still a tendency to regard its interpretation as highly specialized and outside the province of the general histopathologist. In this atlas I have tried to lift the veil of neuropathological mystique and to describe and illustrate the basic reactions of muscle cells.

Interpretation of the biopsy depends not only upon recognition of morphological abnormalities, but upon understanding why they occur. Throughout the atlas I have attempted to correlate morphological changes with pathogenetic mechanisms. Undoubtedly new ideas will emerge from the current research activities in this field and simplistic theories will be expanded or discarded.

Diseased muscle cells, as any other cell type, show only limited morphological changes. However bizarre, very few of these changes, if any, are pathognomonic of a single disease. The exact significance of microscopic findings is to a large extent determined by their clinical context. Thus, although this is an atlas, it is definitely not designed to promote 'spot' histological diagnoses. I have aimed to provide a guide to pathological reactions of muscle which will be useful to the practising histopathologist and all students of neuro-muscular disease. I hope that recognition of the lack of specificity of individual morphological features will encourage the close clinico-pathological correlation which is essential for every correct diagnosis and for greater understanding of the complex neuro-muscular diseases.

Acknowledgements

I would like to express my thanks to everyone who has helped me to prepare this atlas. I am particularly grateful to Dr Dennis Harriman, who not only provided me with examples of malignant hyperpyrexia myopathy, but also was responsible initially for teaching me how to perform muscle biopsies and to interpret enzyme histochemistry. I am indebted to Dr Brian Lake who provided me with material from several of the rarer disorders of childhood, to Dr Sebastian Lucas for examples of parasitic myopathy and to Dr Peter Dennis for a case of a fibromatosis. My special thanks are due to Ms Maureen Taylor, without whose technical expertise a muscle biopsy service would never have been established in Cambridge; to Mr Graham Gatward for the preparation of sections for electron microscopy; to Mr Chris Burton for photographic advice and to Mrs Peggy Shipp for the arduous task of typing the manuscript. I am also extremely grateful to Dr Derek Wight for helping me to win my battle with the word processor and to my family for their patience and tolerance.

Technical Methods and Normal Parameters

Introduction

The application of histochemical techniques to skeletal muscle heralded a new era in muscle pathology. Whilst fibres appear uniform in formalin-fixed, paraffin-embedded tissue, in frozen sections enzyme histochemistry reveals a heterogeneous fibre population. Both physiological and pathological changes may be selective for one or other fibre type. The identification of different fibre types has therefore enhanced our understanding of skeletal muscle pathology and provided a valuable diagnostic tool. Electron microscopy, measurements of fibre size and biochemical analysis may give additional information. Muscle biopsy is a relatively simple procedure, but to obtain the maximum information it is essential firstly to select the most appropriate site for biopsy and secondly to handle the specimen correctly. Rough treatment of the fresh specimen, or misguided fixation, can destroy important diagnostic clues and introduce spectacular artifacts (Figures 1.1 and 1.2).

Clinicopathological Correlation

Muscle biopsy is only one of the essential investigations of patients with muscle disease and it must not be examined in isolation. Pathological changes can only be assessed properly with a knowledge of the patient's history, including family history and any drug history and the findings of a clinical, particularly neurological, examination. Changes in the biopsy should also be correlated with the results of electromyographic (EMG) examination and serum enzyme estimations, particularly the creatine phosphokinase (CPK). Thus when muscle biopsy is contemplated the need for close liaison between clinician and pathologist cannot be overemphasized.

Biopsy Site

Even progressive diseases which ultimately produce generalized weakness and wasting usually show early selectivity of certain groups. Ideally the muscle chosen for biopsy should be clinically involved, but not so severely wasted that it will be extensively replaced by fatty and fibrous connective tissue. The biopsy should be taken from the belly of the muscle and not close to the tendinous insertion as increased connective tissue and split fibres, which can mimic a myopathy, are normal findings in this location (Figure 1.3). Most of the larger limb muscles are accessible to biopsy, but the larger superficial proximal limb muscles, deltoid and quadriceps femoris are probably the easiest and safest

to biopsy, particularly with a blind needle biopsy, as there is little danger of damaging major nerves or blood vessels. Fortuitously these muscles are involved in many disorders, including Duchenne muscular dystrophy, congenital myopathies and polymyositis. However in others, such as myotonic dystrophy or Charcot–Marie–Tooth disease, a lower leg muscle may be more appropriate. In a few rare myopathies ophthalmoplegia is the paramount clinical sign, but biopsy of a proximal limb muscle will frequently establish the diagnosis. It is often useful to perform the EMG prior to muscle biopsy. EMG abnormalities may provide helpful guidance to an appropriate site for biopsy. This is particularly true of conditions like polymyositis where muscle involvement can be patchy and difficult to ascertain solely by clinical examination. The biopsy should never be taken from the exact point at which an EMG needle has been inserted as artifactual changes may be confused with genuine pathology. As most muscle diseases display at least approximate symmetry it is reasonable to carry out EMG studies on one side only and reserve the opposite limb for biopsy. Blood for CPK estimation should be collected before a biopsy as a temporary rise will probably follow.

Motor End-point Biopsy

Histological study of the terminal innervation by vital staining or silver impregnation can yield additional diagnostic information (Figure 1.4). It particularly assists the differentiation of chronic denervating and myopathic disease. Motor endplates are generally clustered near the midpoint of a muscle and at this point maximal twitch to minimal electrical stimulus is obtained. The site is first located by stimulation through the skin and then a fine electrode is applied to the surface of the exposed muscle.

Biopsy Technique and Handling the Specimen

The techniques of biopsy and of handling the specimen are the keys to successful results from a muscle biopsy. Muscle biopsy can be obtained by open biopsy through a small skin incision or by needle biopsy[1,2]. Needles of different gauges are available, suitable for patients of different ages with varying muscle bulk (Figure 1.5). There are advantages and disadvantages of both methods and which is most appropriate is best decided in the individual case. Needle biopsy is the quickest, easily performed in outpatients and more than one site can be examined in a stoical patient. The disadvantages are that the sample is tiny, difficult to orientate and even in experienced hands muscle is not always obtained.

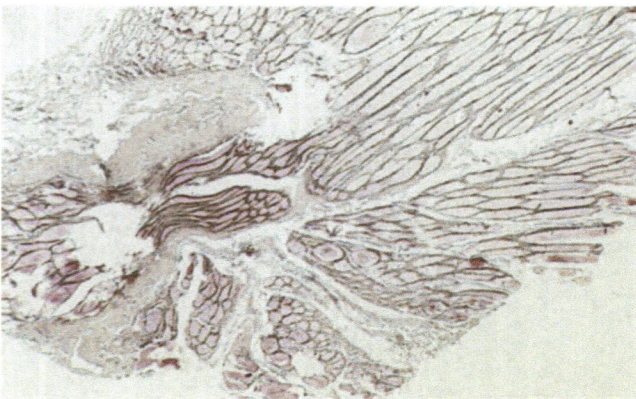

Figure 1.1 Crush artifact. The specimen has been severely distorted by rough surgical handling. Correct orientation is impossible and the fibres appear to be all different shapes and sizes. In this preparation the shape of fibres is revealed by the connective tissue framework.   Gordon and Sweet's stain for reticulin × 30

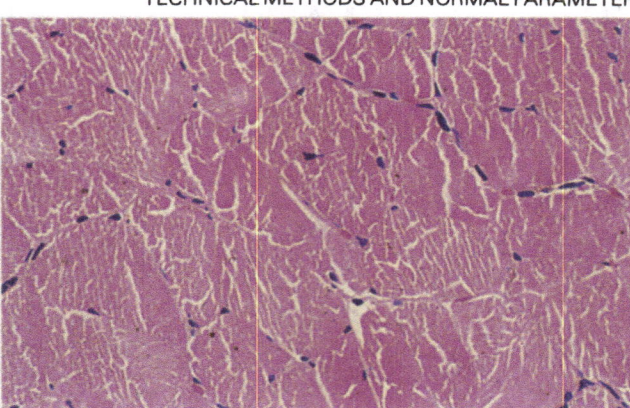

Figure 1.2 Formalin fixed muscle. The cytoplasm appears 'cracked', an artifact which obscures cytoplasmic detail.   H & E × 180

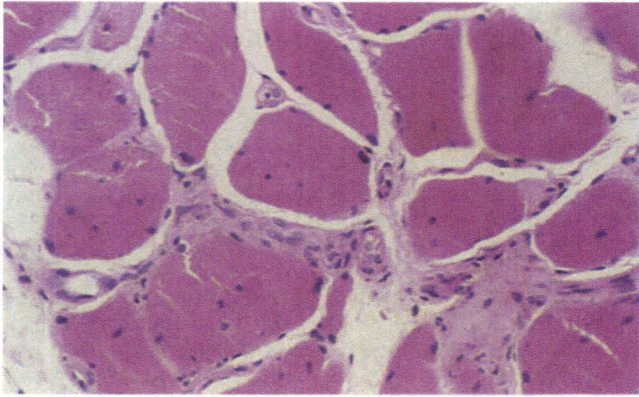

Figure 1.3 Tendon insertion of a limb muscle, showing variation in fibre size, central nuclei and interstitial fibrosis. This is a completely normal appearance at this site.   H & E × 180

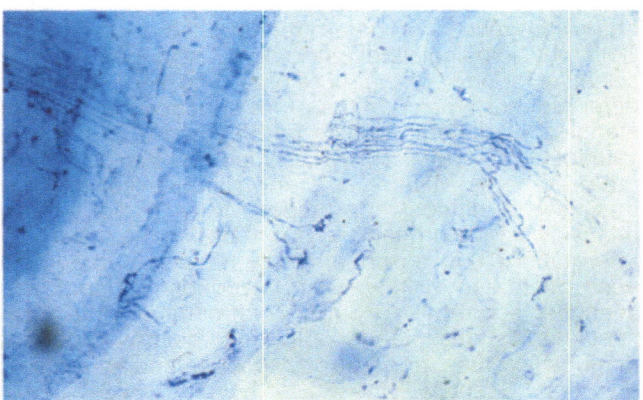

Figure 1.4 Nerve endings obtained by motor end point biopsy and demonstrated by methylene blue vital staining. Nerve endings will rarely be found in a biopsy, unless the motor end point is first identified by electrical stimulation.   Methylene blue vital staining × 75

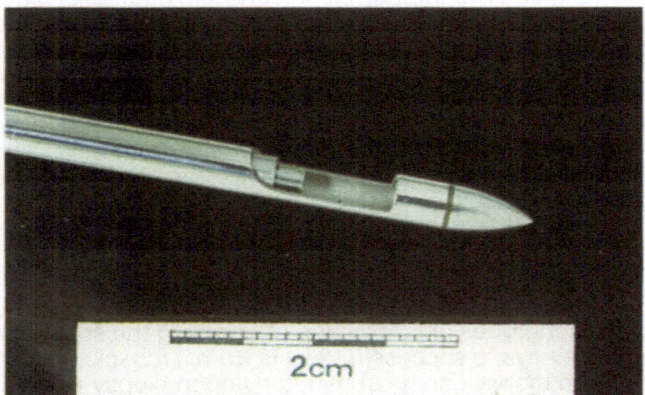

Figure 1.5 Bergström muscle biopsy needle. A small skin incision is made with a scalpel and the needle is firmly pushed into muscle with the window closed. Once inserted into the muscle the window is opened by withdrawing the inner cylinder and the muscle bulges into the gap. The inner cylinder, which has a cutting edge, is then pushed quickly downward, biting off a small piece of muscle. The central rod, shown in the picture, is used to dislodge the specimen and is only inserted after the needle has been withdrawn

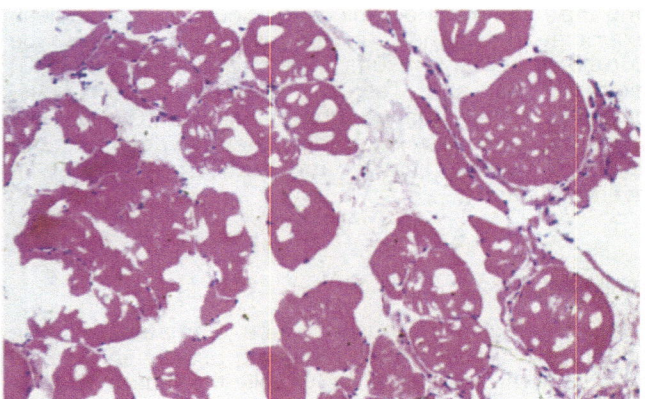

Figure 1.6 Ice crystal artifact in muscle which has been frozen slowly in liquid nitrogen. There is gross distortion of fibre architecture and the appearance can mimic a vacuolar myopathy. Compare this with the muscle that has been snap frozen in isopentane, shown in Figure 1.7.   H & E × 180

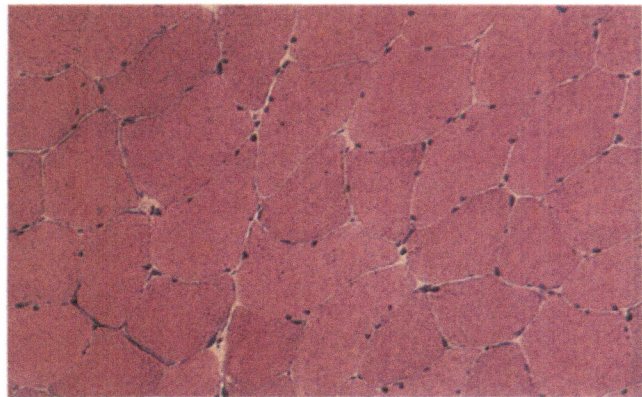

Figure 1.7 Normal adult muscle. There is little variation in size and shape of fibres. The sarcolemmal nuclei are relatively inconspicuous and situated peripherally. The fibres in a fascicle fit closely together with no intervening fibrous connective tissue. In a good frozen section it may be possible to distinguish type 1 and 2 fibres even with an H & E stain as type 1 fibres are more darkly stained. H & E × 180, cryostat section

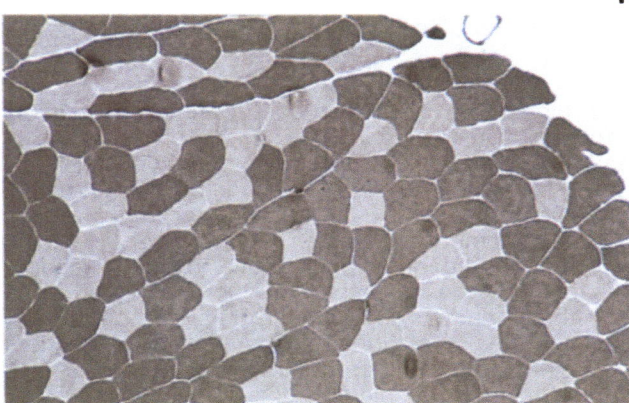

Figure 1.8 Myofibrillar (myosin) ATP-ase with preincubation at pH 9.4. Normal adult muscle showing clear differentiation of type 1 fibres (light) and type 2 fibres (dark). × 75 serial sections shown in Figures 1.9 and 1.10

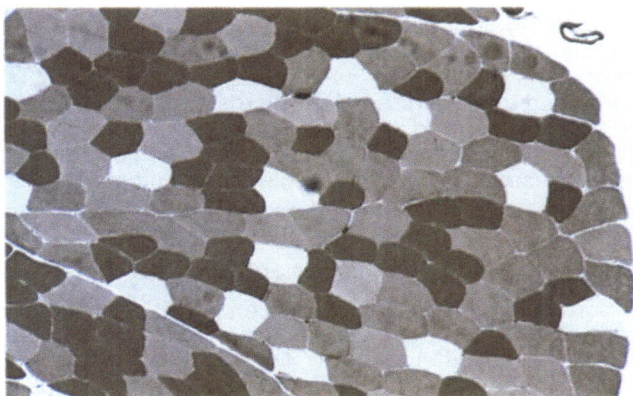

Figure 1.9 Myofibrillar ATP-ase with preincubation at pH 4.6 permits a subdivision of type 2 fibres into type 2A (light) and type 2B (grey). Type 1 fibres are darkly stained. × 75

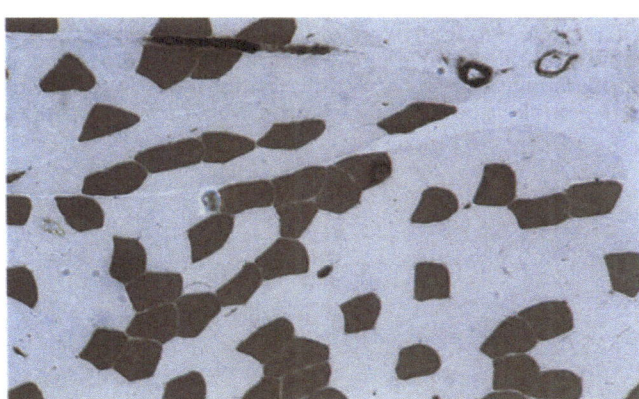

Figure 1.10 Myofibrillar ATP-ase with preincubation at pH 4.3. There is a reversal of the reaction shown in Figure 1.8. Type 1 fibres are strongly reactive and stain darkly, whereas type 2 show no activity and are pale. × 75

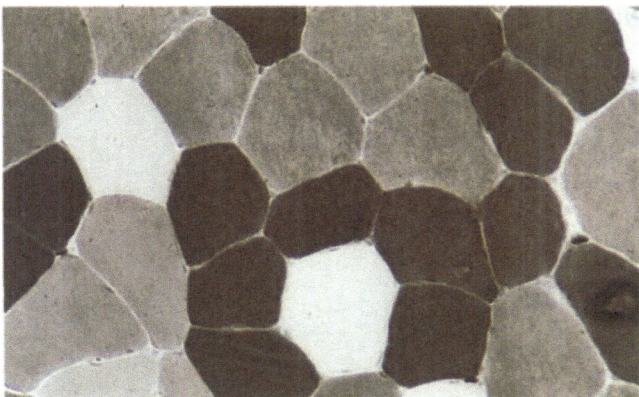

Figure 1.11 The normal mosaic pattern created by the different fibre types in normal human limb muscle. Fibres from at least 3 separate motor units are shown in this section. The intermingling of fibres from adjacent motor units is responsible for the normal mosaic pattern. Myosin ATP-ase at pH 4.6, × 180

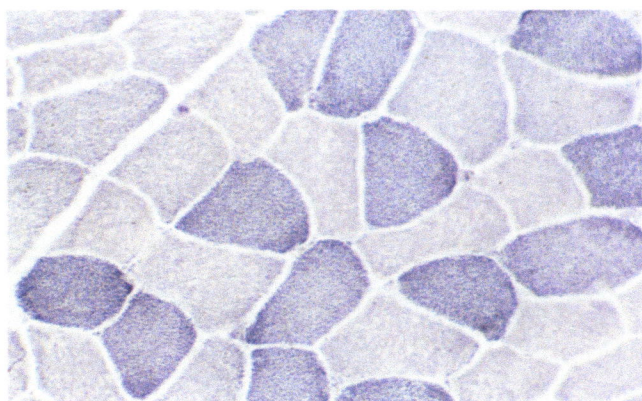

Figure 1.12 Oxidative enzyme activity. NADH-TR reaction. Type 1 fibres show greatest activity and are more darkly stained. Type 2 fibres have less activity and are light. NADH-TR × 180

Open biopsy has the advantages of ensuring that the specimen is definitely muscle and provides a larger sample that is easy to orientate. It will, however, leave a small scar which is undesirable particularly in a growing child. Open biopsy is essential if motor endplates are sought. Both methods are easily performed under local anaesthetic. A general anaesthetic is rarely needed, perhaps only on occasion in young children. The anaesthetist and surgeon should be aware of the risk, albeit remote, of malignant hyperpyrexia in a patient with an undiagnosed muscle disorder (see chapter 10).

In an open biopsy diathermy is usually unnecessary and should certainly be avoided close to the surface of the muscle. Ideally the surgeon should remove about three small cylinders of muscle (each approximately 0.3 × 1.5 cm). These are readily obtained if the course of the muscle fascicles is defined before cutting into the muscle. Small cylinders are easier to handle and to orientate than a large chunk and indeed huge pieces and large incisions are quite unnecessary. Some operators prefer to clamp the two ends of the specimen before excision[3]. This method has certain advantages, in that the muscle can be frozen whilst held in the clamp and is thus maintained at *in vivo* resting length. However it does usually require a slightly longer incision and with care equally good results can be obtained with simple excision.

Once it is obtained the viable muscle should be handled as little as possible before freezing because the naturally irritable tissue will tend to hypercontract. A very thin cylinder should be first removed and fixed for electron microscopy. The specimen for histochemistry should be orientated to produce a block from which true transverse sections can be obtained (Diagram 1.1). A rapid freezing method is required to prevent the formation of ice crystals which grossly distort the fibres and sometimes mimic a genuine vacuolar myopathy (Figures 1.6 and 1.7).

Direct immersion in liquid nitrogen, widely used for general surgical biopsies, such as breast, is not suitable for skeletal muscle. A technique that is generally successful for open biopsy specimens, and that also avoids hypercontraction, is to transfix the muscle cylinder with two fine needles (e.g. intramuscular injection needles) inserted into a piece of rubber, and immerse the whole specimen in isopentane, cooled almost to freezing point (Diagram 1.2). The muscle will freeze instantly and afterwards must only be handled with cold instruments. If it is touched by hand, or even with instruments at room temperature, it will thaw slightly and the results will be far from perfect. Tiny specimens obtained by needle biopsy must usually be orientated under a dissecting microscope and then can be frozen supported in a viscous freezing medium, such as OCT. It is advisable always to freeze and keep aside a separate small piece for possible biochemical analysis.

Biopsy – Routine Techniques and Normal Parameters

In normal human muscle various enzyme histochemical reactions reveal different staining intensities in individual fibres. These differences in enzyme profile correlate with different physiological properties. The simplest classification, which has gained wide acceptance, is based on the myofibrillar ATP-ase reaction[4,5] (Figures 1.8–1.10). This enzyme exhibits variable pH sensitivity. At alkaline pH there are two clearly defined fibre populations. The lighter-staining fibres with least

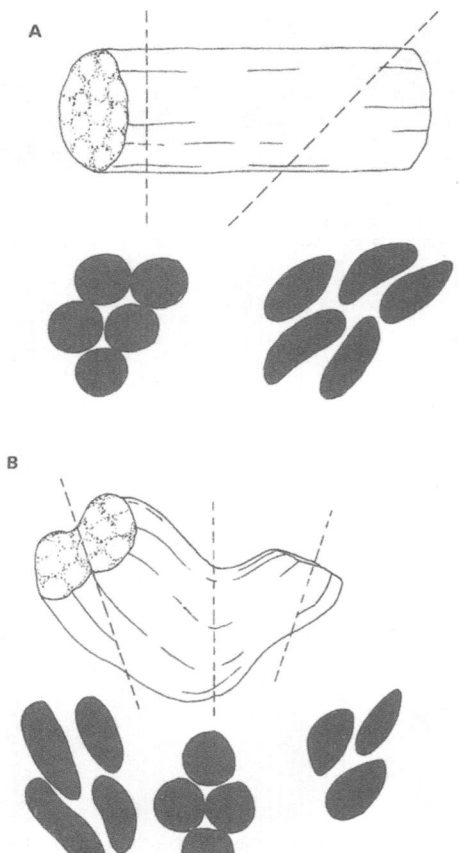

Diagram 1.1 These diagrams illustrate the need to obtain true transverse sections in order to make measurements and comparisons of fibre diameters. **A:** Slanted sections through a cylinder of muscle produce elongated and oval outlines; **B:** when the specimen is not correctly orientated and a curled cylinder is sectioned, all manner of shapes and sizes of fibres will appear.

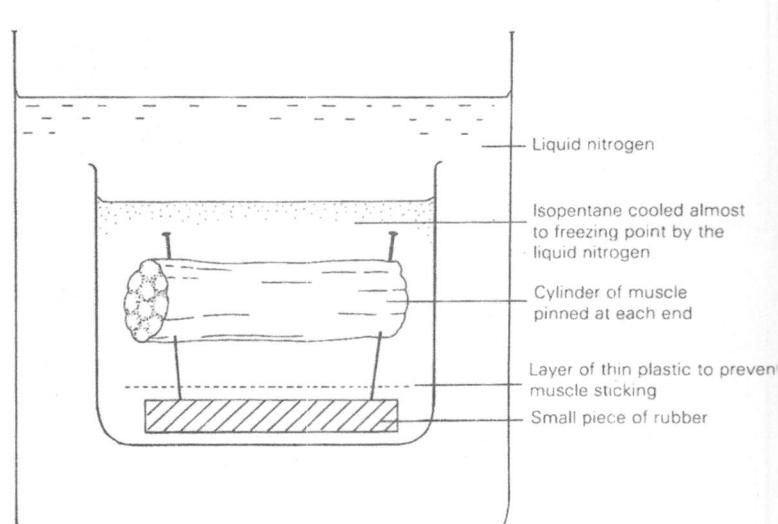

Liquid nitrogen

Isopentane cooled almost to freezing point by the liquid nitrogen

Cylinder of muscle pinned at each end

Layer of thin plastic to prevent muscle sticking

Small piece of rubber

Diagram 1.2 Rapid freezing method

activity are slow-twitch fibres, also termed type 1 (Figure 1.8). The darker-staining fibres with greater activity are fast-twitch – type 2 fibres. Type 1 fibres are also strongly reactive with oxidative enzymes, such as NADH-TR, but show a weaker reaction with PAS and phosphorylase. Type 2 fibres show a reversal of these activities. Type 2 fibres can be further subdivided with pH modification of the ATP-ase reaction (Figure 1.9). Thus type 2 fibres which lose activity at pH 4.8–4.6 are type 2A, whereas others which maintain activity down to pH 4.3 are type 2B. Type 2A have a greater oxidative capacity and are sometimes referred to as fast-oxidative-glycolytic, and 2B as fast glycolytic. The fatiguability of the different fibre types correlates with oxidative capacity, high oxidative capacity conferring greater resistance to fatigue[6]. In the neonate an additional fibre type can be identified showing myo-fibrillar ATP-ase activity over a wide range, pH 10–4.3. These have been called type 2C fibres, but in reality are undifferentiated fibres, which mature in the first year of life[7]. Very few are found in normal adult muscle. Undoubtedly this classification is an oversimplification[8], nevertheless it reflects different physiological and pathological states, is readily reproducible and therefore of considerable diagnostic value.

It has become increasingly apparent that fibre typing, beginning in the last 3 months of gestation and completed in the first year, is not immutable. This property of muscle fibres is not intrinsic, but dictated by the electrical input from the motor nerve[9]. Cross-innervation experiments in animals have revealed that a change in innervation can induce fibre type conversion[10]. This phenomenon may occur naturally in man when reinnervation takes place after injury or during a chronic neurogenic disease. Muscle fibres also exhibit great plasticity in response to exercise and hormonal stimuli, such as thyroid hormones[8,11]. Metabolic adaptations are reflected by changes in the enzyme profile. It is uncertain whether complete fibre type conversion can be induced by physical training, but there may be a shift in fibre type proportions as demonstrated by the routine histochemical techniques[12].

The muscle fibres supplied by a single motor nerve form a functional unit, THE MOTOR UNIT. The component fibres contract synchronously and show uniform histo-chemical reactions[13]. The fibres of individual motor units are not tightly clumped together, but interdigitate with those of adjacent units (see Diagram 1.3). In human limb muscles all three fibre types (i.e. Type 1, 2A and 2B) are normally present and the intermingling of the motor units creates a mosaic histochemical pattern (Figure 1.11). This is the normal picture in all human limb muscles. Large groups, i.e. more than about 25 fibres, of uniform type, are usually patho-logical and indicate that a change in fibre type has occurred. This is most often a consequence of reinnervation of denervated fibres. Smaller uniform groups are not always of pathological significance. The preponderance of one or other fibre type does vary between different muscles and between the same muscles of different individuals[14,15]. In muscles with a marked predominance of one fibre type (e.g. the soleus muscle may contain 80% of type 1 fibres), larger numbers of the dominant fibre will lie in closer apposition than in muscles with equal fibre type proportions. Sections of whole muscles at post-mortem have shown there is considerable variation in the composition of different parts of a muscle[16]. The sig-nificance of fibre type grouping is best determined by comparison with the surrounding pattern. Interpretation may be difficult in a tiny biopsy[17].

Further Staining Reactions

The reactions for oxidative enzymes, such as NADH-TR and succinic dehydrogenase, not only distinguish fast and slow fibres, but also highlight cell organelles, particularly mitochondria and display the orderly cyto-architecture[5] (Figures 1.12 and 1.13). The periodic Schiff stain (PAS) is used to detect glycogen (Figure 1.14), and lipid droplets can be demonstrated with the Oil red O stain (Figure 1.15). Gormori's trichrome method[18] applied to unfixed frozen sections is particularly valuable for the demonstration of cytoarchi-tectural disturbances with an increase in the intermyo-fibrillar constituents, such as mitochondria or inclusions such as nemaline rods (Figure 1.16). Histochemical methods are available for demonstration of myophos-phorylase and phosphofructokinase[5], but these are not essential routine requirements (Figures 1.17 and 1.18). These reactions should be performed in anyone with a history of undue fatiguability, and it would seem sensible to perform them in any young patient with an undiagnosed muscle disorder. The histochemical stain for acid phosphatase[5] may elucidate mechanisms of cell degeneration. Acid phosphatase activity correlates with lysosomal activity, which in skeletal muscle includes membranous structures derived from the sarcoplasmic reticulum as well as conventional lysosomes.

Fibre Size

Fibre atrophy and abnormal hypertrophy are important indicators of disease. Fibre size can be accurately assessed from fibre diameter, but only in genuine trans-verse sections taken at right angles to the long axis of the fibre, hence the emphasis on careful orientation of specimen. Slanted sections produce oval and elongated fibre outlines (Diagram 1.1). There is a wide range of normal fibre sizes, dependent on age, sex and physical activity. Fibre diameters gradually enlarge throughout childhood reaching adult proportions in early 'teens[19]. In the normal child type 1, 2A and 2B fibres are fairly uniform in size[20]. In adults, particularly in men, type 2A and 2B fibres are frequently slightly larger than type 1, whereas in women the reverse may be found[21]. However, in a normal muscle, fibres of the same histo-chemical type are approximately equal in size. Fibre size varies between different muscles of the same individual as well as between different people. There are also differences in the diameters of fixed and frozen muscle, with variation according to the technique employed. In general, excess variability of fibre size within a single biopsy is the most significant finding and always patho-logical, whereas variation between different muscle or even sequential biopsies may have other explanations.

Gross abnormalities of fibre size are easily recognized by simple inspection, but more subtle changes can be confirmed by actual measurements of fibre diameters, using a micrometer eyepiece or less laboriously an image analyser. Congenital fibre type disproportion is an example of a myopathy that usually presents in early childhood and has been defined solely on the basis of small type 1 fibres[22].

Electron Microscopy

Electron microscopy can be a useful adjunct to light microscopy, provided its limitations are recognized. A biopsy is only a small sample, but the amount of tissue that can reasonably be examined by EM is comparatively minute. Artifacts, particularly disruption of myofibrils, are easily introduced unless the tissue is

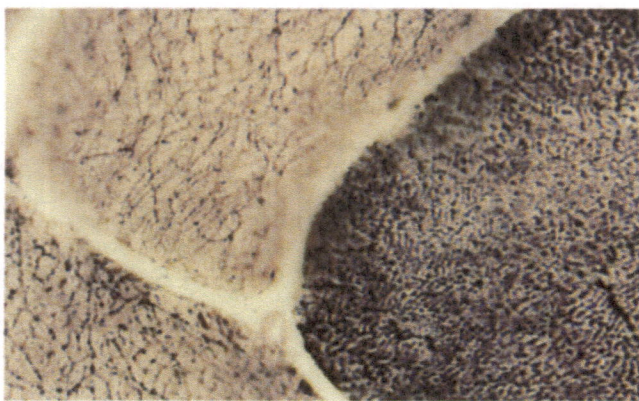

Figure 1.13 Oxidative enzyme activity is predominantly located in the mitochondria. Thus at high magnification these organelles are visible as small darkly stained dots. The intermyofibrillar network, but not the myofibrils, is stained in this reaction, which therefore reveals the orderly cytoplasmic architecture of normal fibres. NADH-TR × 750

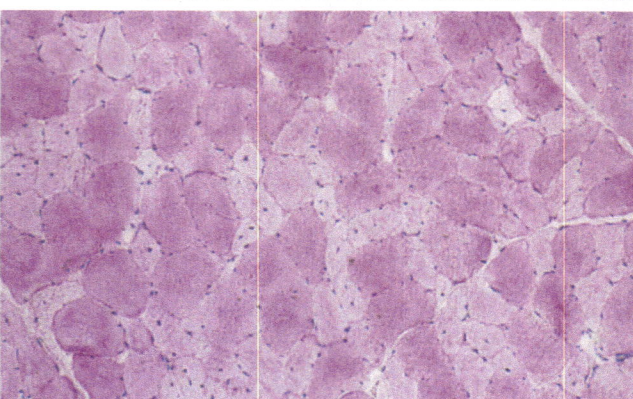

Figure 1.14 Periodic acid Schiff (PAS) stain for glycogen. Glycogen content is greatest in type 2 fibres, stained deep pink. This biopsy is from a case of myotonic dystrophy, in which the type 1 fibres are uniformly smaller than type 2 and also contain central nuclei. A great increase in cytoplasmic glycogen may be demonstrable in certain glycogen storage disorders. PAS × 75

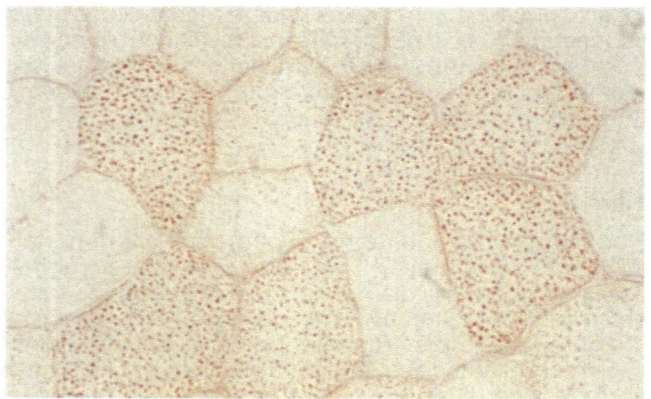

Figure 1.15 Oil red O stain for neutral lipid. Lipid droplets are stained red. In normal muscle only faint, minute dots are visible in type 1 fibres. This biopsy shows an abnormal accumulation of lipid in a patient with carnitine deficiency. Increased lipid is also seen in patients receiving steroid therapy and in myopathy associated with chronic alcoholism. Oil red O × 300

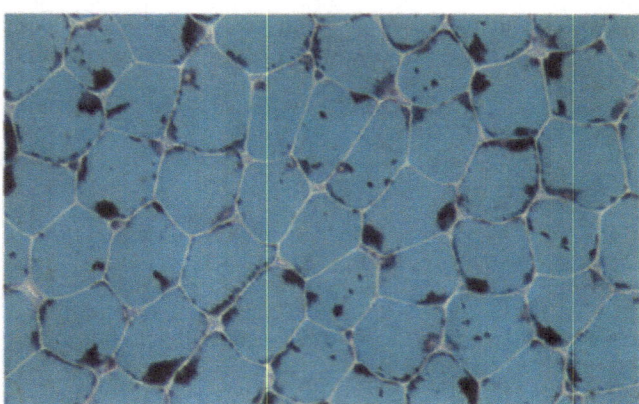

Figure 1.16 Gomori's trichrome method applied to cryostat sections. Intermyofibrillar constituents stain purplish-red. This biopsy shows an accumulation of nemaline rods in a child with a nemaline myopathy. These abnormal cytoplasmic bodies are barely visible with haematoxylin and eosin and are not revealed by the histochemical stains. Gomori's trichrome × 180

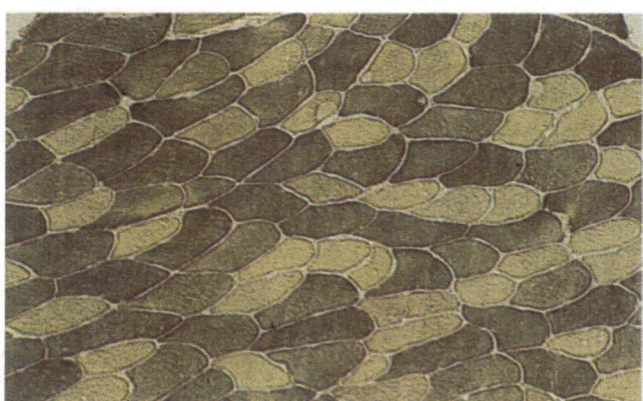

Figure 1.17 Histochemical demonstration of myophosphorylase. Activity is greatest in type 2 fibres, which show bluish-grey cytoplasm. A negative result is obtained in patients with McArdle's disease – myophosphorylase deficiency. × 75

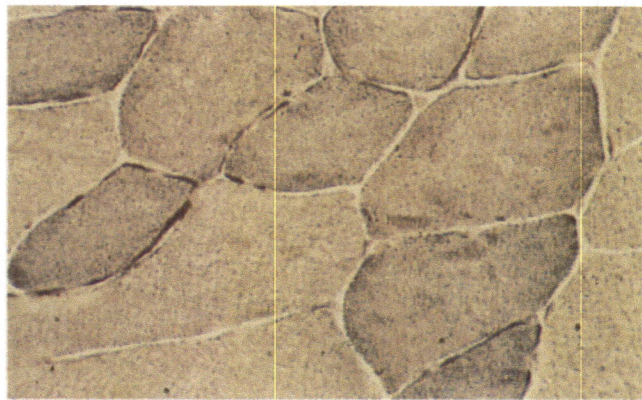

Figure 1.18 Histochemical demonstration of phosphofructokinase. The reaction is strongest in type 2 fibres (bluish-grey). This histochemical method is not a routine requirement. A negative result is obtained in patients with phosphofructokinase deficiency. The clinical picture of this disorder is very similar to McArdle's disease. The possibility should be considered in anyone with a history of undue fatiguability. × 300

very carefully fixed. Most light microscopic changes are not specific for any one disease and this is even more true at the subcellular level. There are fine structural differences between fast- and slow-twitch fibres in man. The Z bands are wider and there is a greater mitochondrial volume. However the differences are not so great as to make fibre typing at the ultrastructural level a practical possibility[23]. Despite these limitations the discovery of morphological abnormalities in cell organelles may assist in diagnosis. For example in certain metabolic disorders mitochondria are large and misshapen. In a few cases, deficiency of a specific mitochondrial enzyme has been proven by biochemical analysis[24].

Biochemical Analysis

This is not a routine requirement. It is only necessary when the clinical and pathological findings suggest a metabolic myopathy. A few of the rare enzyme deficiencies, for example myophosphorylase and phosphofructokinase deficiency, can be diagnosed from a negative histochemical reaction in tissue sections. For other glycogen storage diseases, such as acid maltase deficiency, and disorders of lipid metabolism, such as carnitine palmitoyl transferase deficiency, no such methods are available and these enzymes must be estimated by biochemical analysis of frozen tissue. Unfortunately some of the more recently identified mitochondrial enzyme defects, e.g. cytochrome oxidase deficiency, cannot be detected in a frozen specimen and further fresh tissue must be obtained. Almost certainly further enzyme deficiencies involving muscle have yet to be discovered.

Biopsy – Pathological Changes

Muscle, as all tissue, shows only limited responses to disease. Morphological changes are rarely disease-specific. The diagnosis rests upon the summation of changes in fibre size and fibre type distribution, abnormalities of cell architecture and changes in the interstitium, particularly inflammation and fibrosis. The pathologist must interpret these findings against the background of wide normal variation. Traditionally muscle disorders are categorized as NEUROGENIC when changes in muscle are secondary to disease of the lower motor neuron, and MYOPATHIC when the muscle cell itself is the primary pathological target. This is undoubtedly an oversimplification of the complex interrelationship between motor nerve and muscle. It is, for example, difficult to classify some of the more recently identified congenital myopathies, in which abnormal neurotrophic influences are suspected, but definite pathological changes have not been identified in the neuron. Nevertheless it is still a useful concept with good clinico-pathological and EMG correlation.

References

1. Edwards, R. H. T., Maunder, C., Lewis, P. D. and Pearce, A. G. E. (1973). Percutaneous needle biopsy in the diagnosis of muscle diseases. *Lancet*, **2**, 1070–71

2. Edwards, R. H. T. and Maunder, C. (1977). Muscle biopsy. *Hospital Update*, **3**, 569–81

3. Harriman, D. G. F. (1976). Muscle. In Blackwood, W. and Corsellis, J. A. N. (eds.) *Greenfield's Neuropathology* (London: Edward Arnold), 3rd edn.

4. Brooke, M. H. and Kaiser, K. K. (1974). The use and abuse of muscle histochemistry. *Ann N. Y. Acad. Sci.*, **228**, 121–44

5. Filipe, M. I. and Lake, B. D. (1983). Enzymes. In *Histochemistry in Pathology*. (Edinburgh: Churchill Livingstone), pp. 318–32

6. Kugelberg, E. and Lindgren, B. (1979). Transmission and contraction fatigue of rat motor units in relation to succinate dehydrogenase activity of motor unit fibres. *J. Physiol. (Lond.)*, **288**, 285–300

7. Colling-Saltin, A.-S. (1978). Enzyme histochemistry on skeletal muscle of the human foetus. *J. Neurol Sci.*, **39**, 169–85

8. Saltin, B., Henriksson, J., Nygaard, E., Andersen, P. and Jansson, E. (1977). Fibre types and metabolic potentials of skeletal muscle in sedentary man and endurance runners. *Ann N. Y. Acad. Sci.*, **301**, 3–29

9. McArdle, J. J. and Sansone, F. M. (1977). Re-innervation of fast and slow twitch muscle following nerve crush at birth. *J. Physiol. (Lond.)*, **271**, 567–86

10. Buller, A. J., Eccles, J. C. and Eccles, R. M. (1960). Interactions between motor neurons and muscles in respect of the characteristic speeds of their responses. *J. Physiol. (Lond.)*, **150**, 417–39

11. Wiles, C. M., Young, A., Jones, D. A. and Edwards, R. H. T. (1979). Muscle relaxation rate, fibre type composition and energy turnover in hyper- and hypo-thyroid patients. *Clin. Sci.*, **57**, 375–84

12. Andersen, P. and Henriksson, J. (1977). Training induces changes in the subgroups of human type II skeletal muscle fibres. *Acta Physiol. Scand.*, **99**, 123–5

13. Edstrom, L. and Kugelberg, E. (1968). Histochemical composition, distribution of fibres and fatigueability of single motor units. *J. Neurol. Neurosurg. Psychiatry*, **31**, 424–33

14. Edgerton, V. R., Smith, J. L. and Simpson, D. R. (1975). Muscle fibre type populations of human leg muscles. *Histochem. J.*, **7**, 259–66

15. Lexell, J., Downham, D. and Sjöström, M. (1983). Distribution of different fibre types in human skeletal muscles. *J. Neurol. Sci.*, **61**, 301–14

16. Hendriksson-Larsén, K. B., Lexell, J. and Sjöström, M. (1983). Distribution of different fibre types in human skeletal muscles: 1. Method for the preparation and analysis of cross sections of whole tibialis anterior. *Histochem. J.*, **15**, 167–78

17. Mahon, M., Toman, A., Willan, P. L. T. and Bagnall, K. M. (1984). Variability of histochemical and morphometric data from needle biopsy specimens of human quadriceps femoris muscle. *J. Neurol. Sci.*, **63**, 85–100

18. Drury, R. A. B. and Wallington, E. A. (1967). Gomori's rapid one step trichrome stain. In Carleton's *Histological Technique*. (London: Oxford University Press), 4th edn., p. 169

19. Dubowitz, V. and Brooke, M. H. (1973). *Muscle Biopsy: a Modern Approach*. (London: Saunders)

20. Brooke, M. H. and Engel, W. K. (1969). The histographic analysis of human muscle biopsies with regard to fibre types: 4. children's biopsies. *Neurology*, **19**, 591–605

21. Brooke, M. H. and Engel, W. K. (1969). The histographic analysis of human muscle biopsies with regard to fibre types: 1. Adult male and female. *Neurology*, **19**, 221–33

22. Brooke, M. H. (1973). Congenital fibre type disproportion. In Kakulas, B. A. (ed.) *Clinical Studies in Myology*. International Congress series No. 295. (Amsterdam: Excerpta Medica), pp. 147–59

23. Jerusalem, F., Engel, A. G. and Peterson, H. A. (1975). Human muscle fibre fine structure: morphometric data on controls. *Neurology*, **25**, 127–34

24. Tassin, S. and Brucher, J. M. (1982). The mitochondrial disorders: pathogenesis and aetiological classification. *Neuropathol. Appl. Neurobiol.*, **8**, 251–63

Skeletal muscle is composed of highly adaptable cells, responding to physiological stimuli and alterations in the internal environment by both metabolic and structural changes. The same changes occur, and are sometimes very conspicuous, in muscle diseases.

Adaptation to Exercise

Muscle responds to physical training by hypertrophy, but fast and slow twitch fibres respond differently to exercise. Type 1 fibres are the first to be recruited in any low intensity dynamic exercise, such as marathon running or swimming, which relies upon oxidative metabolism. Fast twitch type 2 fibres are preferentially recruited in short bursts of high intensity activity, such as weight lifting or sprinting, largely fuelled by anaerobic glycolysis. Endurance training, therefore, produces enlargement of type 1 fibres, whereas maximal contractions induce type 2 hypertrophy. In addition, there is some plasticity of fibre type according to demand. Exercise may not bring about the complete conversion of type 1 and type 2 fibres that is achieved by cross-innervation, but there is metabolic adaptation of the type 2 fibre subgroups. Endurance training increases oxidative capacity and converts 2B fibres to 2A[1]. Conversely, high intensity training increases glycolytic activity and the proportion of 2B fibres[2]. It seems that athletic potential in a particular sport may be genetically determined, through the relative proportions of type 1 and type 2 fibres, whilst specific training improves performance by inducing both hypertrophy and modification of the subtypes. Hypertrophied fibres are also commonly found in the biopsy of many chronic neuromuscular diseases, because surviving fibres in a wasted muscle are overloaded. When many fibres have been lost, all available motor units are recruited in the attempt to maintain mobility and both type 1 and type 2 fibre hypertrophy develop.

Immobility

As increased activity leads to hypertrophy, so any prolonged period of immobilization causes shrinkage. Again, different responses are seen in the different fibre types. Disuse atrophy in the bed-bound patient is reflected in selective type 2 fibre atrophy[3], particularly 2B atrophy. This is also seen to a mild extent with the decline of physical activities that generally accompanies old age[4] and in the legs of patients restricted by osteoarthrosis of the hips[5]. It is also a problem for the astronauts who experience weightlessness. Slow twitch type 1 motor units are recruited first in any low intensity exercise, but type 2 fibres are used to the greatest extent in maximal contractions and are therefore underemployed in the inactive patient. Severe type 2 fibre atrophy may occur in the limbs of the patient with spastic paresis due to an upper motor neuron lesion[6,7,7a]. This may be accompanied by mild type 1 hypertrophy, because the hypertonic state is associated with almost continual stimulation of the low threshold slow twitch motor units. Conversely, type 1 atrophy is associated with the sort of immobilization that prevents tonic contractions. It can be produced experimentally by tenotomy[8], and has been described in man after knee injuries which cause joint fixation. In progressive muscle diseases, compensatory hypertrophy is seen as long as the patient is mobile; once this becomes impossible the immobility of the chairbound patient will contribute to further deterioration. In disuse atrophy, non-specific degenerative changes, such as breakdown and disorganization of myofibrils, eventually occur[3,9].

Ageing

In addition to the type 2 fibre atrophy attributed to immobility, various degenerative and denervating changes have been cited as effects of ageing. However, it seems unlikely that any are specific or inevitable. Poor nutrition, ischaemic limbs and co-existent disease may all compound the decrease in fibre size. In addition to a tendency to type 2 fibre atrophy, a shift in composition, to an increased proportion of slow twitch fibres is reported[4]. Ageing muscle fibres, as many other cell types, contain increased amounts of lipofuschin pigment. Mild denervation atrophy is sometimes found, particularly in distal limb muscles, and may well be due to entrapment neuropathy[10], rather than neuronal loss in the spinal cord.

Reactions to Injury – Necrosis and Regeneration

The most severe consequence of skeletal muscle injury is fibre necrosis. However, due to the great length of individual cells, injury is often focal and produces only segmental necrosis. Traumatic injury and acute ischaemia are possible causes, but this change is a final common pathway of many muscle diseases, including Duchenne dystrophy and polymyositis. In the necrotic zone striations are lost and the cytoplasm appears structureless (Figures 2.1 – 2.3). The stumps of the undamaged portion of the parent fibre become separated by formation of new plasma membrane (Figure 2.2). Mononuclear phagocytic cells rapidly invade the necrotic segment and ingest cytoplasmic debris (Figures 2.4 and 2.5). Clumps of disorganized

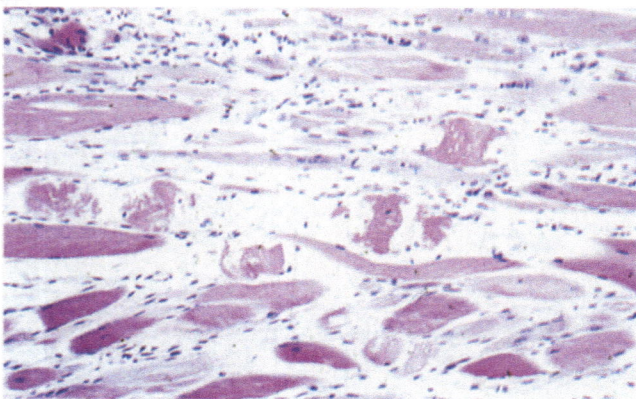

Figure 2.1 Eosinophilic contraction bands, produced by clumped myofibrils in hypercontracted fibres, intervening segments of amorphous pale staining cytoplasm. This region of the fibre is irreversibly damaged. This biopsy was taken from a swollen, traumatized muscle in a child's foot. H & E × 75

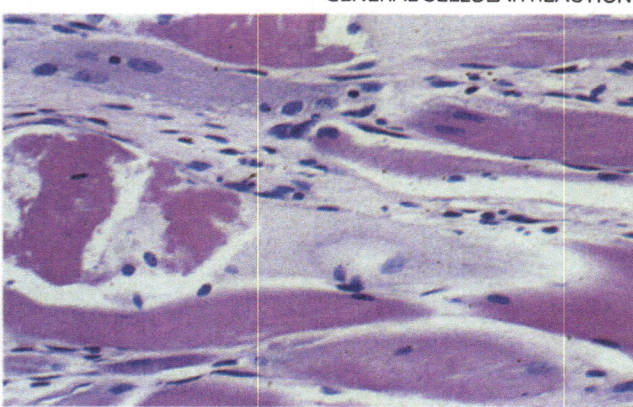

Figure 2.2 Injured segment, containing contraction bands and pale, structureless cytoplasm, becomes separated from remaining viable portion of the muscle fibre. H & E × 300

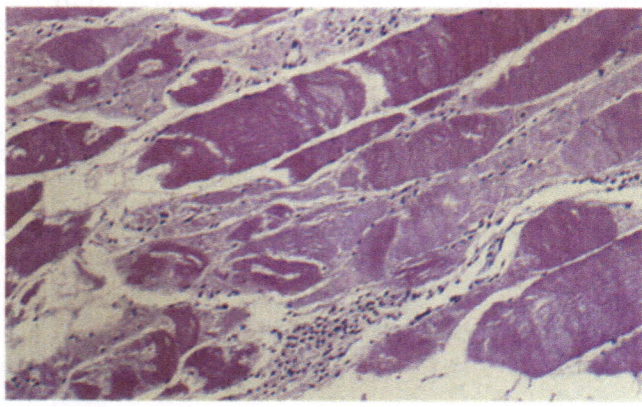

Figure 2.3 Necrotic muscle in the anterior compartment syndrome. Blotchy, purple muscle, removed surgically, after incision of the tight fascia of the anterior tibial compartment, for relief of severe muscle pain and swelling. Several muscle fibres show homogeneous pale staining cytoplasm and others contain deeply eosinophilic clumped cytoplasm. There is an early inflammatory cell response. H & E × 180

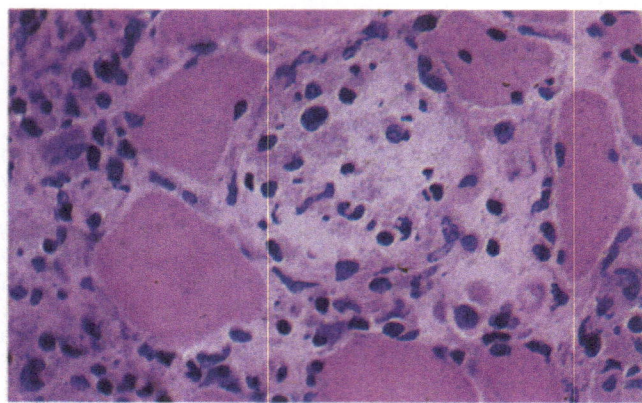

Figure 2.4 Pale staining cytoplasm of a necrotic fibre filled with phagocytes which remove the necrotic debris from the injured muscle fibre. H & E × 300

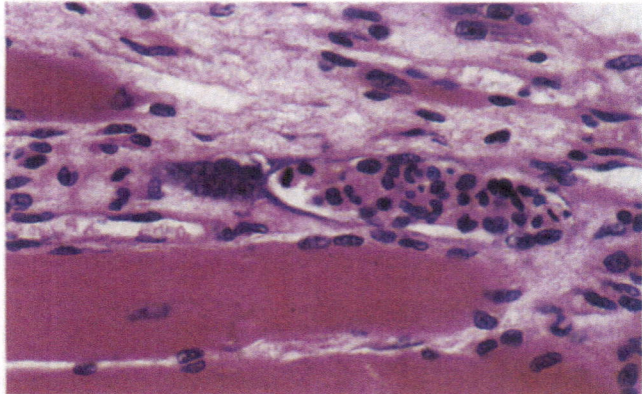

Figure 2.5 A necrotic segment filled with phagocytes. Adjacent to this there is a cluster of large nuclei, which probably indicate myoblasts fusing to form a myotube. H & E × 300

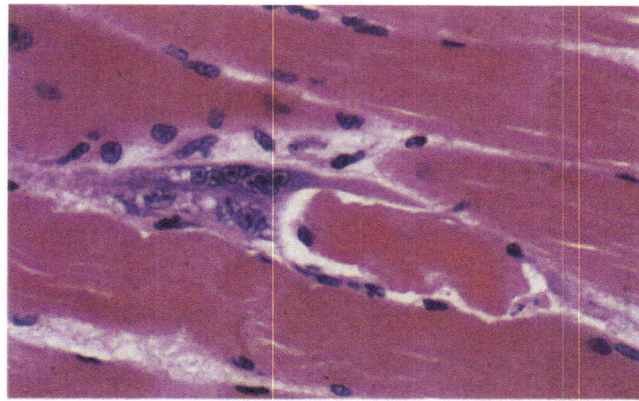

Figure 2.6 Basophilic myotubes have formed and are beginning to encircle a residual remnant of eosinophilic, degenerating cytoplasm from the necrotic segment. H & E × 300

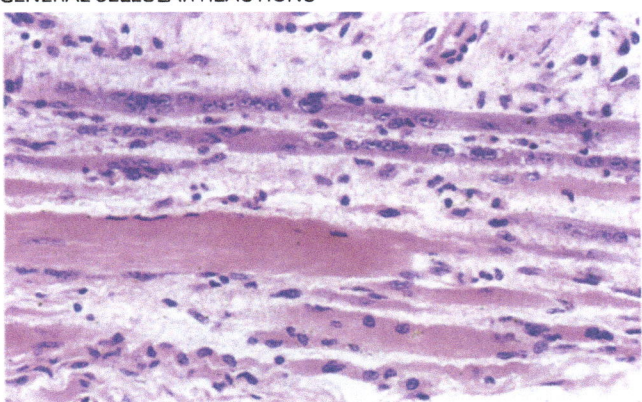

Figure 2.7 Thin regenerating myotubes, which have columns of large central nuclei and basophilic cytoplasm. The myotubes grow along the basement membrane and collagen scaffold of the original fibre. H & E × 180

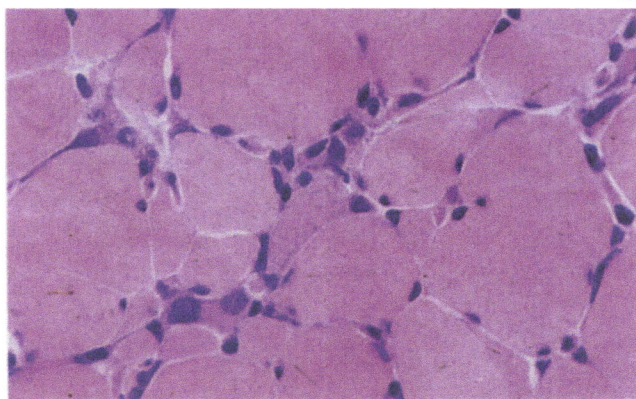

Figure 2.8 Basophilic, regenerating fibres in polymyositis. Necrosis and regeneration are very commonly found in polymyositis and dermatomyositis. (Same case shown in Figures 2.9 and 2.10. H & E × 300

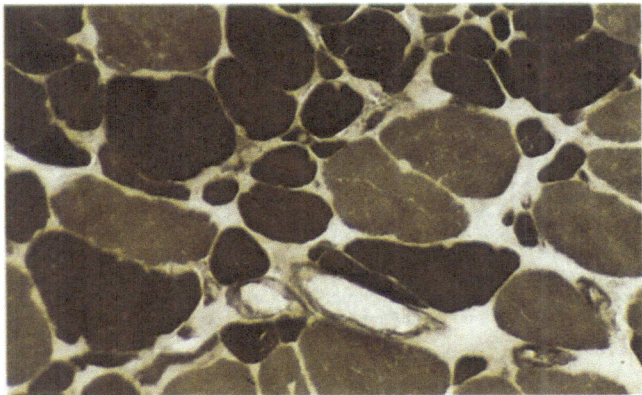

Figure 2.9 Regenerating, immature 2C fibres, which show myosin ATP-ase activity at both alkaline and acid pH. Comparison with Figure 2.10 reveals that several of the tiny fibres, which are dark in this preparation at pH 9.4, still show moderate activity at pH 4.1. ATP-ase pH 9.4 × 300

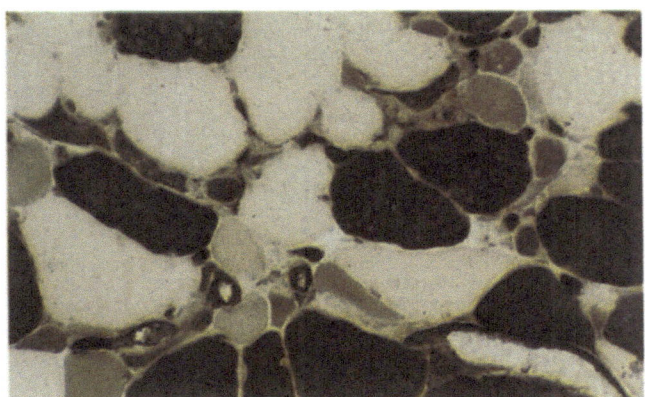

Figure 2.10 Type 2C fibres. Serial section to Figure 2.9. Small, type 2C fibres appear grey. Type 1 fibres are dark, type 2A and 2B are light. ATP-ase pH 4.1 × 300

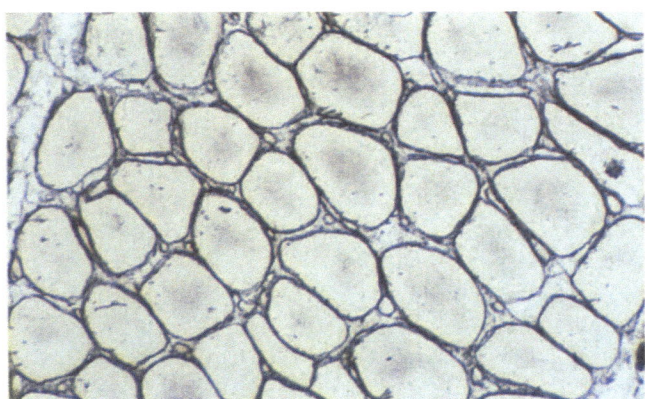

Figure 2.11 Connective tissue framework. Each muscle fibre has a basement membrane, but is also encased by a reticulin network, composed of fine collagen fibrils. Preservation of this framework after injury guides the regenerating myotubes to restore normal architecture. Gordon and Sweet's method for reticulin × 180

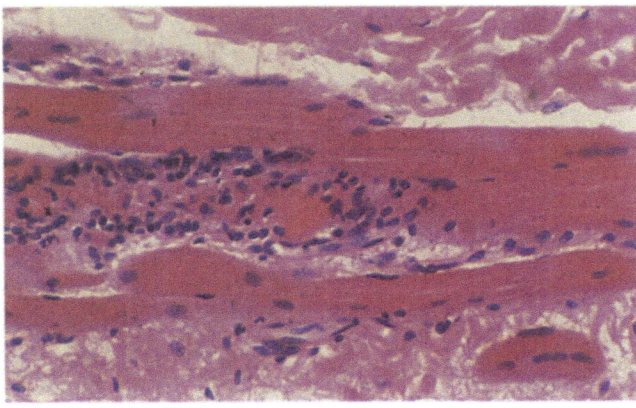

Figure 2.12 Segmental necrosis in Duchenne muscular dystrophy is a major pathological finding and particularly common in the early years. This muscle from a 3-year-old boy shows an eosinophilic necrotic segment, invaded by mononuclear phagocytes. H & E × 180

Electron Micrographs

The sequence of fine structural changes that take place during muscle fibre necrosis and regeneration are illustrated in rat muscle 3–4 days after a light, crushing injury. The changes in man are essentially similar.

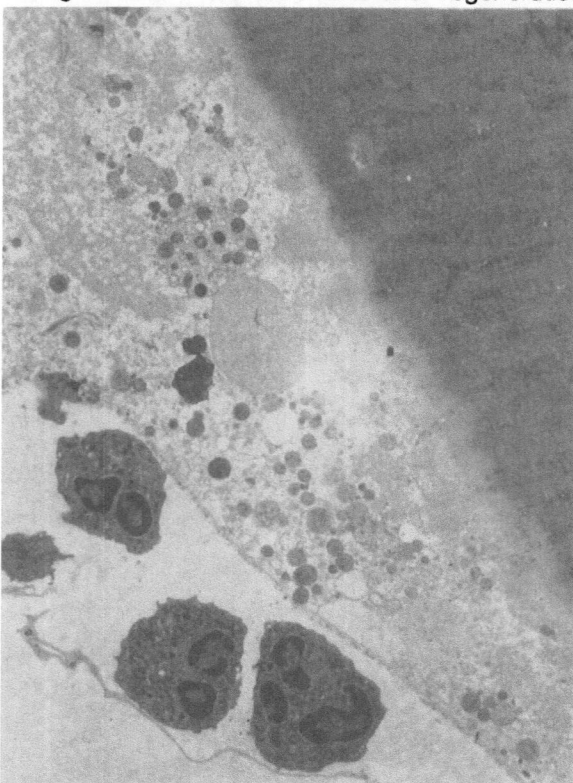

Figure 2.13 Polymorphoneutrophil leukocytes close to the sarcolemma of a necrotic fibre. The peripheral cytoplasm is devoid of myofibrils and contains lysosomes and swollen mitochondria. The inner myofibrils are clumped and appear almost structureless. EM × 1900

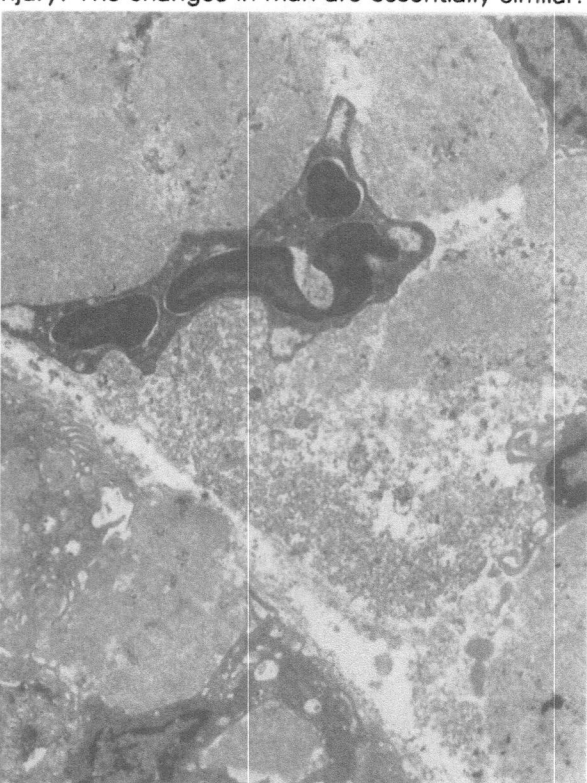

Figure 2.14 Polymorphoneutrophil leukocyte invading a necrotic fibre. The polymorph can be recognized from its lobated nucleus. Mononuclear macrophages are also visible. The cell structure is disintegrating. Only clumps of disorganized myofilaments are recognizable. EM × 3400

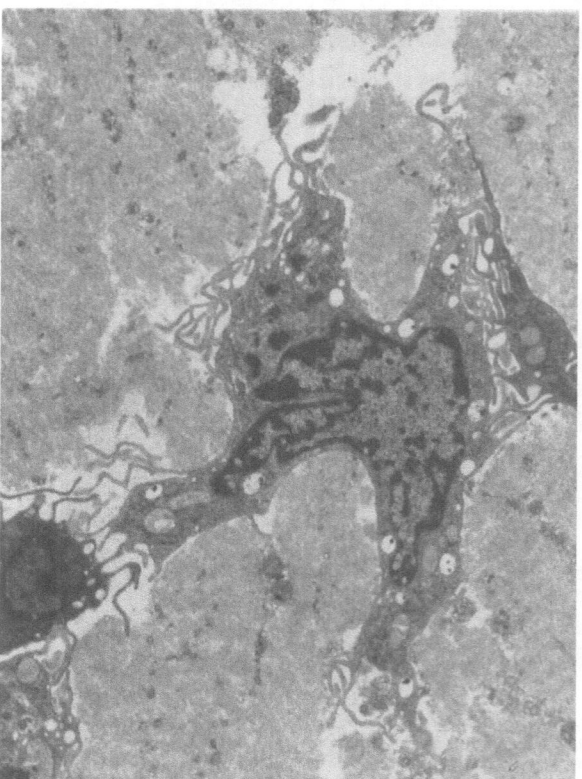

Figure 2.15 Macrophages, with complicated cell processes extending amongst the clumped disorganized myofilaments in the cytoplasm of the necrotic cell. EM × 3400

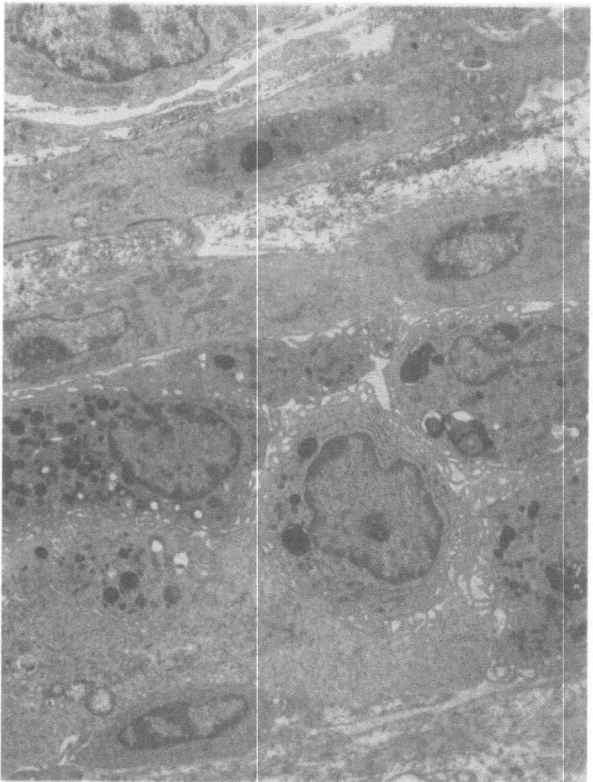

Figure 2.16 A necrotic fibre filled with macrophages, recognized by complex cytoplasmic processes and also the numerous secondary lysosomes, derived from phagocytosis of cellular debris. Two elongated myoblasts have grown alongside the phagocytes and appear to be fusing to form a myotube. The myoblasts are enclosed within the basement membrane and collagen scaffold of the original cell. EM × 1900

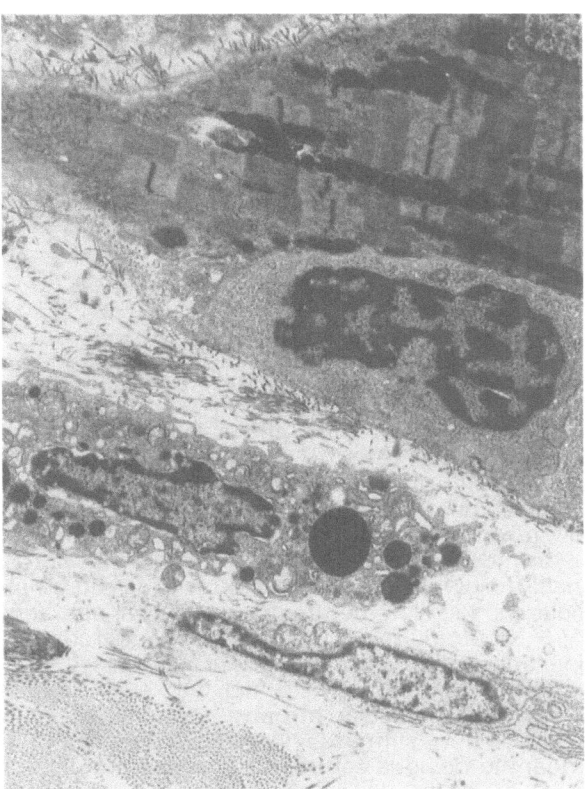

Figure 2.17 Activated mononuclear satellite cell alongside a mature fibre. A macrophage, or fibrohistiocyte, containing many lysosomes is present in the interstitium. EM × 3400

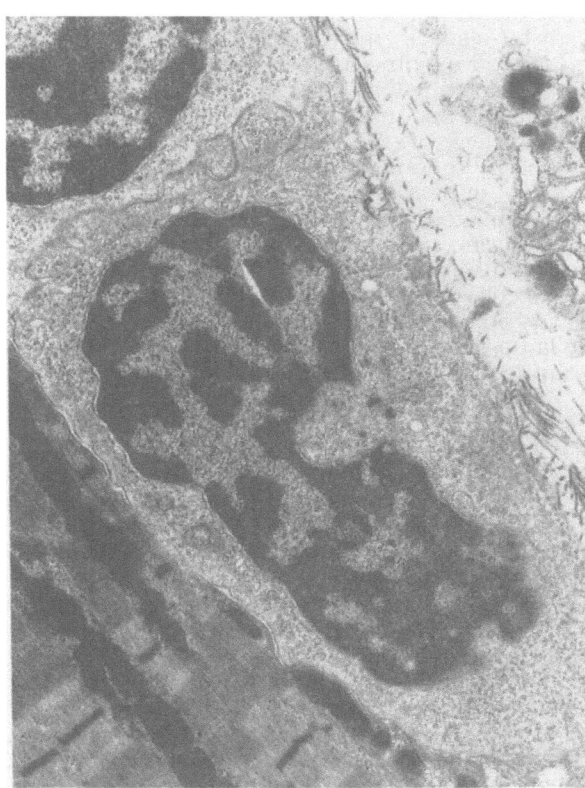

Figure 2.18 The satellite cells, from which regeneration and growth occur, can be seen to have separate cell membranes from the parent fibre, although enclosed with the same basement membrane. The cytoplasm contains ribosomes, but no myofilaments. EM × 7100

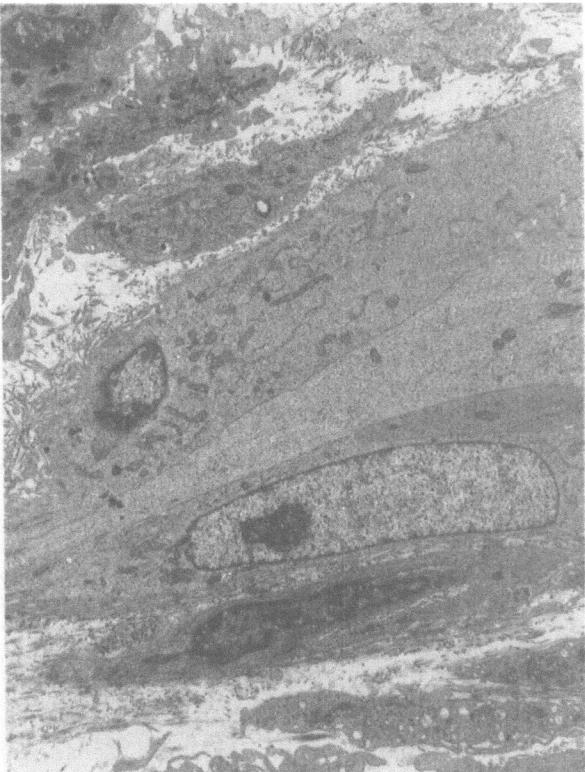

Figure 2.19 Myotube fusion. The ends of several elongated pale cells, which lie close together, encased by the same basement membrane. EM × 1900

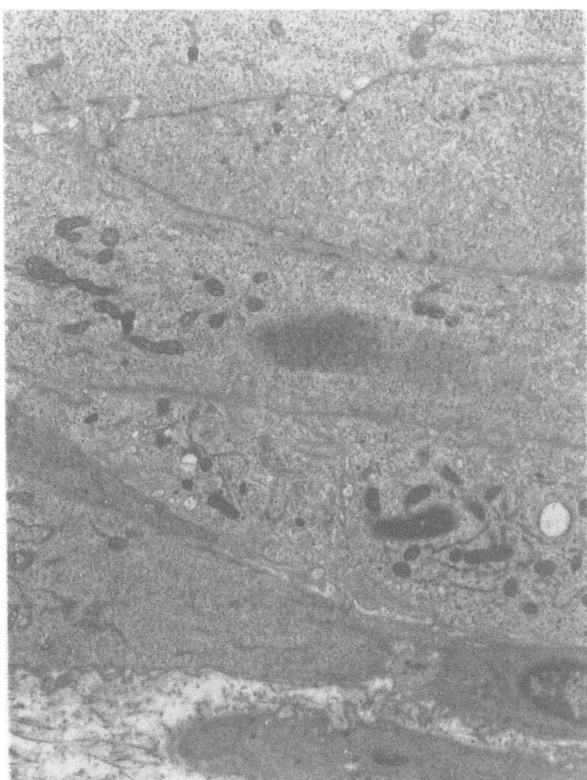

Figure 2.20 Myotube fusion. Elongated cells, with very closely apposed cell membranes and no intervening basement membranes. Fusion of the myotubes eventually reconstitutes the damaged fibre. At this stage the cytoplasm contains ribosomes, mitochondria, rough endoplasmic reticulum but only scanty myofilaments. EM × 3400

myofilaments can be detected in the phagocyte cyto- plasm by electron microscopy. Initially, cytoplasm of the injured segment may appear clumped and eosinophilic, but with dissolution and ingestion of its organelles, it becomes pale and barely stained.

Irrespective of the cause, segmental necrosis is followed by regeneration, which retraces the steps of normal embryogenesis[11] (Figures 2.13–20). Undifferentiated, mononuclear satellite cells lie between the muscle cell basement membrane and the sarcolemma. Injury stimulates the proliferation of satellite cells which migrate from the ends of the parent cell, line up and fuse to form thin, basophilic myotubes, with large vesicular nuclei. Initially, the myotubes grow alongside the disintegrating segment (Figure 2.6) but as the necrotic debris is removed the myotubes fuse together and with the ends of the parent cell to restore normal structure (Figure 2.7). Cytoplasmic diffe- rentiation with formation of myofibrils begins in the myotubes, but the full expression of mature fibre type is not achieved until innervation is re-established. The tiny immature fibres, called 2C fibres, show myosin ATP-ase activity at both acid and alkaline pH (Figures 2.8–2.10). Provided that injury does not destroy the reticulin framework of the muscle, normal fibre archi- tecture is restored (Figure 2.11). When this scaffold is disrupted the fusion of myotubes and parent cells may be haphazard and variously forked or branching fibres may form. The skeletal muscle cell does have con- siderable regenerative capacity, providing viable satellite cells persist, but with sustained or repetitive injury, fibroblastic proliferation may exceed regeneration, and interstitial fibrosis develops. Shortly after injury a few central nuclei may appear in a bulge of cytoplasm at the stump ends of the parent fibre; how- ever, there is no evidence that nuclei in the parent cell can undergo mitotic division and no significant regeneration occurs from this sarcoplasmic bud.

Segmental necrosis is frequently initiated by hyper- contraction, recognized by eosinophilic bands of clumped myofibrils. It seems that this degree of dis- organization is irreversible (Figures 2.1 and 2.2). Hypercontraction precedes necrosis in Duchenne dystrophy[12] (Figure 2.12), and it is also the typical fibre injury of physical overloading. Thus, it may occur with very strenuous activity in normal people[13] and in the overloaded, surviving muscle fibres of chronic neuro- muscular disease.

Ischaemia

Skeletal muscle has a rich blood supply. There is a capillary network surrounding each fibre, most dense around slow, oxidative type 1 fibres. Acute ischaemia producing infarction of a whole muscle is relatively uncommon, but sometimes occurs in the compartment syndromes. The anterior tibial muscles are encased in a tight fascial sheath. Strenuous exercise leads to increased blood flow and the muscle becomes turgid. In some people the tight fascia may impair the venous return, the muscles become oedematous and the rise in pressure in the compartment is sufficient to occlude blood flow. This causes pain and if ischaemia is sustained the muscle becomes infarcted. A similar problem may arise in the post-tibial compartment and I have seen the same phenomenon in the temporal muscles of a middle-aged woman, which literally swelled and became painful as she chewed vigorously. Infarcted muscle undergoes all the changes of necrosis

and regeneration[14]. However, if the blood supply is not restored fairly rapidly there will be repair by fibrosis and not regeneration. Due to good collateral circulation, large muscle infarcts secondary to embolism or vasculitis are uncommon. They may occur in poly- arteritis nodosa and have been described in diabetics with severe peripheral vascular disease[15]. Tiny isch- aemic foci, due to occlusion of arterioles and even small arteries, may explain many of the pathological changes in muscle in juvenile dermatomyositis[16].

Contractures and Arthrogryposis

Acquired contractures frequently result from the combination of immobility, severe muscle atrophy and replacement fibrosis. Thus, they develop late in the course of Duchenne muscular dystrophy and chronic spinal muscular atrophy. The contractures associated with upper motor neuron lesions and spasticity may initially reflect differential increased tone in flexor and extensor muscles, but, here too, atrophy and fibrosis invariably follow. Arthrogryposis refers to a syndrome of multiple congenital contractures of varied aetio- logy[17,18]. Contractures in the neonate result from intra- uterine immobility, but this does not always imply primary muscle pathology. In fact the severe infantile form of spinal muscular atrophy is characterized by floppiness, not stiffness. Arthrogryposis may be secondary to obvious central nervous system disease, causing spasticity. It is sometimes due to muscle atrophy and fibrosis as in congenital muscular dystrophy. It may also result simply from oligo- hydramnios, which limits fetal movement. The muscle can be entirely normal and contractures of this type show the best response to physiotherapy.

Scoliosis and the Rigid Spine Syndrome

These two complex disorders show a clinical deformity that sometimes has a muscular basis.

Scoliosis can be a congenital or acquired spinal deformity. The former may arise from an intrauterine insult to mesenchymal tissue. The latter can be secondary to a variety of progressive wasting muscle diseases, such as severe chronic spinal muscular atrophy or Duchenne dystrophy.

There is also idiopathic, adolescent onset scoliosis, with particular severity in girls[19]. Recent histological studies of muscle have revealed asymmetry and small fibres in both paraspinal and deltoid muscles. It is not clear whether this represents a primary growth dis- turbance in muscle or a neurological disorder with altered proprioceptive input[19].

The rigid spine syndrome is a rare clinical condition of flexion contracture of the spine beginning in infancy or early childhood. It may be associated with scoliosis, joint contractures and mild non-progressive proximal muscle weakness[20]. This picture also probably has a varied pathologic basis. Examination of peripheral muscle has shown varying degrees of fibre type dis- proportion[20,21] and in other cases fibrosis[22,23]. Fibrosis has also been reported in the paraspinal muscles[24], but in general these have not been examined. Cases with skeletal muscle fibrosis are perhaps related to con- genital muscular dystrophy (see Chapter 9).

References

1. Jansson, E. and Kaijer, L. (1977). Muscle adaptation to extreme endurance training in man. *Acta Physiol. Scand.*, **100**, 315–24

2. Prince, F. T. *et al.* (1981). A morphometric analysis of human muscle fibres with relation to fibre types and adaptations to exercise. *J. Neurol. Sci.*, **49**, 165–79

3. Mendell, J. R. and Engel, W. K. (1971). The fine structure of type 2 muscle atrophy. *Neurology*, **21**, 358–65

4. Larsson, L., Grimby, G. and Karlsson, J. (1979). Muscle strength and speed of movement in relation to age and muscle morphology. *J. Appl. Physiol.*, **46**, 451–6

5. Sirca, A. and Susec-Michieli, M. (1980). Selective type 2 fibre atrophy in patients with osteoarthritis of the hip. *J. Neurol. Sci.*, **44**, 149–59

6. Edstrom, L., Grimby, L. and Hannerz, J. (1973). Correlation between recruitment order of motor units and muscle atrophy pattern in upper motor neuron lesion: significance of spasticity. *Experientia*, **29**, 560–1

7. Castle, M. E., Reyman, T. A. and Schneider, M. (1979). Pathology of spastic muscle in cerebral palsy. *Clin. Orthop.*, **142**, 223–33

7a. Scelsi, R., Lotta, S., Poggi, P. and Marchetti, C. (1984). Morphological findings in the anterior tibial muscle of patients with cerebral vascular accidents. *Acta Neuropathol. (Berl).*, **62**, 324–31

8. Jaffe, D. M., Terry, R. D. and Spiro, A. J. (1978). Disuse atrophy of muscle – a morphometric study using image analysis. *J. Neurol. Sci.*, **35**, 189–200

9. Dastur, D. K., Gagrat, B. M. and Manghani, D. K. (1978). Fine structure of muscle in human disuse atrophy. *Neuropathol. Appl. Neurobiol.*, **5**, 85–101

10. Neary, D., Ochoa, J. and Gilliat, R. W. (1975). Subclinical entrapment neuropathy in man. *J. Neurol. Sci.*, **24**, 283–98

11. Sloper, J. C. and Partridge, T. A. (1980). Skeletal muscle regeneration and transplantation studies. *Br. Med. Bull.*, **36**, 153–8

12. Cullen, M. J. and Mastaglia, F. L. (1980). Morphological changes in dystrophic muscle. *Br. Med. Bull.*, **36**, 145–52

13. Hikida, R. S. *et al.* (1983). Muscle fibre necrosis associated with human marathon runners. *J. Neurol. Sci.*, **59**, 185–203

14. Karpati, G., Carpenter, S., Melmed, C. and Eisen, A. A. (1974). Experimental ischaemic myopathy. *J. Neurol. Sci.*, **23**, 129–61

15. Banker, B. Q. and Chester, C. S. (1973). Infarction of thigh muscle in the diabetic patient. *Neurology*, **23**, 667–77

16. Carpenter, S., Karpati, G., Rothman, S. and Watters, G. (1976). The childhood type of dermatomyositis. *Neurology*, **26**, 952–62

17. Dubowitz, V. (1978). Disorders with muscle contracture and joint rigidity. In Schaffer, A. J. and Markowitz, M. (eds.) *Muscle Disorders in Childhood: Major Problems in Clinical Paediatrics Series, pp. 232–244. (Philadelphia: W.B. Saunders)*

18. Krugliak, L., Gadoth, N. and Behar, A. J. (1978). Neuropathic form of arthrogryposis multiplex congenita. *J. Neurol. Sci.*, **37**, 179–85

19. Yarom, R., Wolf, E. and Robin, G. C. (1982). Deltoid pathology in idiopathic scoliosis. *Spine*, **7**, 463–70

20. Mussini, J. M., Gray, F., Hauw, J. J., Piete, A. M. and Prost, A. (1981). Rigid spine syndrome: Histological examination of male and female cases. *Acta Neuropathol. (Berl.)*, Suppl. VII, 331–33

21. Seay, A. R., Ziter, F. A. and Petajan, J. H. (1977). Rigid spine syndrome. *Arch. Neurol.*, **34**, 119–22

22. Dubowitz, V. (1978). Rigid spine syndrome. In Schaffer, A. J. and Markowitz, M. (eds.) *Muscle Disorders in Childhood: Major Problems in Clinical Paediatrics Series*, pp. 239–244. (Philadelphia: W. B. Saunders)

23. Goto, I., Nagasaka, S., Nagara, H., Kuroiwa, Y. (1979). Rigid spine syndrome. *J. Neurol. Neurosurg. Psychiatry.*, **42**, 276–79

24. Goebel, H. H., Lenard, H. G., Gorke, W. and Kunze, K. (1977). Fibre type disproportion in the rigid spine syndrome. *Neuropadiatrie*, **8**, 467–77

Neurogenic muscle diseases are those in which the primary pathology is in the lower motor neuron and changes in the muscle are secondary. A muscle fibre permanently deprived of its motor nerve supply gradually atrophies and shows internal disorganization. Neurogenic diseases can be conveniently divided into three groups according to the site of the primary pathological lesion: (1) anterior horn cell, (2) axon and (3) motor end plate. The distribution of atrophic fibres within a muscle biopsy may give an indication of the site of the motor neuron lesion. Thus, anterior horn cell diseases, e.g. motor neuron disease, are characterized by groups of atrophic fibres reflecting simultaneous atrophy of whole motor units (Diagram 3.1) (Figures 3.1 and 3.2). A lesion of the spinal nerve root can produce a similar picture. Pathological changes in the peripheral nerve distal to points of axonal branching will only affect a small proportion of muscle fibres in any one motor unit. The atrophic fibres are then more widely scattered or within tiny groups of only two or three fibres. Diseases of the motor end plate, of which myasthenia gravis is the most important, do not as a rule produce permanent denervation until the later stages, when the pattern is chiefly one of isolated atrophic fibres.

Morphological Changes in Denervation

Variation in the rate of atrophy has been observed between fast and slow fibres and between different species. However, there is general agreement that in man and other mammals all fibre types atrophy most rapidly in the first 2–3 months after denervation and thereafter quite slowly until a stationary state is reached[1,2]. Chronically denervated fibres may be reduced in calibre to 10–20% of the original[1] (Figure 3.3). When a large motor nerve is completely severed a whole muscle atrophies and although changes may not be entirely uniform, all the muscle fibres show a reduction in diameter whilst retaining their normal rounded contour in transverse section. In contrast, in most of the chronic denervating diseases only a small proportion of muscle fibres are affected initially and the shrinking, denervated fibres assume an angular outline, as though moulded by the adjacent healthy fibres (Figures 3.1 and 3.4). Angular, atrophic fibres are a characteristic feature of denervating disease and grouped atrophy is pathognomonic. The residual innervated fibres may show compensatory hypertrophy (Figure 3.2).

After denervation, muscle cell nuclei may show transient enlargement, but usually remain in their normal peripheral location. A profusion of central nuclei is unusual in denervation, although as the fibre shrinks, so the nuclei come to occupy a larger part of the cross-sectional area. After several months the severely atrophic fibre may consist of only a thin rim of cytoplasm and a cluster of pyknotic nuclei (Figure 3.3). The fate of the denervated cell is variable. Some muscle fibres ultimately degenerate and disappear when additional factors, such as ischaemia, may be responsible. Other severely atrophic fibres survive for long periods, at least 1 year, possibly several years, retaining a few myofibrils in the cytoplasm. Chronic denervation atrophy leads to a corresponding increase in interstitial connective tissue. The endomysium is thickened around atrophic fibres and there is fibrosis of the perimysium. In severely atrophic muscle there is both adipose and fibrous replacement.

Fine Structure

Fine structural changes can be detected within a few days of denervation and progress as the cell atrophies. The subcellular changes have been described in greatest detail in animals and, whilst some contradictory observations may be due to the particular species and muscle examined, most relate to the interval of time following denervation. The essential findings are of myofibrillar atrophy proportional to reduction in fibre size[3]. Loss of myofilaments and disruption of fibrils commence at the periphery and are most severe in type 2 fibres. There is an early increase in size and re-orientation of mitochondria, but after a few weeks these organelles also become smaller. The sarcolemma becomes wrinkled and there may be accumulation of subsarcolemmal lysosomes[4] (Figure 3.23). The sarcoplasmic reticulum is enlarged by focal dilatations and the concentration of this membranous component is actually increased[3]. There is early development of subsarcolemmal ribosomes, probably related to an increased synthesis of acetyl choline receptors[5]. Eventually, in the severely atrophic fibre there is considerable reduction in all of these cell organelles.

Staining Reactions

In early denervation, increased ribosomes may impart faint basophilia with H & E. Small, angular fibres that stain deeply with the NADH-TR reaction are characteristic of denervation (Figure 3.4). These may be derived from both type 1 and type 2 fibres. Tetrazolium, the blue-coloured, reaction product, binds to mitochondria and also to sarcoplasmic reticulum and the transverse tubular system. The relative increase in these organelles at the expense of myofibrils is probably responsible for

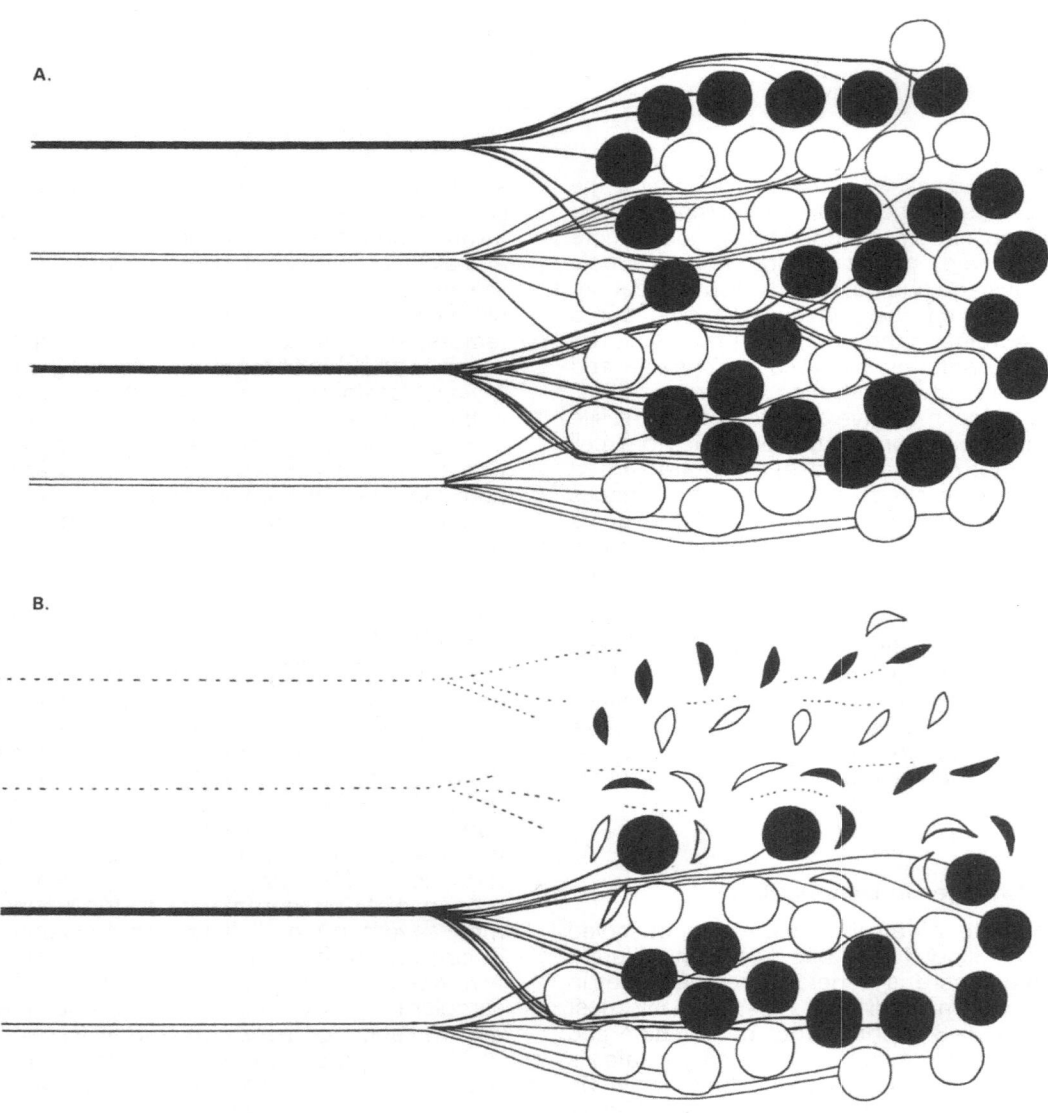

Diagram 3.1   A. The normal motor unit. Fibres within individual motor units show uniform histochemical reactions. Fibres of adjacent motor units intermingle to give a mosaic pattern. **B.** Grouped atrophy. Denervation atrophy due to anterior horn cell disease involves whole motor units.

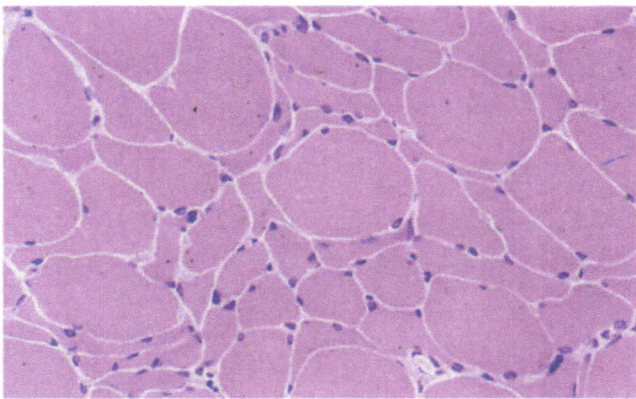

Figure 3.1 Small group atrophy in deltoid muscle of 56-year-old man with motor neuron disease. Angular atrophic fibres contrast with larger, rounded, mildly hypertrophied fibres.   H & E × 180

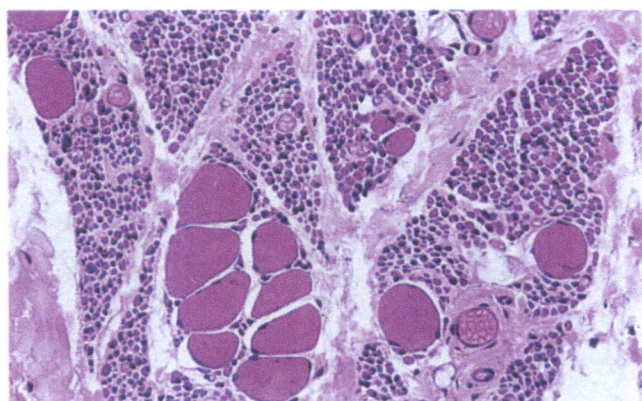

Figure 3.2 Large group atrophy in quadriceps muscle of 3-year-old boy with chronic spinal muscular atrophy. Whole fascicles composed of atrophic fibres indicate loss of many contiguous motor units. The few residual innervated fibres are greatly hypertrophied.   H & E × 75

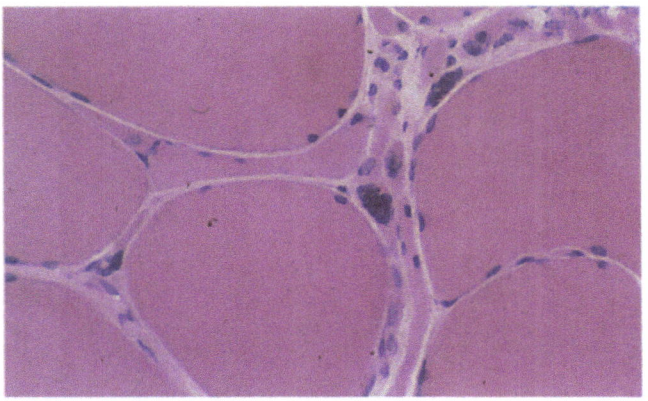

Figure 3.3 A small group of severely atrophic, denervated fibres in chronic spinal muscular atrophy. The tiny fibres consist of a few pyknotic nuclei and rim of cytoplasm, indicating long standing denervation. They are easily over-looked amidst normal-sized or hypertrophied fibres.   H & E × 450

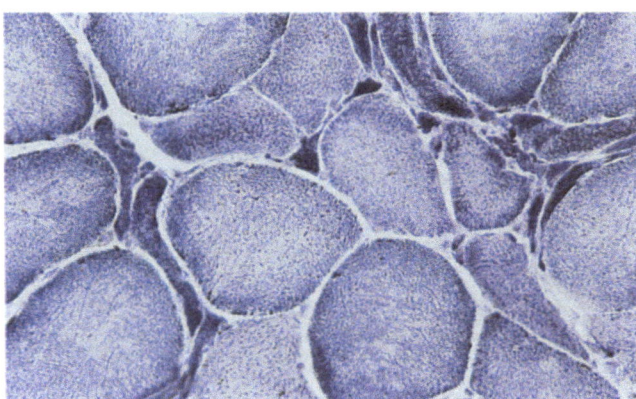

Figure 3.4 A group of angular, atrophic, denervated fibres in motor neuron disease stained darkly with the NADH-TR reaction. Tetrazolium, the blue reaction product, binds to mitochondria and the sarcotubular system. The relative increase in these organelles, at the expense of myofibrils, may explain increased intensity of reaction in the denervated fibre.   NADH-TR × 300

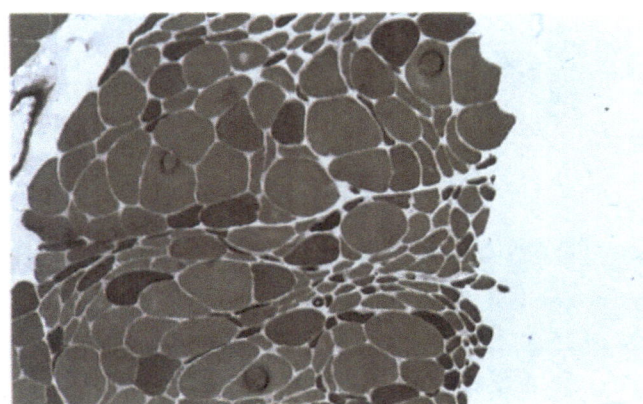

Figure 3.5 Small group, denervation atrophy in gastronemius muscle of 15-year-old boy with distal, chronic spinal muscular atrophy. Atrophic fibres are both type 1 and type 2.   ATP-ase pH 9.4 × 75

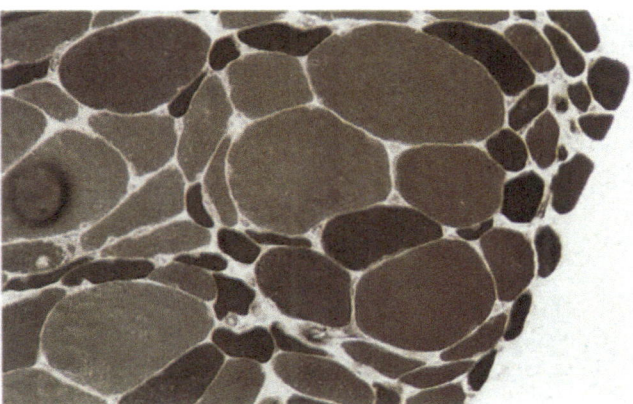

Figure 3.6 Small group, denervation atrophy. Same case as Figure 3.5. Type 1 fibres (light) are clearly distinguished from type 2 fibres (dark) even in the smallest, most severely atrophic fibres.   ATP-ase pH 9.4 × 300

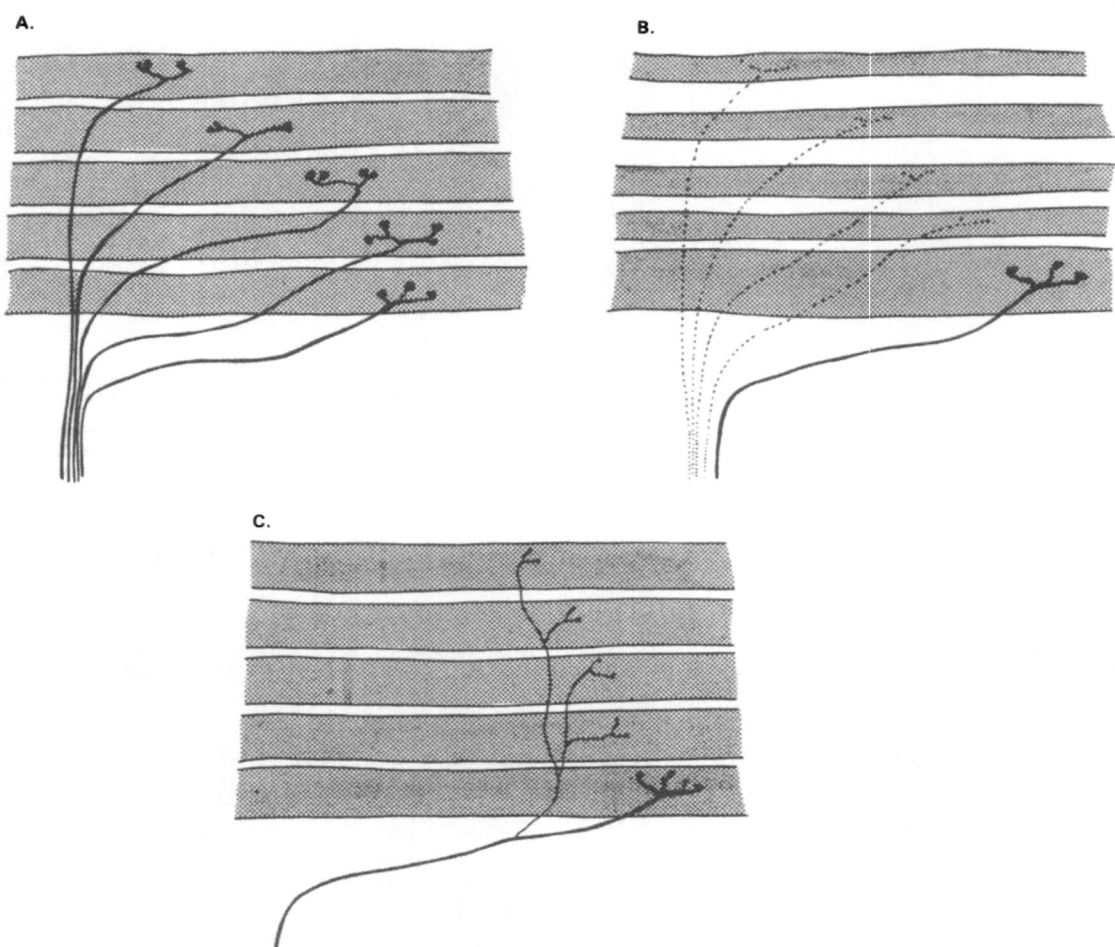

Diagram 3.2   Re-innervation by collateral axonal sprouting **A.** Normal arrangement of terminal innervation. Preterminal axons are unbranched. Single motor end plate on each fibre. **B.** Denervation. Degeneration of several terminal axons. **C.** Re-innervation by sprouting from a surviving healthy axon.

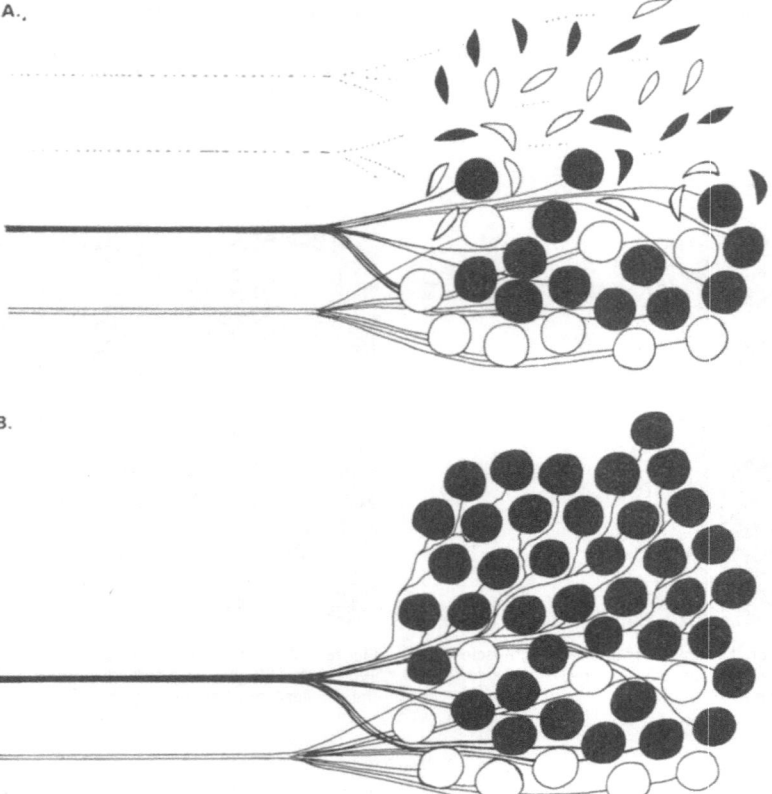

Diagram 3.3   A. Grouped atrophy due to denervation. Atrophic fibres retain original fibre type. **B.** Type grouping produced by re-innervation. Preterminal sprouting by preterminal healthy axons is responsible for re-innervation and may bring about a change in fibre type. New enlarged motor units are seen as clumps of uniform fibre type, replacing the original mosaic pattern.

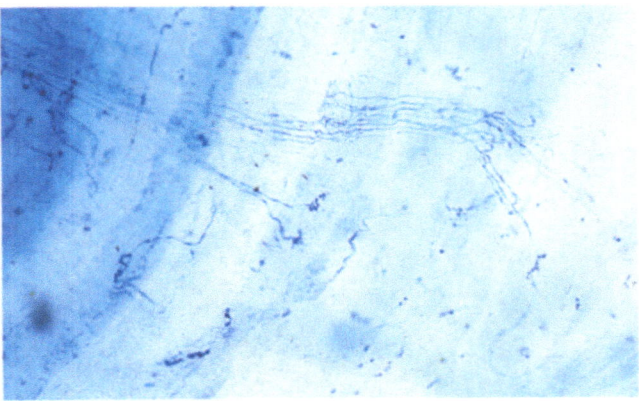

Figure 3.7 Normal terminal innervation. Spray of subterminal axons. Each terminates in one motor end plate (occasionally two) on different muscle fibres. Methylene blue vital staining × 75

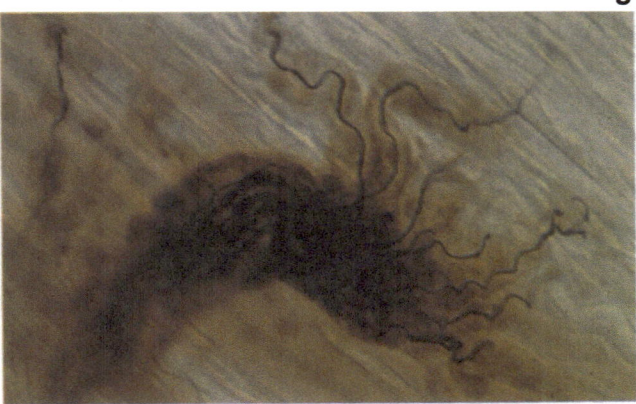

Figure 3.8 Normal terminal innervation. Spray of subterminal axons separating as they approach the motor end plates. Schofield's silver method × 180

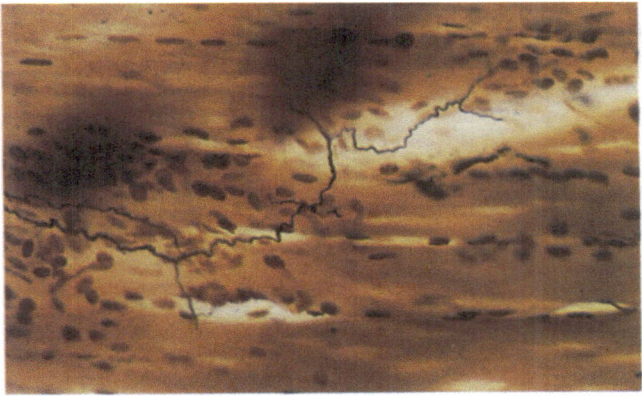

Figure 3.9 Collateral re-innervation in chronic spinal muscular atrophy. Preterminal axon branches several times to give rise to separate motor end plates on at least three different muscle fibres. Schofield's silver method × 180

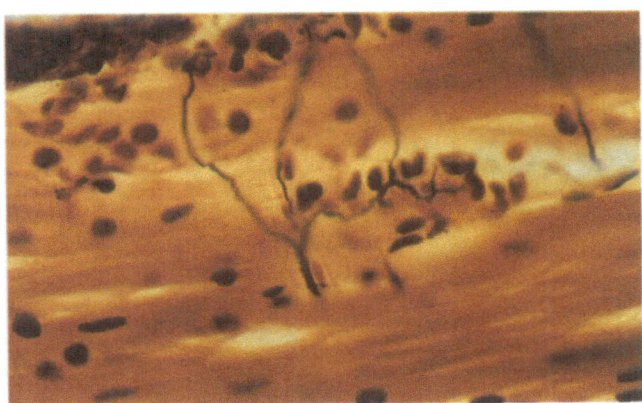

Figure 3.10 Collateral sprouting. Fine branches arising from a preterminal axon, indicating re-innervation. Schofield's silver method × 300

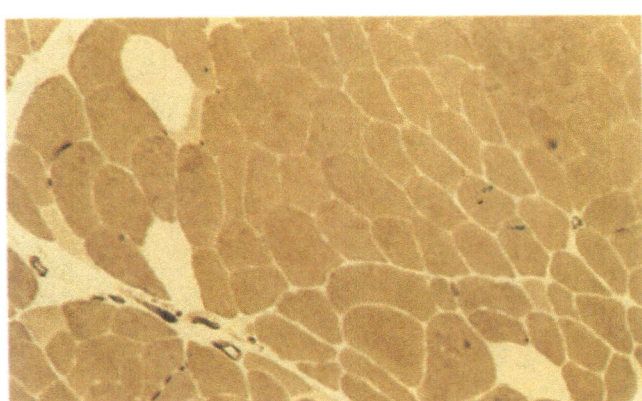

Figure 3.11 Type grouping in deltoid muscle of elderly man with motor neuron disease. The normal mosaic pattern is replaced by a large group of uniform type 1 fibres, indicative of re-innervation, creating new enlarged motor units. ATP-ase pH 9.4 × 75

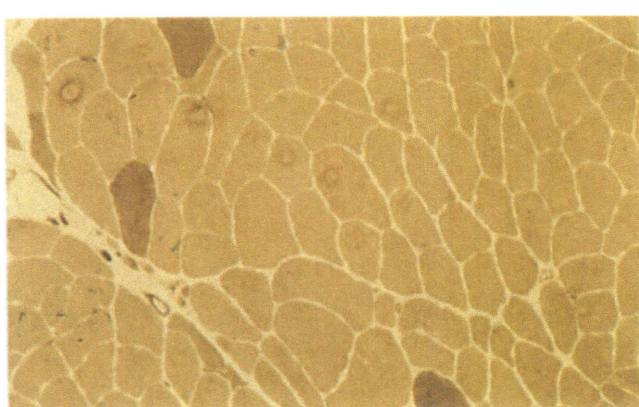

Figure 3.12 Type grouping. Serial section to Figure 3.11. ATP-ase pH 4.6 × 75

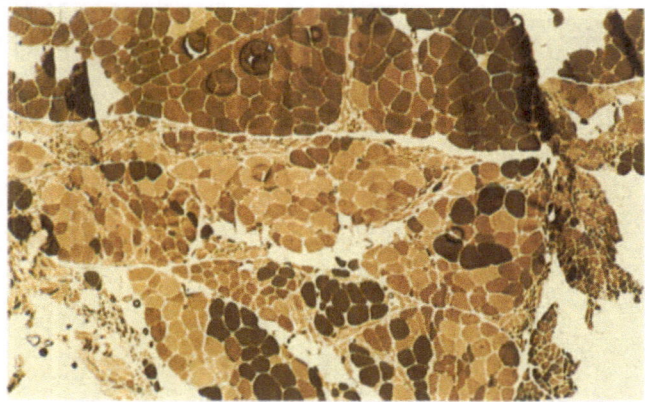

Figure 3.13   Type grouping in chronic spinal muscular atrophy. Small group denervation atrophy is also present. Uniform clumps of type 1 fibres (dark) and type 2 fibres (light and intermediate) indicate re-innervation. Large groups of type 2 fibres are usually found only in the more chronic denervating disorders.   ATP-ase pH 4.6 × 30

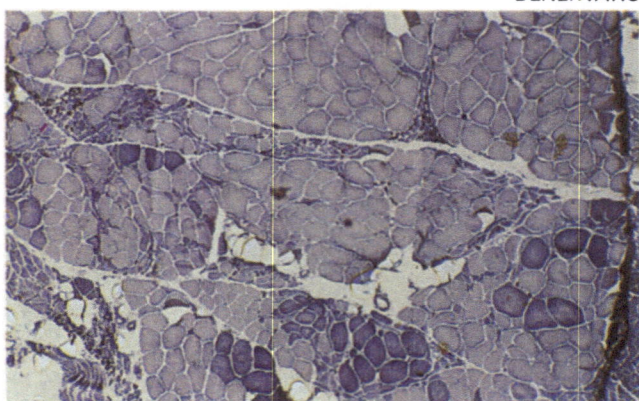

Figure 3.14   Type grouping due to re-innervation. Serial section to Figure 3.13. Type 2 fibres are light, type 1 fibres are dark.   ATP-ase pH 4.6 × 30

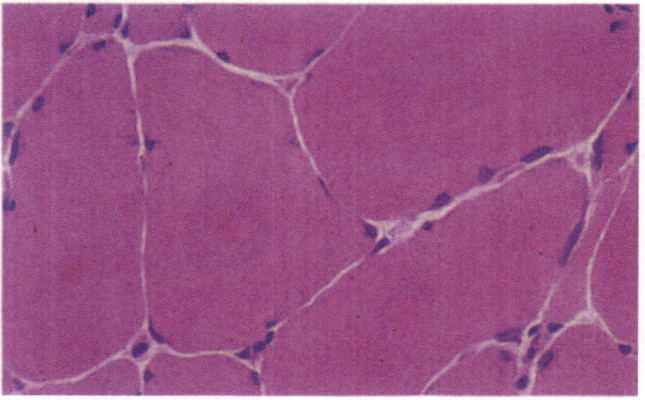

Figure 3.15   Target fibres. Target fibres in type 1 fibres of deltoid muscle of 54-year-old man with motor neuron disease. Target fibres may appear in early denervation or during early re-innervation. There is a central eosinophilic core with peripheral pale staining halo.   H & E × 450

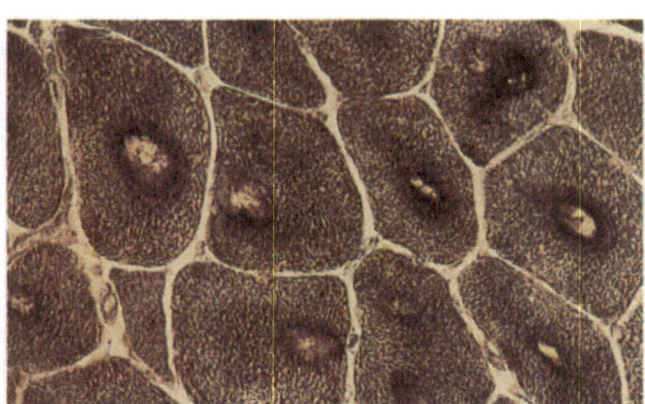

Figure 3.16   Target fibres. The central core is unstained, but the halo has increased enzymic activity.   NADH-TR × 300

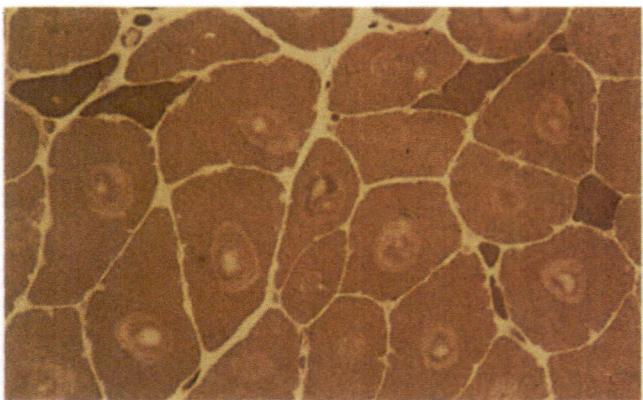

Figure 3.17   Target fibres. Only type 1 fibres contain targets. In this preparation there are four concentric zones, an unstained core, a ring of enzyme activity, a further ring devoid of activity and normal periphery.   ATP-ase pH 9.4 × 300

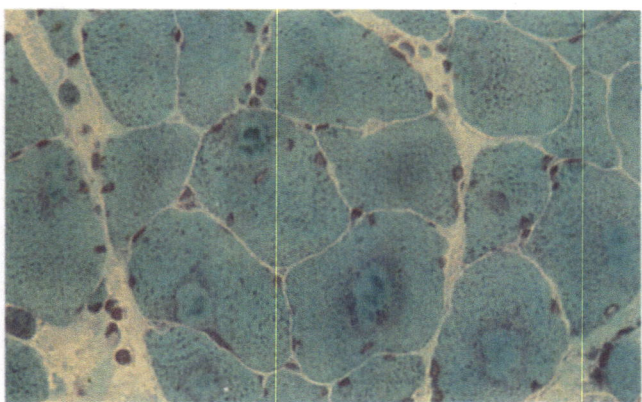

Figure 3.18   Target fibres. Central zone and outer ring have a purplish tinge. Gomori's trichrome × 300

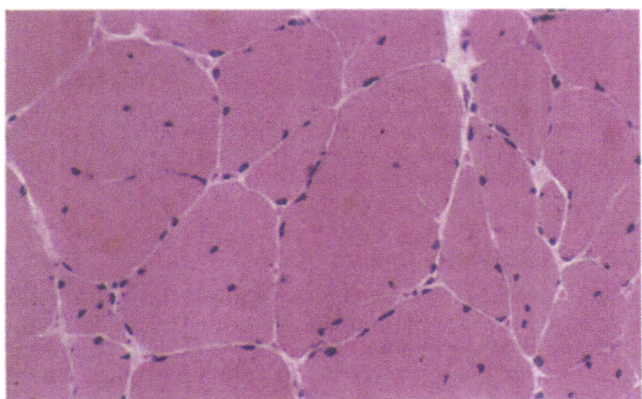

Figure 3.19 Fibre splitting in deltoid muscle of young man with slowly progressive mild form of chronic spinal muscular atrophy. Clefts in hypertrophied fibres are associated with central nuclei. Some fibres also contain small eosinophilic targets.   H & E × 300

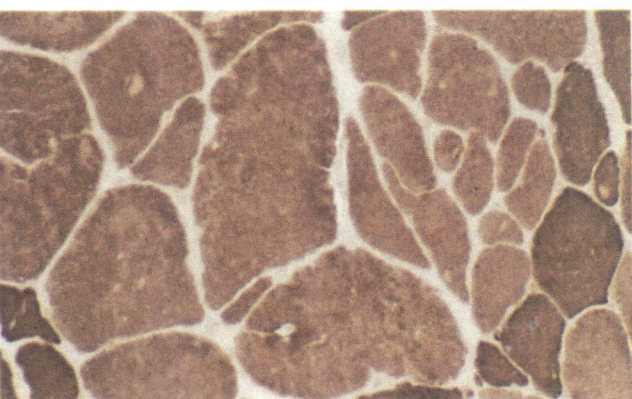

Figure 3.20 Fibre splitting – serial section of that shown in Figure 3.19. Comparison with the H & E section shows that the cluster of tiny type 1 fibres (light) is derived from splitting of larger fibres.   ATP-ase pH 9.4 × 300

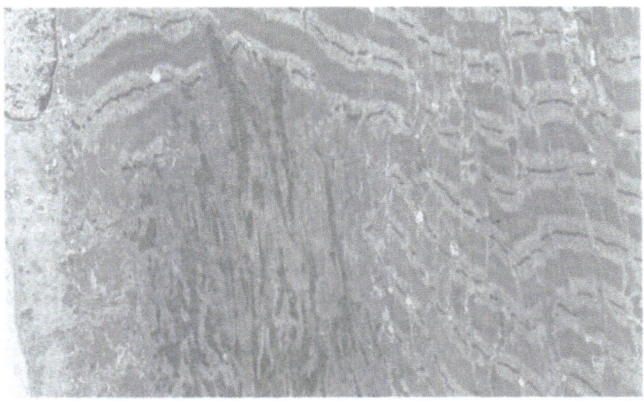

Figure 3.21 Target fibre in motor neuron disease. The central portion of the fibre shows myofilament disorganization, with abundant electron dense Z-band material.   EM × 4500

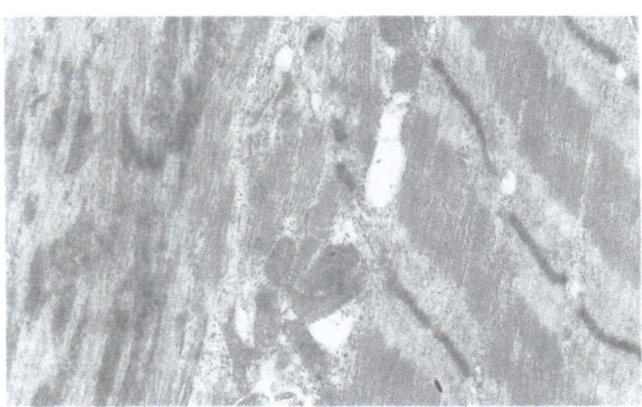

Figure 3.22 Target fibre. Central disorganization, with Z-band smearing. A narrow intermediate zone, with large mitochondria and slight myofilament disarray. Normal peripheral myofibrils.   EM × 11 000

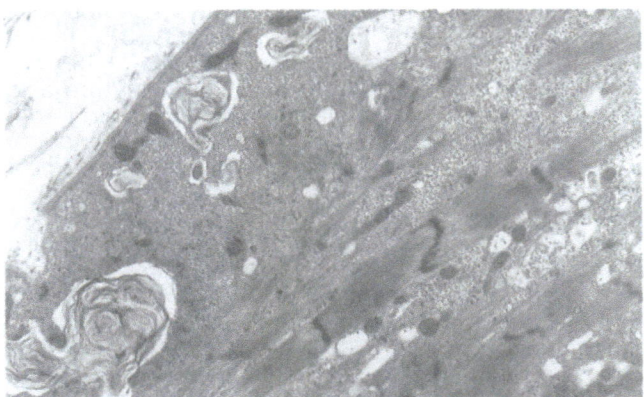

Figure 3.23 Peripheral disorganization in a denervated fibre, in motor neuron disease. There is a decrease and irregular arrangement of myofilaments. Several membranous whorls probably represent lysosomes.   EM × 7100

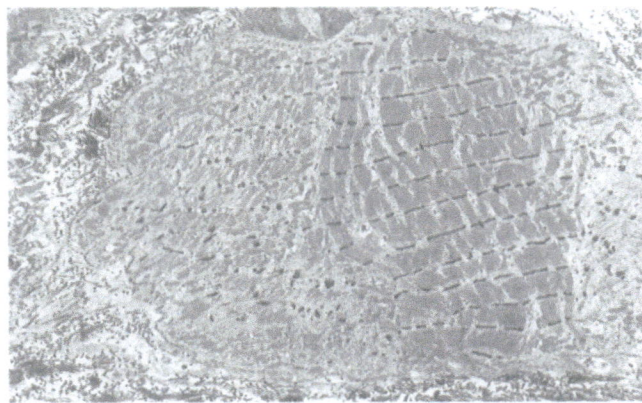

Figure 3.24 Disorganization of normal architecture in chronic, partial denervation. By light microscopy this biopsy from a young man with mild chronic spinal muscular atrophy showed fibre hypertrophy and conspicuous secondary myopathic changes. The abnormal arrangement of myofibrils may be a result of functional overloading of an innervated fibre.   EM × 2500

the intensity of staining. Increased lysosomal activity can be demonstrated with the acid-phosphatase reaction. Myosin ATP-ase remains detectable for a long period, probably many months after denervation and for as long as some myofibrils persist in the cytoplasm. Thus the different fibre types can still be distinguished, even amongst quite severely atrophied fibres (Figures 3.5 and 3.6). All fibre types are affected. Denervating disease rarely produces selective fibre type atrophy.

Re-innervation

In man, denervation is reversible for several months and possibly up to a year after onset[6]. Re-innervation completely restores normal structure and function of the cell.

Normal human muscle fibres do not have multiple innervation. A single motor end plate is formed *in utero* and the cell will not accept further innervation. However, after denervation the whole sarcolemma is again receptive. Re-innervation can take place at the site of the original motor end plate or elsewhere along the sarcolemma and can be mediated by regeneration of the original axon or sprouting from another axon. In disease of the motor end plate, terminal sprouting occurs from the original axon[7]. In anterior horn cell disease, where there is dying back of the axon, collateral sprouting occurs from the preterminal portion of adjacent healthy axons[7] (Diagram 3.2). This neuronal sprouting has been observed within 3 weeks of denervation. The stimulus to both terminal and pre-terminal sprouting probably resides in the denervated muscle cell, which synthesizes extrajunctional acetyl choline receptors. These receptors may in some way provide a chemotactic stimulus to the nearest healthy axon. In animals axonal sprouting and re-innervation can be prevented by pharmacological blockade of the new acetyl choline receptors[8].

When an axon is severed, sprouts also appear from the nodes of Ranvier close to the proximal cut end. As this may be some considerable distance from the muscle fibre, it suggests another mechanism is operating. In the intact cell, retrograde axonal transport possibly inhibits nodal sprouting. Inhibition ceases when the axon is severed.

Terminal and preterminal axon branching can be detected in a biopsy from the innervation zone, the motor end point, by methylene blue vital staining or Schofield's silver impregnation. These methods can be a useful adjunct to histochemistry in the investigation of chronic neuromuscular disease (Figures 3.7 – 3.9). The terminal innervation band is a narrow zone, close to the midpoint of normal human limb muscles, where motor end plates are concentrated[9] (Diagram 3.2). Each anterior horn cell supplies a large number of muscle fibres by successive bifurcation of its axis cylinder. Within the muscle motor neurons lie in tight bundles that branch repeatedly until they approach the innervation zone (Figure 3.7). A spray of short, myelinated, preterminal axons emerges from the bundle and each supplies a single end plate to one muscle fibre (Figures 3.8 and 3.9). The nerve terminal is thin, unmyelinated axon. In man, only a very small percentage of preterminal axons are branched and give rise to two end plates on the same or adjacent fibres. The functional terminal innervation ratio is the ratio of innervated muscle fibres to preterminal axons and in normal human muscle is approximately a 1:1 ratio[9]. After denervation and subsequent re-innervation this ratio may increase. In a biopsy one subterminal nerve fibre innervating three or more muscle fibres is certain evidence of re-innervation (Diagram 3.2) (Figure 3.10).

The Effects of Re-innervation

The consequences of re-innervation are threefold. Firstly, normal structure and contractile activity of the cell can be completely restored. Secondly, enlarged motor units are created by axonal sprouting, which enables one anterior horn cell to supply many additional muscle fibres[10]. These giant motor units can be detected by electromyography. Thirdly, analogous to cross-innervation experiments, a new motor nerve can induce a change in muscle fibre type[11]. This fibre type conversion may initially produce fibres with inter-mediate properties of fast and slow fibres, but ultimately conversion of both fine structure and enzyme profile appears complete. This change is reflected in a biopsy by type grouping (Diagram 3.3). The normal mosaic pattern is replaced by large clumps of uniform fibre type[12]. In normal human limb muscles groups of more than 12 contiguous fibres of the same type are unusual and more than 20 is strong evidence of re-innervation (Figures 3.11 and 3.12). Re-innervation may convert type 1 to type 2 fibres or the reverse. However, type 2 fibre grouping is usually only seen in the most chronic slowly, progressive denervating diseases (Figures 3.13 and 3.14). Type 1 fibre grouping predominates in more rapidly progressing disease and may be a reflection of earlier sprouting from type 1 motor neurons[7] (Figures 3.11 and 3.12). In general, in the most rapidly progressive denervating diseases fibre atrophy is the most significant pathological change. In the more chronic disorders a mixed pattern of grouped atrophy and type grouping is created by successive denervation, re-innervation and further denervation (Figures 3.13 and 3.14). Under these circumstances uniform type groups of atrophic fibres appear as the newly formed motor units are themselves denervated.

Target Fibres

The target is an aptly named cytoarchitectural abnormality, most often found in type 1 fibres in denervating diseases (Figures 3.15 – 3.18). Target fibres are best demonstrated with the NADH-TR or ATP-ase reaction (Figures 3.16 and 3.17). They are also revealed by the trichrome stain (Figure 3.18). In trans-verse section, the fibres appear normal at the periphery but contain a central or eccentric zone devoid of enzyme activity and bounded by a darkly stained rim of increased activity. With H & E the central zone is often eosinophilic and the border pale or faintly basophilic (Figure 3.15). Electron microscopy shows disorientated myofilaments and fibrillary masses of Z-band material in the central zone, but only very scanty mitochondria (Figures 3.21 and 3.22). In the inter-mediate zone there is an accumulation of mitochondria and glycogen. Myofibrils may show Z-band smearing[13]. The outermost zone is entirely normal. The longitudinal extent of the target is very variable.

Variations of this abnormality are fibres with an indistinct dark rim, usually called targetoid and those where it is absent, which are indistinguishable from the cores of central core disease. Transitions between these forms occur and it seems likely that they reflect different stages of the same basic disturbance[14].

In human muscle numerous targets are almost always indicative of a neurogenic disease. Experimental observations have shown the target is a transient and reversible phenomenon[15]. Targets may appear in early denervation and again during re-innervation. They are most often seen in normal size fibres[14]. It seems likely that disorganization of architecture is attributable to temporary excessive irritability of the fibre[16]. In neurogenic disorders target and core-targetoid fibres appear exclusively in type 1 fibres, but the same phenomenon can be produced experimentally in type 2 fibres by tenotomy[15,16].

Secondary Myopathic Changes in Association with Chronic Partial Denervation

In denervating diseases increasing functional stresses are applied to residual innervated fibres. In chronic, slowly progressive conditions this not only induces considerable functional hypertrophy, but may also be responsible for a variety of architectural abnormalities and even degenerative changes in the fibres. Thus moth-eaten fibres and other disturbances of myofibrillar arrangement appear (Figure 3.24). In very large fibres central nuclei are common and their appearance may precede fibre splitting (Figure 3.19). Longitudinal clefts lined by plasma membrane extend into the cytoplasm (Figure 3.20) creating abnormal branched fibres or sometimes completely separate fragments, which will atrophy unless they are innervated[17,18]. The split fibres can be identified in transverse section by the separate fragments which fit together as pieces of a jigsaw and show the same histochemical reaction (Figures 3.19 and 3.20). Functional overloading can also cause segmental necrosis, which is followed by phagocytosis and regeneration. In the biopsy of chronic partial denervation these secondary myopathic changes may be superimposed upon the basic pattern of group atrophy and type grouping.

References

1. Sutherland, S. (1978). Morphological changes in striated muscle due to denervation. In *Nerves and Nerve Injuries* (pp 229–47) (Edinburgh: Churchill Livingstone)

2. Tomanek, R. J. and Lund, D. L. (1973). Degeneration of different types of skeletal muscle fibres. I. Denervation. *J. Anat.*, **116**, 395–407

3. Engel, A. G. and Stonnington, H. H. (1974). Morphological effects of denervation of muscle. A quantitative ultrastructural study. *Ann. N. Y. Acad. Sci.*, **228**, 68–88

4. Cullen, M. J. and Pluskal, M. G. (1977). Early changes in the ultrastructure of denervated rat skeletal muscle. *Exp. Neurol.*, **56**, 115–31

5. Gauthier, G. F. and Dunn, R. A. (1973). Ultrastructural and cytochemical features of mammalian skeletal muscle fibres following denervation. *J. Cell Sci.*, **12**, 525–47

6. Sutherland, S. (1978). The capacity of human muscles to function efficiently following re-innervation after prolonged denervation. In *Nerves and Nerve Injuries*, 2nd Edn., pp. 312–16. (Edinburgh: Churchill Livingstone)

7. Duchen, L. W. (1975). Pathology of the innervation of skeletal muscle. In Harrison, C. V. and Weinbren, K. (eds.) *Recent Advances in Pathology 9*, pp. 217–48. (Churchill Livingstone)

8. Pestronk, A. and Drachman, D. B. (1978). Motor nerve sprouting and acetyl choline receptors. *Science*, **199**, 1223–5

9. Coers, C. and Woolf, A. L. (1959). Normal histology of the intramuscular nerves and nerve endings. In *The Innervation of Muscle. A Biopsy Study*, pp. 12–41. (Oxford: Blackwell Scientific Publications)

10. Kugelberg, E., Edstrom, L. and Abbruzzesse, M. (1970). Mapping of motor units in experimentally re-innervated rat muscle. *J. Neurol., Neurosurg. Psychiatry.*, **33**, 319–29

11. Romanul, F. C. A. and van der Meulen, J. P. (1966). Reversal of enzyme profiles of muscle fibres in fast and slow muscles by cross innervation. *Nature (Lond.)*, **212**, 1369–70

12. Edstrom, L. and Kugelberg, E. (1969). Histochemical mapping motor units in experimentally re-innervated skeletal muscle. *Experientia*, **25**, 1044–5

13. DeCoster, W., De Reuck, J. and Vander Eecken, H. (1976). The target phenomenon in human muscle. A comparative light microscopic, histochemical and electron microscopic study. *Acta Neuropathol. (Berl.)*, **34**, 329–38

14. Schmitt, H. P. (1979). Quantitative analysis of the size distribution of target and targetoid fibres employing the method of Daeves and Beckel for mixed distributions. *Acta Neuropathol. (Berl.)*, **45**, 215–20

15. DeReuck, J., DeCoster, W. and Vander Eecken, H. (1977). The target phenomenon in the rat muscle following tenotomy and neurotomy. Comparative light microscopic and histochemical study. *Acta Neuropathol. (Berl.)*, **37**, 49–53

16. DeReuck, J., DeCoster, W. and Vander Eecken, H. (1977). Development and inhibition of the target phenomenon in tenotomised rat muscle. *Acta Neuropathol. (Berl.)*, **40**, 179–81

17. Schwartz, M. S., Sargeant, M. and Swash, M. (1976). Longitudinal fibre splitting in neurogenic muscular disorders. Its relation to the pathogenesis of 'myopathic' change. *Brain*, **99**, 617–36

18. Swash, M., Schwartz, M. S. and Sargeant, M. K. (1978). Pathogenesis of longitudinal splitting of muscle fibres in neurogenic disorders and in polymyositis. *Neuropathol., Appl. Neurobiol.*, **4**, 99–115

Motor Neuron Disease

The most severe denervating disorders are those due to degeneration and loss of motor nerve cells. Poliomyelitis is an example of acute anterior horn cell disease attributable to the cytopathic effects of the virus, but is unlikely to require diagnostic muscle biopsy. In the more chronic disorders pathological changes beginning in the nerve cell body are frequently followed by gradual 'dying back' of the axon. These diseases include the spinal muscular atrophies and motor neuron disease. Pathologically, certain chronic peripheral neuropathies may also be anterior horn cell diseases, but, because they also show peripheral demyelination, they will be described separately (Chapter 6).

Motor neuron disease (MND) is a disease of middle to old age with male predominance (M:F = 2:1), characterized by progressive, widespread degeneration of motor nerve cells. The disease affects anterior horn cells, brainstem nuclei and Betz cells in the cerebral cortex. The disease is by no means rare and has world-wide distribution. The majority of cases are sporadic, although familial forms exist, most with dominant inheritance and sometimes onset in the late twenties or early thirties[1,2]. Clinically, the combination of upper and lower motor neuron lesions is characterized by wasting and fasciculation of limb muscles associated with spasticity and brisk reflexes. The upper limbs are usually affected first and the lesions may be asymmetrical. The first signs often appear in the distal, small muscles of the hand, but in most cases the disease progresses quite rapidly to a global weakness. The duration from clinical onset to death rarely exceeds 3 years. A more rapid downhill course may follow early bulbar involvement, because difficulty in swallowing leads to aspiration pneumonia and early death. In rare familial cases the disease is only slowly progressive over a period of 10 years or more. Various clinical patterns occur dependent on the maximal site of neuron loss. Amyotrophic lateral sclerosis describes a form where corticospinal tract signs predominate, whereas progressive muscular atrophy and progressive bulbar palsy refer to dominant lower motor neuron lesions of the limbs and medulla, respectively. There is no cardiac involvement in MND. In the common sporadic cases there is no sensory loss. The extraocular muscles and autonomic nervous system are spared.

There are three isolated geographical locations with an extraordinarily high incidence of the disease. One is the little Pacific island of Guam where MND accounts for 10% of deaths amongst the Chamorro people, another is the Kiwi peninsula of Japan and the third is in New Guinea[3]. Although genetic susceptibility seems likely, a clear pattern of Mendelian inheritance has not been demonstrated. Specific environmental factors have been sought, and a neurotoxic effect of manganese in drinking water is suggested[4].

Investigations have revealed increased concentrations of manganese[5] and other metals, particularly lead, in the spinal cord of MND patients[6]. However, the findings are variable and may represent accumulation in already degenerate neurons[7].

Neurotropic viruses have often been proposed as the cause of MND, but there are no consistent positive findings. Several reports have suggested that patients with residual damage due to poliomyelitis are more susceptible to MND[8,9], but polio virus has not been isolated from neural tissue, virus particles have not been identified by electron microscopy and transmission experiments have been unsuccessful. A pathogenetic role for viruses cannot be completely dismissed. Certain viral antigens, polio, measles and herpes have been identified by direct immunofluorescence in the jejunal mucosa of MND patients, but rarely in controls[10]. The antigens may only be markers of defective immunity as impaired T cell function has also been demonstrated in MND[11]. There is circumstantial evidence for immuno-pathological activity. An unusually high incidence of HLA-A2, A3 and A28 has been reported[12]. Immune complexes have occasionally been detected in serum in glomeruli[13]. Diluted serum from patients with MND but not from other chronic neurological disorders, including spinal muscular atrophy, has been shown to be selectively toxic to mouse anterior horn cells in culture[14]. The aetiology of MND is still obscure and probably multifactorial. A variety of insults may culminate in neuron degeneration with advancing age.

Postmortem Findings

Postmortem studies in MND show shrunken anterior spinal nerve roots. Macroscopically there is extensive loss of anterior horn cells, particularly in the lumbar and cervical enlargements[15]. Residual neurons may show degenerative changes and occasionally neuronophagia, but inflammatory cell infiltration is rare. Somatic motor neurons innervating skeletal muscles are diffusely involved in MND except at the rostral and caudal extremities of the neuraxis[16]. Thus, although motor nuclei of the trigeminal and facial nerves may be affected, the oculomotor, trochlear and aducens nuclei are spared and also neurons of the sacral anterior horn responsible for innervation of external sphincters of the anus and urethra[17]. Unlike storage diseases, which usually show universal neuronal involvement, in MND, cell dropout is patchy. Even in severely affected zones, occasional cells are spared. Various fine structural changes have been observed including eosinophilic cytoplasmic inclusions in motor nerve cell bodies, which are possibly autophagic vacuoles. There may be accumulations of neurofilaments, called spheroids, in

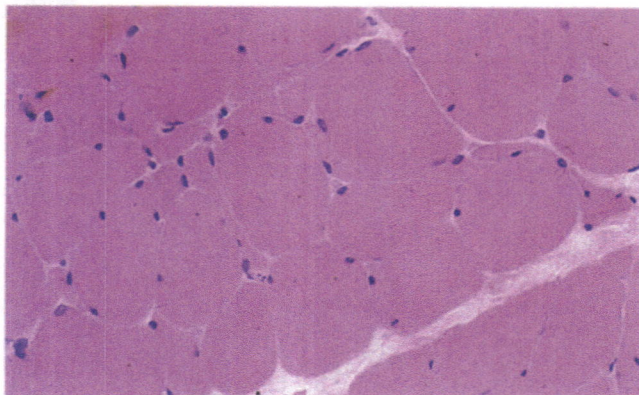

Figure 4.1 Small group atrophy in motor neuron disease. Deltoid muscle of 75-year-old woman with a short history of bulbar weakness and recent evidence of weakness in arms. H & E × 180

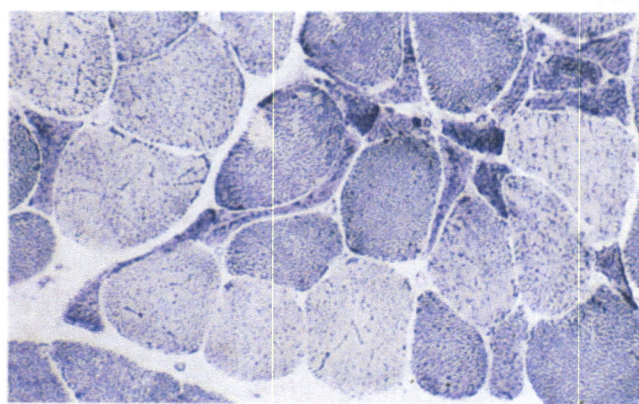

Figure 4.2 Small group atrophy in motor neuron disease. Serial section of Figure 4.1. Atrophic, denervated fibres are darkly stained and thus more readily identified with the oxidative enzyme reaction. NADH-TR × 180

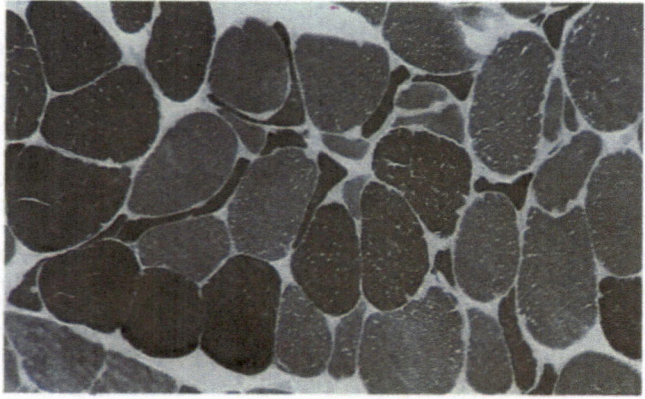

Figure 4.3 Small group atrophy in motor neuron disease. Serial section of Figures 4.1 and 4.2. Atrophic, denervated fibres are both types 1 and 2. ATP-ase pH 9.4 × 180

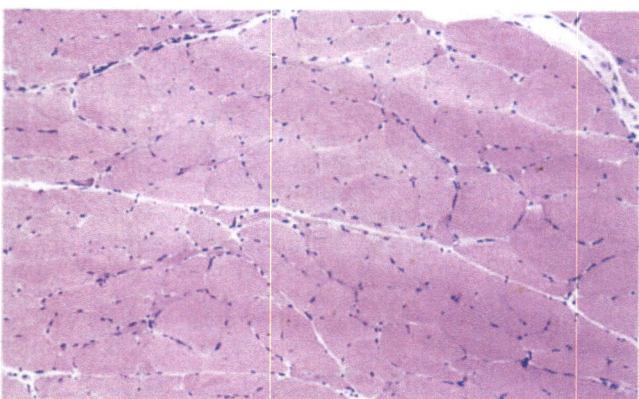

Figure 4.4 Small group atrophy in motor neuron disease. Quadriceps muscle of 58-year-old man. Atrophic fibres are easily overlooked in H & E sections. H & E × 75

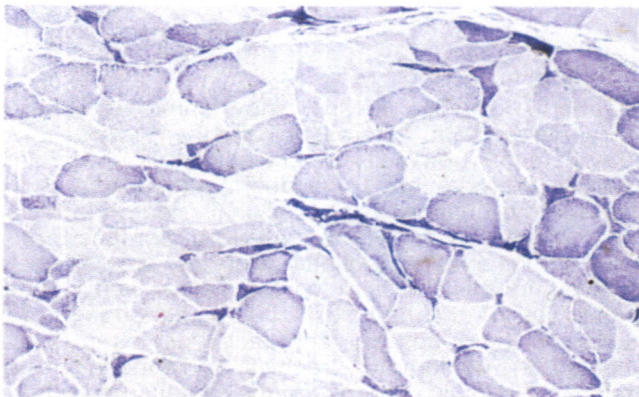

Figure 4.5 Small group atrophy in motor neuron disease. Serial section of Figure 4.4. Atrophic fibres, darkly stained with the oxidative enzyme reaction are easily identified, even at low magnification. NADH-TR × 75

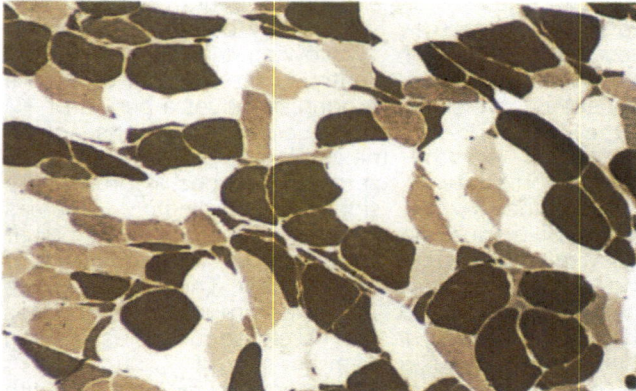

Figure 4.6 Small group atrophy in motor neuron disease. Serial section of Figures 4.4 and 4.5. Atrophic, denervated fibres are both types 1 and type 2. ATP-ase pH 4.6 × 75

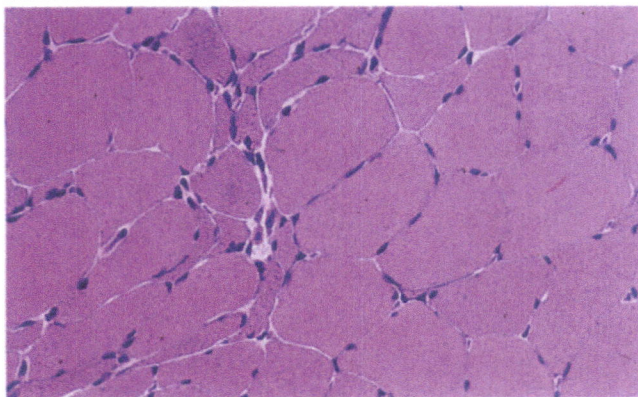

Figure 4.7 Small group atrophy in motor neuron disease. Atrophic denervated fibres have faintly basophilic cytoplasm. This may be due to increased ribosomal activity and also to loss of myofibrils.   H & E × 180

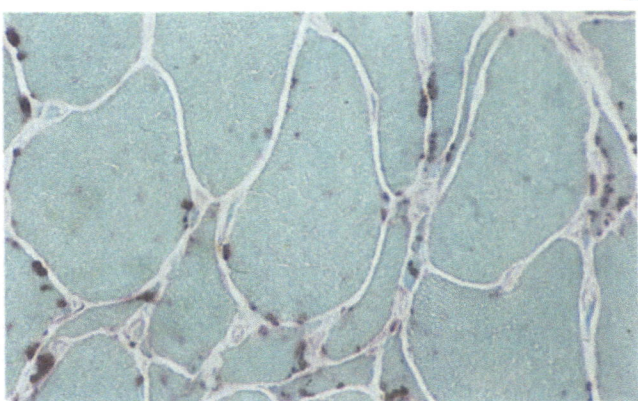

Figure 4.8 Atrophic, denervated fibres show some increase in acid-phosphatase activity, located in lysosomes. Secondary lysosomes, which correlate with lipofuschin pigment, are always present in ageing muscle cells, but denervated fibres also show an increase in primary lysosomal enzyme activity. Acid phosphatase × 300

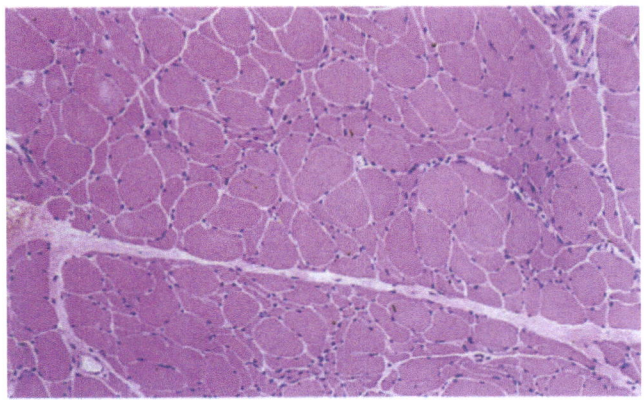

Figure 4.9 Small group atrophy in deltoid muscle of 55-year-old man with weakness of all limbs. A distinctive picture of clusters of angular atrophic fibres, which contrast with the mildly hypertrophied innervated fibres. H & E × 75

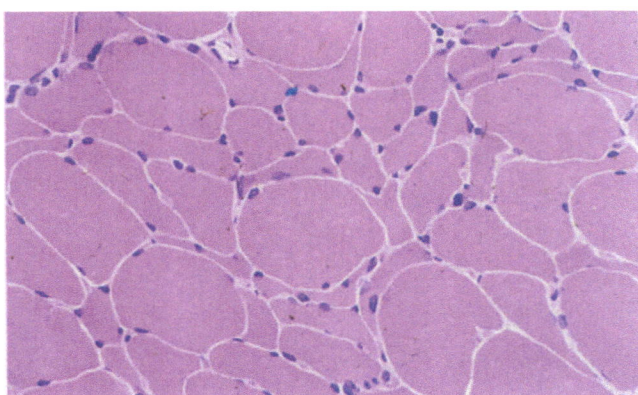

Figure 4.10 Small group atrophy. Angular denervated fibres appear moulded by hypertrophic innervated fibres.   H & E × 180

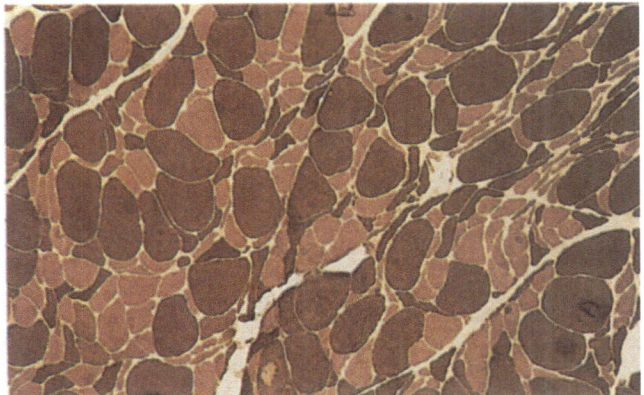

Figure 4.11 Compensatory hypertrophy in motor neuron disease. Deltoid biopsy from a 48-year-old woman with a 9-month history of lower limb weakness. Fasciculation noted in deltoids. Atrophic fibres are both type 1 and type 2, but the majority of hypertrophied fibres are type 2 (dark). In early MND, many innervated type 2 motor units are still present and respond to overloading by compensatory hypertrophy.   ATP-ase pH 9.4 × 75

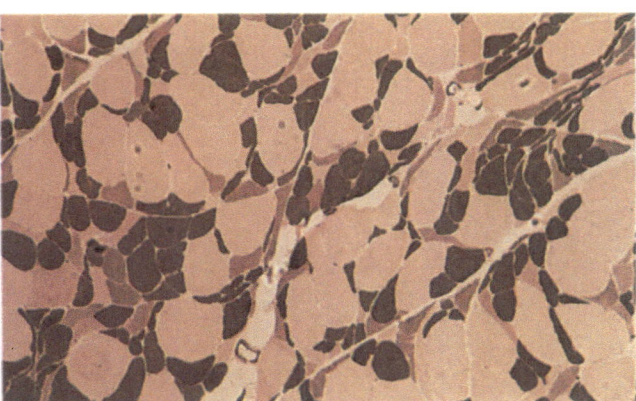

Figure 4.12 Compensatory hypertrophy in motor neuron disease. Serial section to Figure 4.11. Type 2A fibres appear light, type 2B intermediate and type 1 dark.   ATP-ase pH 4.6 × 75

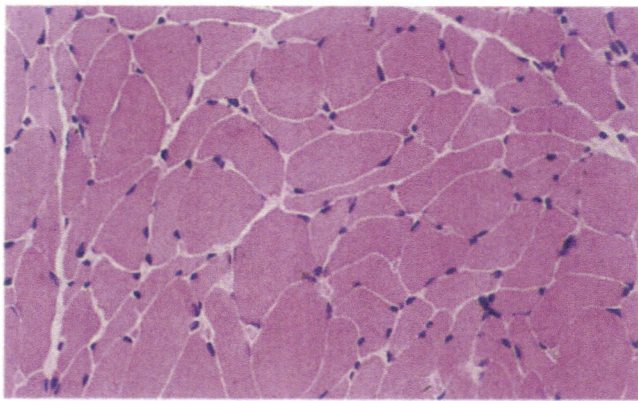

Figure 4.13 Selective type 2 fibre atrophy is revealed by histochemistry, but with H & E the pattern could be mistaken for denervation atrophy. Biceps muscle of 67-year-old woman with 8-year history of a connective tissue disease, with seronegative arthritis, raised ESR and antinuclear factor. Mild progressive proximal muscle weakness. (Same cases shown in Figures 4.15 and 4.16.) H & E × 180

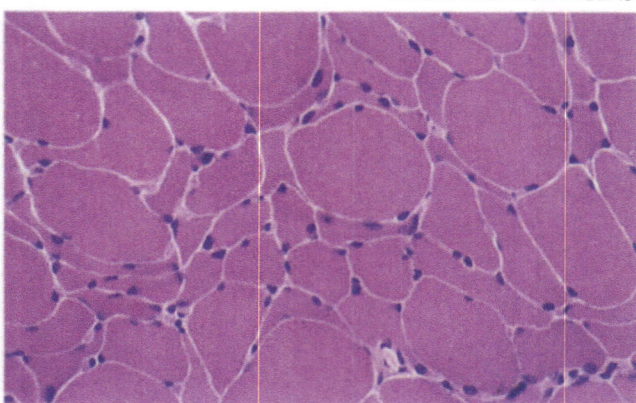

Figure 4.14 Denervation atrophy in motor neuron disease for comparison with Figure 4.13. H & E × 180

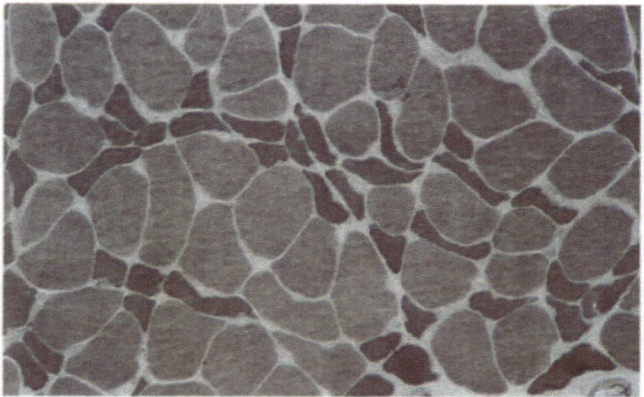

Figure 4.15 Serial section to Figures 4.13 and 4.14 showing selective type 2 atrophy (dark fibres). This pattern contrasts with denervation atrophy, which characteristically involves both type 1 and type 2 fibres. ATP-ase pH 9.4 × 180

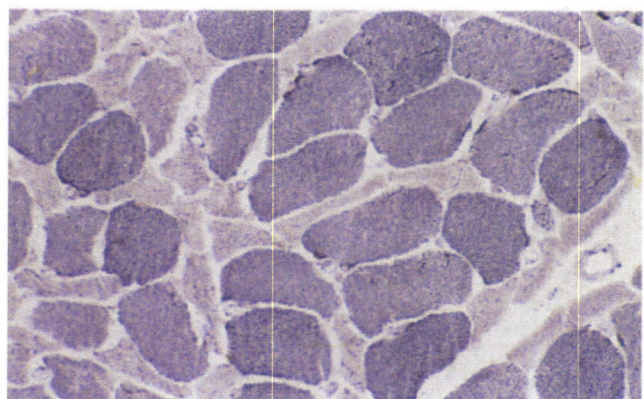

Figure 4.16 Serial section to Figure 4.13 reveals selective type 2 atrophy. NADH-TR × 180

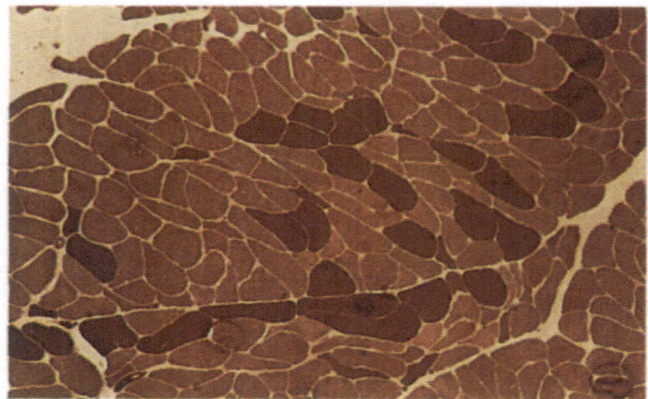

Figure 4.17 Type grouping in motor neuron disease in deltoid muscle of 56-year-old woman with 4-month history of increasing weakness of lower limbs. Fasciculations observed in both legs and arms. The normal mosaic pattern has disappeared. The majority of fibres are type 1 fibres (light), with a few remaining type 2 fibres (dark). The change is due to re-innervation of denervated fibres by type 1 motor neurons and conversion of many type 2 fibres to type 1. ATP-ase pH 9.4 × 75

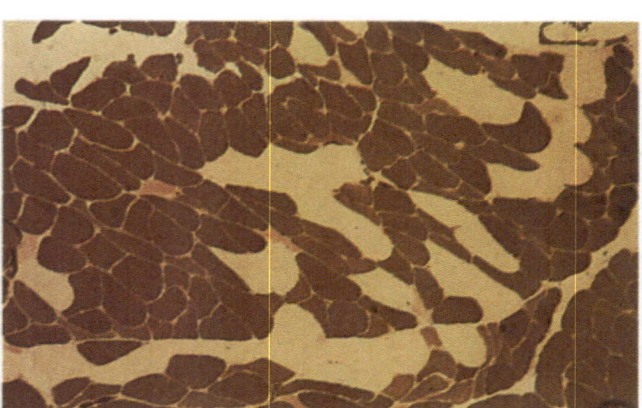

Figure 4.18 Type grouping in motor neuron disease. Serial section to Figure 4.17. Type 1 fibres are dark. Type 2 fibres are light. ATP-ase pH 4.3 × 75

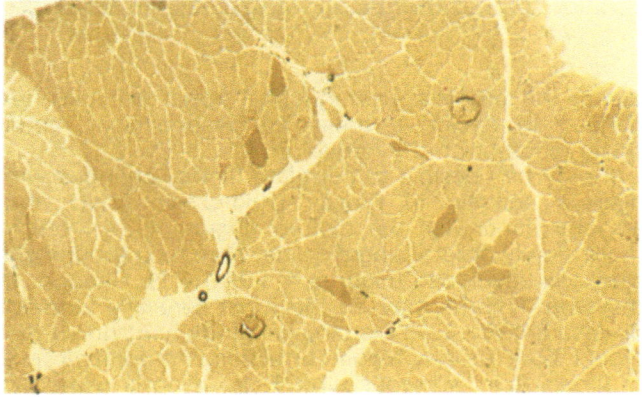

Figure 4.19 Type grouping in motor neuron disease. Deltoid muscle of 54-year-old man with 3-year history of gradually increasing, asymmetrical weakness of legs and arms. Whole fascicles are composed of type 1 fibres, with very few residual type 2 fibres. Type grouping in MND is usually of type 1 fibres. (Same case shown in Figures 4.20 and 4.21.) ATP-ase pH 9.4 × 30

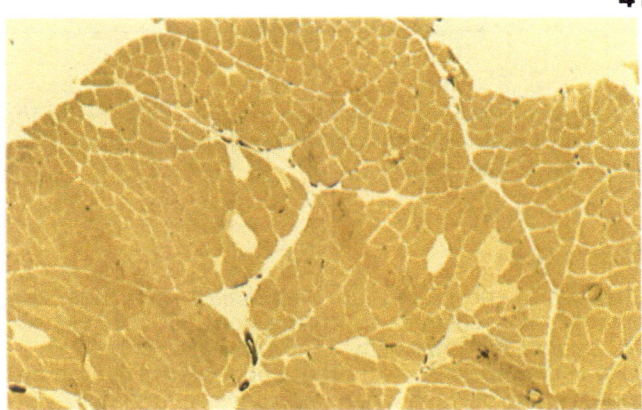

Figure 4.20 Type grouping. Serial section to Figure 4.19. ATP-ase pH 4.2 × 30

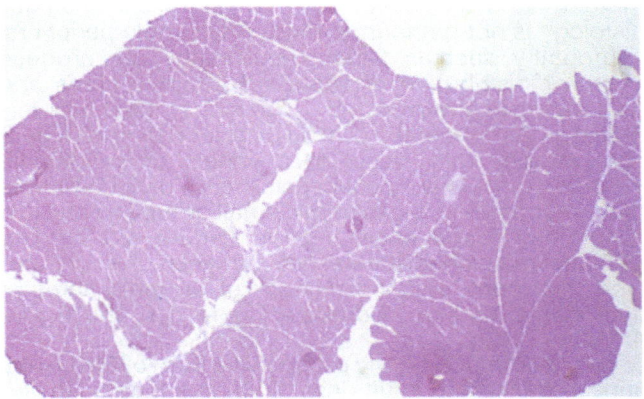

Figure 4.21 Serial section to Figures 4.19 and 4.20. The evidence of denervation and subsequent re-innervation cannot be obtained from an H & E section. H & E × 30

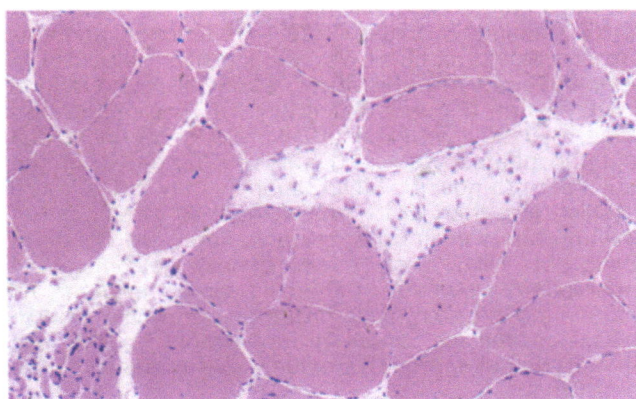

Figure 4.22 Two pale staining, necrotic fibres in unusually slowly, progressive motor neuron disease. Deltoid muscle of a 75-year-old man with gradual deterioration in walking over 5 years, proximal and distal wasting. A group of severely atrophic, denervated fibres is also present. Minor myopathic changes such as this may appear, but are never very great, in classical motor neuron disease. H & E × 180

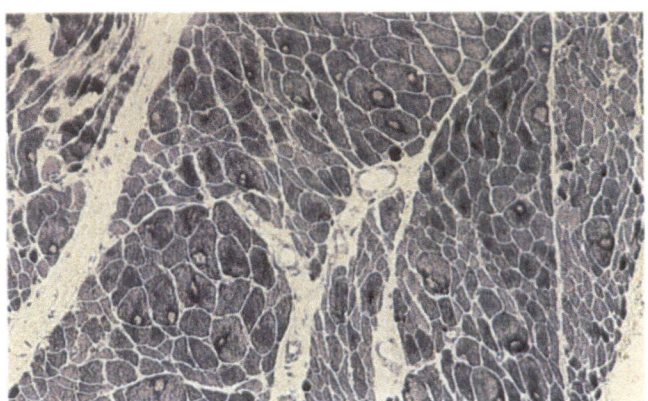

Figure 4.23 Target fibres in deltoid muscle of 64-year-old man with motor neuron disease. NADH-TR × 75

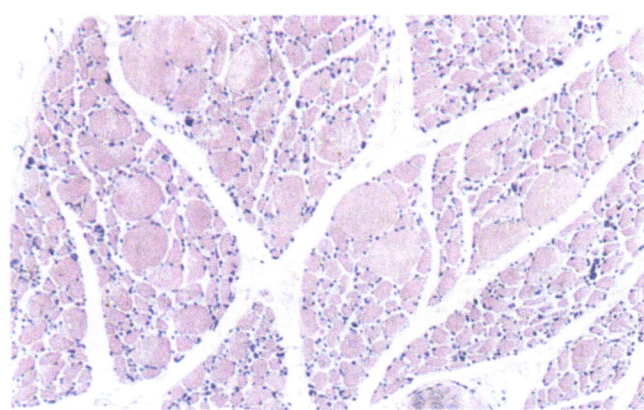

Figure 4.24 Severe neurogenic atrophy in motor neuron disease. Biceps muscle of a 67-year-old woman with rapidly progressing generalized weakness and wasting. H & E × 75

the proximal axon[16]. The changes are not specific for MND and may reflect intracellular disorganization from a variety of causes.

Muscle Biopsy

Changes in the biopsy are dependent upon both the severity of involvement of the muscle selected for biopsy and the chronicity of the disease. Clinical difficulty in diagnosis is most often encountered early in the course of the disease when histological changes may be relatively minor. Established motor neuron disease is clinically unmistakable and has an equally characteristic biopsy picture of rapidly progressing denervation. Some cases may reveal evidence of re-innervation and secondary myopathic changes which imply a slower progression.

The earliest signs of denervation are very small groups (3–4) of angular atrophic fibres (Figures 4.1–4.6). The tell-tale atrophic fibres are easily missed without a careful search. These small fibres are usually darkly staining with the NADH-TR reaction and this histochemical reaction is particularly valuable in detecting a few atrophic fibres, easily missed in routine H & E section (Figures 4.2 and 4.5). The denervated fibres may be faintly basophilic and show increased acid-phosphatase activity (Figures 4.7 and 4.8). In the very early stages of MND, biopsy may be a more sensitive test than EMG, but it must be stressed that small numbers of angular atrophic fibres are not diagnostic of MND, or even definite evidence of denervation. However, if there is clinical evidence of denervation in one muscle group and only suspicion of disease elsewhere, small group atrophy in the less affected muscles provides evidence of multisegmental denervation.

When the muscle biopsied is definitely weak, the histological evidence of denervation is unmistakable. Small group atrophy is obvious and the remaining fibres show varying degrees of compensatory hypertrophy (Figures 4.9 and 4.10). Initially, this enlargement is greater in type 2 fibres (Figures 4.11 and 4.12). Measurement of fibre diameters reveals a twin-peaked histogram. The angular atrophic fibres frequently appear to have been moulded by the adjacent rounded, hypertrophied fibres. The ATP-ase reaction always shows atrophy of both type 1 and type 2 fibres, although either may predominate. If there is selective fibre type atrophy, particularly type 2 atrophy, the diagnosis of denervation is in doubt (Figures 4.13–4.16). This histochemical method may also reveal type grouping, where large clumps of uniform fibre type provide evidence of re-innervation (Figures 4.17–4.21). Initially re-innervation is responsible for type groups of normal sized or hypertrophied fibres, but with the inevitable progress of denervation the new motor units are themselves denervated, creating groups of uniform atrophic fibres. In classical MND the type grouping is most often of type 1 fibres (Figures 4.19 and 4.20).

At all stages of MND inflammatory changes are rare. Isolated, tiny foci of interstitial chronic inflammatory cells are found very occasionally and do not negate the diagnosis, but if there is any more obvious inflammatory cell infiltration MND is an unlikely diagnosis. Even in the most chronic cases showing secondary myopathic changes, inflammatory cells are scarce (Figure 4.22). Target fibres are sometimes found in MND, occasionally in profusion (Figure 4.23). As in other neurogenic conditions the targets appear in type 1 fibres, but it is often difficult to decide if these are evidence of recent denervation or of re-innervation.

It may be possible to correlate biopsy changes with disease activity. In rapidly progressive MND fibre atrophy dominates the picture (Figure 4.24), but in more slowly progressing disease, fibre type grouping is also well developed (Figures 4.19–4.21). Changes in the type 1 fibres may be the most sensitive index of disease activity. One histological study has shown that type 1 fibre atrophy alone correlates with total atrophy of the muscle, whereas type 1 grouping is related to long duration[18]. In the exceptional and usually familial cases of long duration, secondary myopathic effects appear (Figure 4.22). Despite this, the background of small group atrophy and type grouping is still clear.

The Differential Diagnosis

In the biopsy of established MND the loss of many motor units is distinctive. However, in the earlier stages histology is not pathognomonic. Any simple peripheral neuropathy, such as diabetic neuropathy, can produce a similar distribution of scattered atrophic fibres and minimal small group atrophy. The biopsy must be interpreted in the light of the clinical picture. Selective type 2 fibre atrophy may occur in a variety of conditions, including cachexia, polymyositis and carcinomatous neuromyopathy and can mimic small group atrophy in a haematoxylin and eosin section (Figure 4.13). The ATP-ase reaction distinguishes between this uniform type 2 atrophy and the mixture of atrophic fibres in neurogenic disease. (Compare Figure 4.5 and Figure 4.15.)

The uncommon slowly progressive form of MND may appear identical to adult onset SMA in a biopsy. In life, the pyramidal tract signs of MND may be the only distinguishing feature. Cervical and lumbar disc disease can usually be identified by myelography, but mild spondylosis is relatively common in the elderly and may co-exist with MND. Disc lesions may be responsible for chronic denervation atrophy, but in contrast with MND the changes are usually mild. Type groups of atrophic fibres indicating progressive denervation are far more likely to indicate MND. Fasciculations and cramps are common in MND but these signs alone are not pathognomonic of a progressive disorder. They may occasionally develop after poliomyelitis or other virus infections without progressive muscle wasting. Biopsy has revealed evidence of mild, chronic, partial denervation[19]

References

1. Horton, W. A., Eldridge, R. and Brody, J. A. (1976). Familial motor neuron disease. *Neurology*, **26**, 460–5

2. Alberca, R., Castilla, J. M. and Gil-Peralta, A. (1981). Hereditary amyotropic lateral sclerosis. *J. Neurol. Sci.*, **50**, 201–6

3. Gajdusek, D. C. and Salazar, A. M. (1982). Amyotrophic lateral sclerosis and parkinsonian syndromes in high incidence among the Auyu and Jakai people of West New Guinea. *Neurology*, **32**, 107–26

4. Yase, Y. (1972). The pathogenesis of amyotrophic lateral sclerosis. *Lancet*, **2**, 292–6

5. Miyata, S. *et al.* (1983). Increased manganese level in spinal cords of amyotrophic lateral sclerosis determined by radiochemical neutron activation analysis. *J. Neurol. Sci.*, **61**, 283–93

6. Kurlander, H. M. and Patten, B. M. (1979). Metals in spinal cord tissue of patients dying of motor neuron disease. *Ann. Neurol.*, **6**, 21–6

7. Mandybur, T. I. and Cooper, G. P. (1979). Increased spinal lead content in amyotrophic lateral sclerosis – possibly a secondary phenomenon. *Med. Hypotheses*, **5**, 1313–15

8. Campbell, A. M. G., Williams, E. R. and Pearce, J. (1969). Late motor neuron degeneration following poliomyelitis. *Neurology*, **19**, 1101–6

9. Norris, F. H. (1975). Recent advances in motor neuron diseases. In Bradley, W. G., Gardner-Medwin, D. and Walton, J. N. (eds.) (1975). *Recent Advances in Myology, International Congress Series.* pp. 522–36. (Amsterdam: Excerpta Medica)

10. Pertschuk, L. P. *et al.* (1979). Jejunal mucosa in motor neurone disease and other chronic neurological disorders. In Behan, P. O. and Clifford Rose, F. (eds.) *Progress in Neurological Research.* pp. 44–61. (Tunbridge Wells: Pitman Medical Publishing)

11. Behan, P. O. *et al.* (1977). Possible persistent virus in motor neurone disease. *Lancet*, **2**, 1176

12. Behan, P. O., Dick, H. M. and Durward, W. F. (1977). Histocompatibility antigens associated with motor neurone disease. *J. Neurol. Sci.*, **32**, 213–17

13. Oldstone, M. B. A., Perrin, L. H., Wilson, C. B. and Norris, F. H. (1976). Evidence for immune complex formation in patients with amyotrophic lateral sclerosis. *Lancet*, **2**, 169

14. Wolfgram, F. and Myers, L. (1973). Amyotrophic lateral sclerosis; effects of serum on anterior horn cells in tissue culture. *Science*, **179**, 579–80

15. Tsukagoshi, H. *et al.* (1980). Mophometric quantitation of cervical limb motor cells in various neuromuscular diseases. *J. Neurol. Sci.*, **47**, 463–72

16. Iwata, M. and Hirano, A. (1979). Current problems in the pathology of amyotrophic lateral sclerosis. In Zimmerman, H. M. (ed.) *Progress in Neuropathology.* Vol. 4, pp. 277–98. (New York: Raven Press)

17. Mannen, T., Iwata, M., Toyokura, Y. and Nagashima, K. (1977). Preservation of a certain motor neuron group of the sacral cord in amyotrophic lateral sclerosis – its clinical significance. *J. Neurol., Neurosurg. Psychiatry.*, **40**, 464–9

18. Patten, B. M., Zito, G. and Harati, Y. (1979). Histological findings in motor neuron disease. Relation to clinically determined activity, duration and severity of disease. *Arch. Neurol.*, **36**, 560–4

19. Fetell, M. R. *et al.* (1982). A benign motor neuron disorder; delayed cramps and fasciculation after poliomyelitis or myelitis. *Ann. Neurol.*, **11**, 423–7

The spinal muscular atrophies are a group of inherited disorders characterized by degeneration of anterior horn cells (Figure 5.1) and progressive muscle weakness. Pearn[1] has defined seven separate SMA syndromes on a clinical and genetic basis, of which acute infantile and chronic childhood SMA form the majority. In recent years adult onset SMA has been identified as a major cause of the limb girdle syndrome[2]. The carrier frequency for one of the SMA genes is estimated to be 1 in 40 Caucasians. Most types show autosomal recessive inheritance[1,3]. Muscle biopsy and EMG are important diagnostic investigations which provide evidence of denervation. However EMG may be particularly difficult to perform in the very young infant. The serum creatine phosphokinase (CPK) is usually in the normal range, except in the more chronic syndromes when the level may be moderately raised.

Acute infantile SMA (SMA type I or Werdnig–Hoffmann disease) has been identified as a single nosological entity[4]. Onset of clinical weakness is always before 6 months of age, 95% before 4 months and in 30% is antenatal, as judged by diminished fetal movements[4]. The condition is one of the many causes of a floppy infant, but gross weakness and global paresis, as opposed to mere hypotonia, create a distinctive clinical picture. The disease is always fatal by 3 years. The risk in a subsequent pregnancy is one in four, but if a sibling is unaffected at 6 months, normal development can be predicted[5].

Chronic childhood SMA is a separate progressive disorder, also determined in the majority by a single autosomal recessive gene[6]. In comparison with the acute form, chronic childhood SMA does not of itself cause death before 18 months of age and has a wide spectrum of clinical manifestations[7]. The median age at death exceeds 10 years and a few patients survive beyond the third decade. Onset is usually before 3 years, occasionally in the first 6 months (severe chronic SMA, type 2). Most patients with this early onset and generalized disease become severely incapacitated[8]. In a group of 18 cases reported by Pearn less than 25% were able to sit unsupported and none were able to walk[9]. Such patients develop gross deformities, including scoliosis and chest deformities which increase susceptibility to pneumonia and early death. Not all patients are as severely affected. A minority with early onset do manage to walk, but this ability is rarely maintained beyond 10 years (intermediate chronic SMA)[10]. The clinical spectrum also encompasses a small group who present later in childhood (3–14 years), have mild weakness and show only slow progression (mild SMA, type 3, Kugelberg–Welander disease)[9]. These children are able to walk, generally remain mobile for many years, and may have almost normal life expectancy. Children with chronic childhood SMA, unlike those with Duchenne muscular dystrophy are usually of normal intelligence.

In the absence of a family history, chronic childhood SMA, with onset in the first 6 months, may be confused with acute infantile SMA. Muscle biopsy reveals similar changes and is of little value in making the distinction, which is important because of the considerable difference in prognosis. Most cases can be differentiated clinically, because only the acute form shows such profound generalized weakness at onset[5].

Family studies in chronic childhood SMA have shown that whilst the majority of affected siblings follow a similar pattern, in a minority there is marked discordance in clinical severity and age of death[6]. This familial variation forms the basis of the single gene hypothesis. Thus, although the risk of further affected children is one in four, it is impossible to predict the clinical course with certainty. In general, the later the onset, the slower the progression of the disease. There is possibly a female sparing effect[10]. In familial cases with early onset, the sex incidence is equal, but male siblings tend to be more severely affected. In families with the very mild form there is a preponderance of affected males, suggesting their female, heterozygote siblings do not always manifest clinical disease. A small percentage of mild, late onset cases may differ and show autosomal dominant inheritance.

The serum creatine phosphokinase is usually normal in acute infantile SMA and the most severe form of chronic childhood SMA. A moderately raised CPK may be found in less severely affected cases, when it correlates with secondary myopathic changes. A large survey found an elevated CPK in 53% of those who had walked at some stage, but only 25% of those who had never walked[8]. A normal or only slightly raised CPK gives diagnostic support to SMA as opposed to a muscular dystrophy, where high levels are usual.

Adult Onset SMA

Adult onset SMA (also called SMA type 4) is a separate condition and not a variant of the childhood form[11]. It is a relatively benign condition, which although moderately incapacitating, usually does not shorten life. These patients have a normal childhood. Onset is insidious between 15 and 50 years. Muscle weakness is nearly always symmetrical with proximal selectivity and preservation of distal muscles. The clinical progression is very slow with periods of arrest. Until recently almost any slowly progressive limb girdle syndrome was labelled as a muscular dystrophy, but it is now recognized that most are examples of SMA. In a series of nine patients described by Pearn no patient could walk unaided after 20 years, but only one was wheelchair-bound[11]. Inheritance is usually autosomal recessive, but dominant and rare X-linked forms are described[1]. The differential diagnosis includes familial motor neuron disease. The latter is distinguished by pyramidal signs, is often asymmetrical and shows a more rapid progression. Rare variants of adult SMA are families with bulbar involvement[12] and those with striking asymmetry[13]. The continued absence of pyramidal involvement may be the only distinction from MND.

SMA Associated with Hypertrophy of the Calves

This is another relatively benign but rare sex-linked autosomal recessive form of SMA[14]. Onset is in either the first or second decade. All patients have been able to walk, at least in the early years. Hypertrophy of the calves is not usually seen in young children. In 23 recorded cases it appeared between 9 and 39 years and was considered to be a genuine hypertrophy compensating for weakness in other muscles[15]. The hypertrophy may disappear after prolonged immobility. Clinically this form of SMA may be indistinguishable from Becker's dystrophy. The serum creatine kinase is, at least, mildly elevated in all cases.

Distal SMA

Distal SMA is a rare disorder in which both autosomal dominant and recessive inheritance have been reported[16]. The selective involvement of distal limb muscles provides a striking contrast to the proximal weakness of the commoner forms of SMA. This is one of the causes of peroneal muscular atrophy and patients develop the so-called 'inverted champagne bottle' appearance of the legs. Although onset is usually in childhood and may even be infantile, unlike chronic childhood SMA this is a benign very slowly progressive condition compatible with a normal life span. The differential diagnosis includes various distal myopathies and the hereditary sensory and motor chronic peripheral neuropathies (see Chapter 6) in which peroneal muscular atrophy is associated with distal sensory impairment. An apparently unique kindred has recently been described showing dominantly inherited distal SMA and vocal cord paralysis[17]

Muscle Biopsy in SMA

The muscle biopsy changes in acute infantile and severe chronic childhood SMA are indistinguishable and the two disorders must be separated by age of onset, clinical evaluation and any family history. The key pathological feature is a striking, severe grouped atrophy (Figures 5.2–5.4). Whole fascicles may be composed of uniformly tiny, rounded fibres, sometimes smaller than intrafusal fibres (Figure 5.3). The myosin ATP-ase reaction usually shows a normal chequerboard distribution of type 1 and type 2 fibres in the atrophic groups (Figures 5.5 and 5.6). Against the background of large group atrophy there are clumps of normal size or grossly hypertrophied fibres (Figures 5.2 and 5.4). These larger fibres are often of uniform type and may demonstrate an abnormal enzyme profile. Frequently they appear to be type 1 as judged by the myosin ATP-ase reaction (Figure 5.7), but show a variable reaction with the NADH-TR and phosphorylase reactions (Figures 5.8 and 5.9). Fibres with these intermediate histochemical reactions are possibly undergoing re-innervation changes[18]. Groups of hypertrophied type 2 fibres, as shown by myosin ATP-ase, are most unusual. In the early onset forms of SMA small fibres often have large vesicular nuclei, occasionally centrally located and resembling fetal fibres (Figure 5.10). Such immature fibres suggest prenatal onset of denervation[19] This is supported by identification of large amounts of fetal myosin[20].

The clinically intermediate form of childhood SMA also cannot be reliably separated from the most severe by muscle biopsy. The extent of atrophy in small biopsy is no reflection of the overall severity of the disease, best judged on clinical grounds[21] (Figure 5.11). However, children with intermediate SMA tend to show a greater degree of re-innervation (Figure 5.12). Thus larger areas of type 1 fibre grouping may correlate with a more benign course, although eventually all these children become severely disabled (Figures 5.13 and 5.14).

Differential Diagnosis of SMA type 1 and type 2

The classic changes are unmistakable and pathognomonic. When examined in early childhood these forms of SMA are not associated with the secondary myopathic changes of necrosis, fibre splitting or significant fibrosis and are thus unlikely to be confused with congenital muscular dystrophy, or Duchenne dystrophy. The congenital myopathies also usually show distinctive histological abnormalities. However, occasionally in the neonate it may be difficult to differentiate acute spinal muscular atrophy from congenital fibre type disproportion, if the full-blown large group atrophy has not developed[21]. The neonatal biopsy may reveal a normal mosaic pattern in which the fibres are universally small, but the type 1 fibres are obviously smaller than type 2 (Figure 5.11). Follow-up has shown this picture soon becomes converted to the characteristic SMA histology. At the early stage a careful search will usually reveal both a few large type 1 fibres and scattered small type 2 fibres. Failing this, accurate measurement of fibre diameters establishes that in SMA both type 1 and type 2 fibres are abnormally small, whereas in congenital fibre type disproportion although type 1 fibres are small, the type 2 fibres are normal sized or enlarged. Dubowitz recommends that congenital fibre type disproportion should not be diagnosed if there is any evidence of type 2 atrophy[21]. In late survivors of severe chronic and intermediate childhood SMA the picture may again be difficult to interpret and overlaps with the late onset forms (Figures 5.13 and 5.14).

Muscle Biopsy in Mild Chronic Childhood SMA, (Kugel–Welander Disease), Adult Onset and Distal SMA

The mild form of chronic childhood SMA can usually be distinguished from severe and intermediate disease in the early childhood biopsy. Late onset SMA shows similar changes. Denervation produces small group atrophy, occasionally large groups but the chronic, benign course correlates with over-riding evidence of re-innervation and compensatory hypertrophy (Figures 5.13–5.30). Characteristically secondary myopathic changes appear and become more obvious in long-standing disease (Figures 5.16–5.18). Angular atrophic fibres are usually present (Figures 5.19–5.21, 5.27–5.30), but occasionally the atrophic fibres are

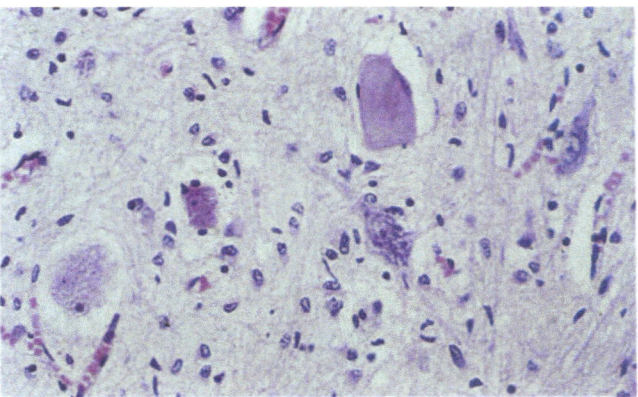

Figure 5.1 Anterior horn cell degeneration in acute infantile SMA. Spinal cord of male infant who died at 3 months. Swollen, chromatolytic and shrunken neurons, but no inflammation.   H & E × 180

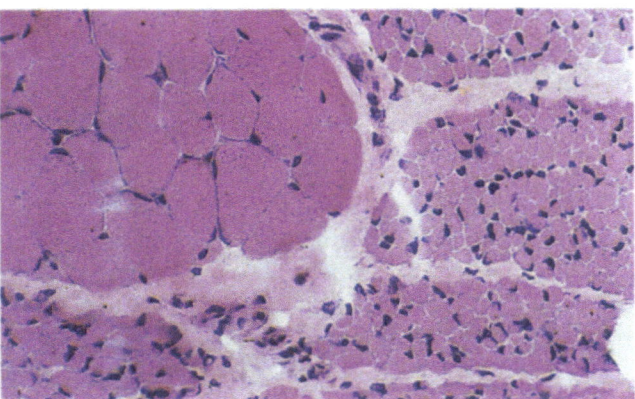

Figure 5.2 Large group atrophy in quadriceps muscle of 9-month-old male infant with severe chronic SMA. Hypotonia, poor muscle bulk and delay in reaching motor milestones. 3-year-old brother similarly affected. The biopsy shows whole fascicles composed of tiny, rounded atrophic fibres. An innervated fascicle shows compensatory hypertrophy.   H & E × 180

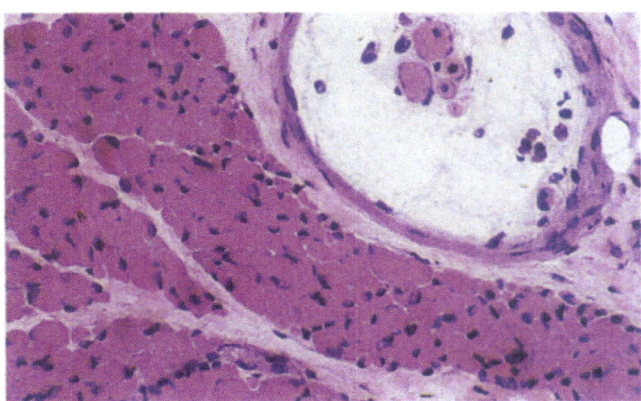

Figure 5.3 Large group atrophy in quadriceps muscle of 4-year-old girl with intermediate chronic SMA. Extrafusal fibres are as small as, or even smaller than, fibres of the muscle spindle. Extrafusal fibres are normally much larger.   H & E × 180

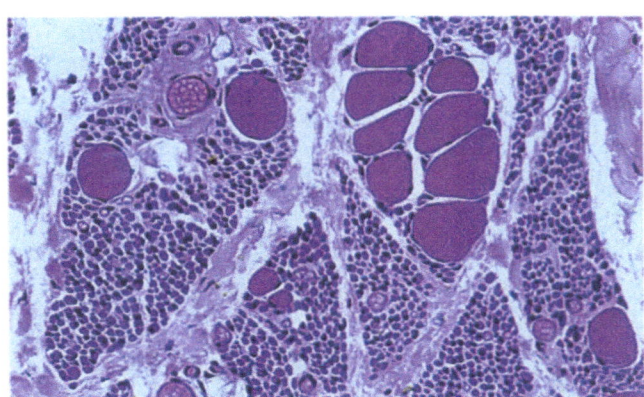

Figure 5.4 A group of grossly hypertrophied fibres against the background of large group atrophy, in quadriceps muscle of 3-year-old boy with chronic SMA of intermediate severity. Despite hypotonia and proximal weakness he was able to run with a rolling gait. (Same case is shown in Figures 5.5–5.8.)   H & E × 75

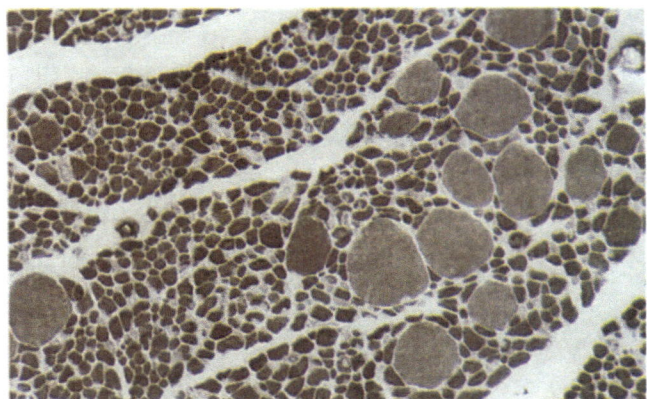

Figure 5.5 Atrophic fibres showing normal chequerboard pattern of type 1 and type 2 fibres in intermediate chronic SMA. Hypertrophied fibres are all type 1 (light).   ATP-ase pH 9.4 × 75

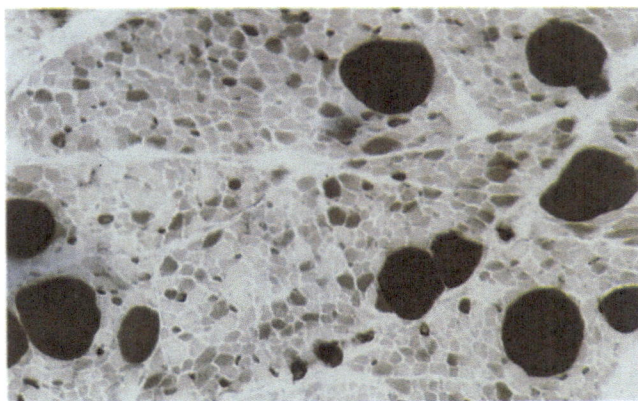

Figure 5.6 Chronic SMA of intermediate severity. Atrophic fibres are type 1 and type 2, but hypertrophied fibres are only type 1 (dark).   ATP-ase pH 4.6 × 75

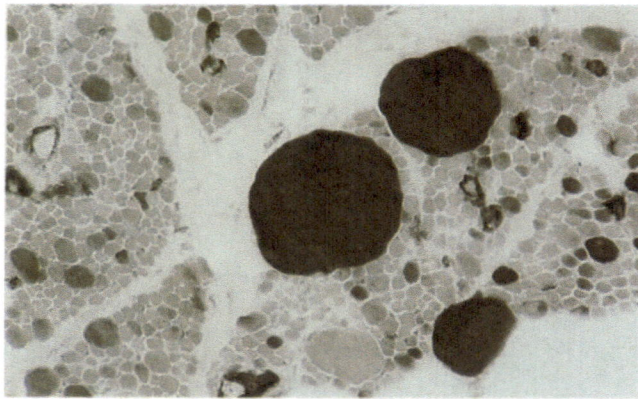

Figure 5.7 Chronic SMA of intermediate severity. Severely atrophic fibres contrast with a few grossly hypertrophied fibres. With the myosin ATP-ase reaction the hypertrophied fibres appear to be type 1 (dark). ATP-ase pH 4.3 × 180

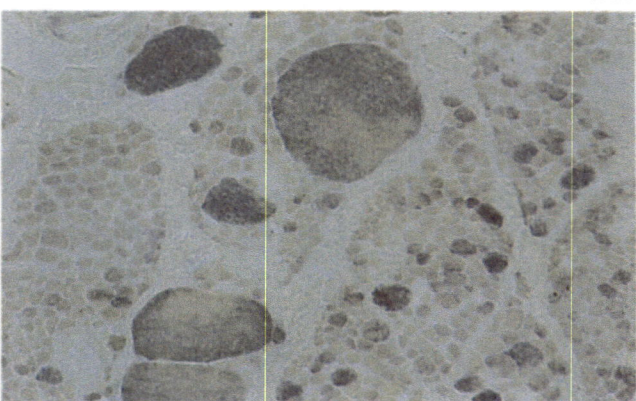

Figure 5.8 Chronic SMA of intermediate severity. Hypertrophied fibres, which are type 1 with the myosin ATP-ase reaction, show moderate phosphorylase activity. This mixed enzyme profile may be due to re-innervation. Phosphorylase × 180

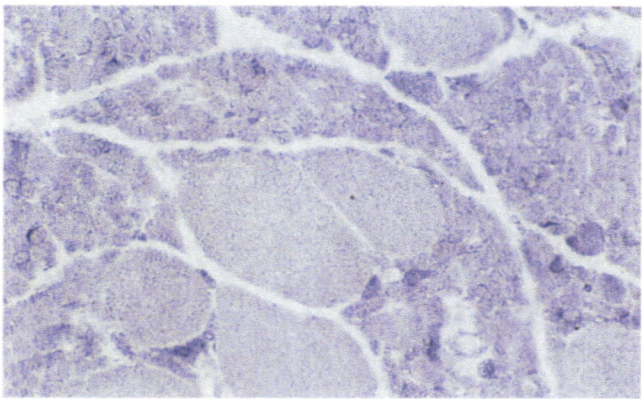

Figure 5.9 Chronic SMA of intermediate severity. Quadriceps muscle of a 4-year-old girl with hypotonia and proximal weakness, but able to walk. Hypertrophied fibres, which are type 1 with myosin ATP-ase show only a weak oxidative enzyme reaction. Type 1 fibres normally show strong oxidative enzyme activity. This mixed enzyme profile may be due to re-innervation. NADH-TR × 180

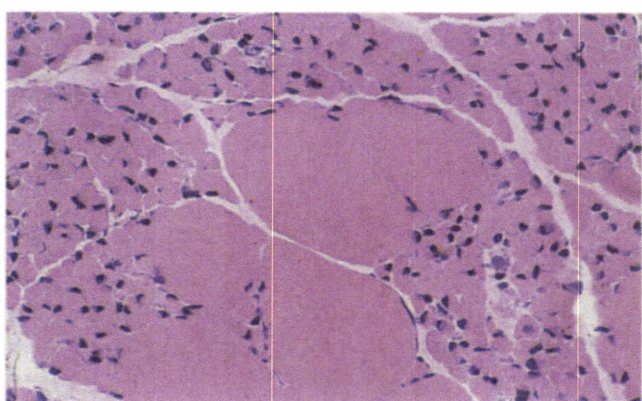

Figure 5.10 Chronic SMA of intermediate severity. Serial section of Figure 5.9. Rounded atrophic fibres have relatively large nuclei, suggesting immaturity. H & E × 180

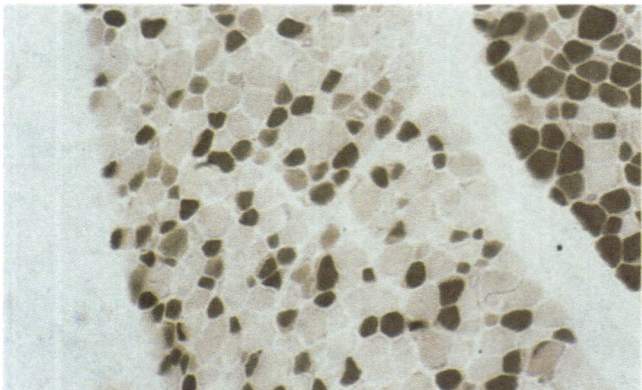

Figure 5.11 Severe chronic SMA. Quadriceps muscle of 9-month-old male infant with similarly affected older brother. Part of this biopsy shows a mosaic distribution pattern with almost selective type 1 atrophy (dark fibres). When this is the only finding, it may be confused with congenital fibre type disproportion. Some larger type 1 fibres in the top right-hand corner indicate the true diagnosis. Elsewhere in this biopsy there was a fascicle of severely hypertrophied fibres. See Figure 5.2. H & E × 180

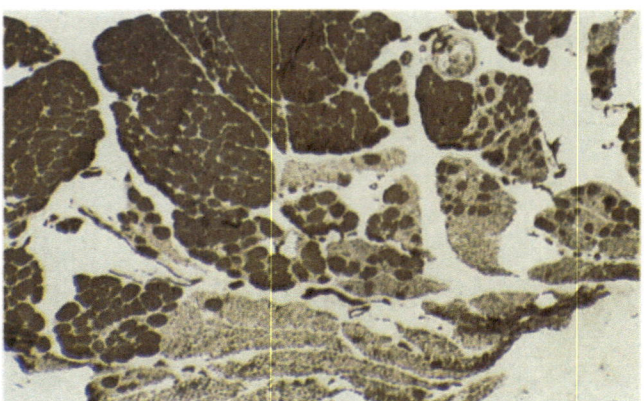

Figure 5.12 Severe chronic SMA with evidence of re-innervation. Quadriceps muscle of a 16-month-old male infant. Delay in motor development first recognized at 9 months. At almost 3 years he is able to sit unaided and stand with support, but is unable to walk. Muscle biopsy shows large groups of type 1 fibres due to re-innervation. ATP-ase pH 4.6 × 30

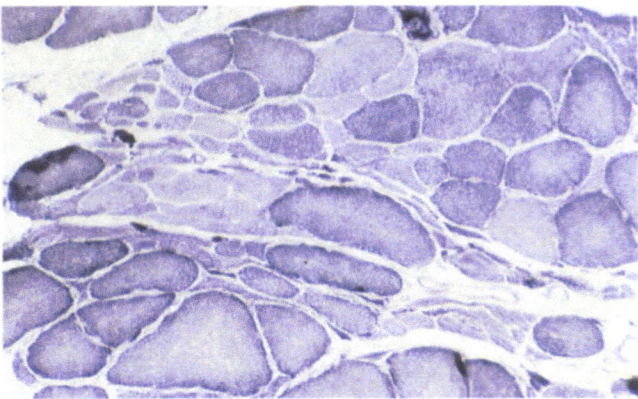

Figure 5.13 Chronic SMA of intermediate severity. Deltoid biopsy of a 22-year-old man. He walked at 16 months, but had never been able to skip or run. His condition deteriorated during childhood and he became wheelchair-bound at 11 years. At 22 years his disease had been static for several years. Wasting was most severe in proximal muscles. CPK – mildly elevated. EMG – myopathic in some muscles, but also evidence of denervation. Biopsy includes some grouped atrophic fibres, also many large fibres and small rounded fibres, which may be the result of fibre splitting. (Same case shown in Figures 5.14–5.18.)   NADH-TR × 180

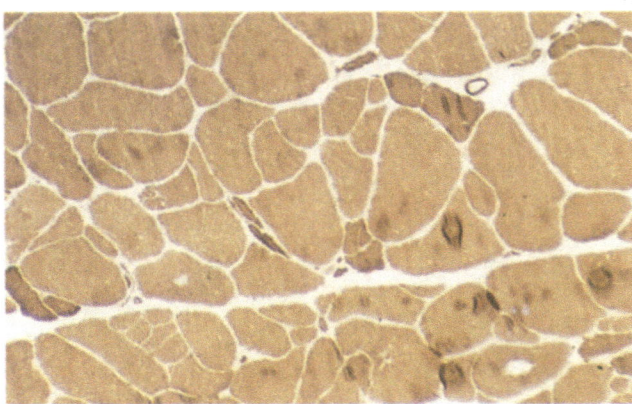

Figure 5.14 Chronic SMA. There is a marked type 1 fibre predominance, attributable to re-innervation.   ATP-ase pH 9.4 × 180

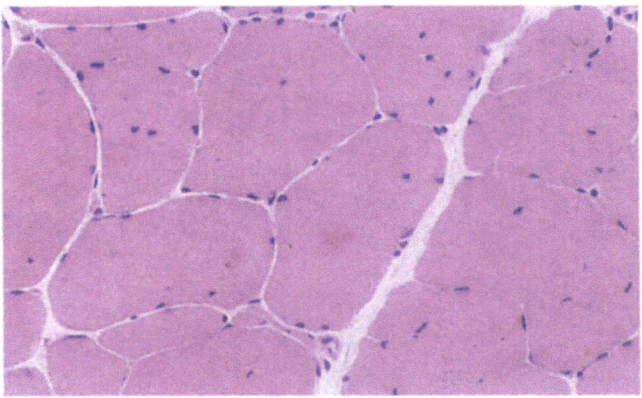

Figure 5.15 Chronic SMA. Large fibres contain central nuclei and comparison with Figure 5.16 suggests most of the small fibres represent split fibres. A large central fibre contains an eosinophilic target. This biopsy contained frequent target fibres, which provided histological confirmation of denervating disease.   H & E × 300

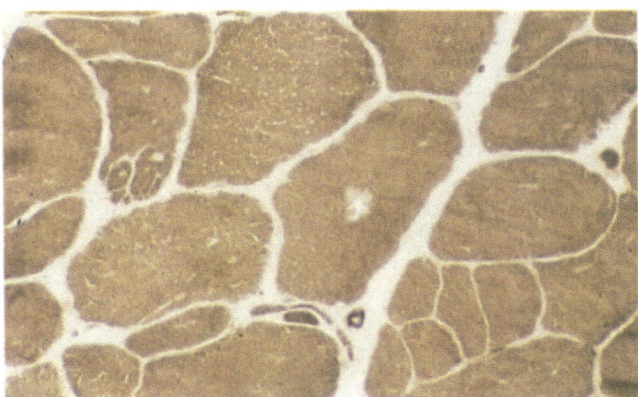

Figure 5.16 Chronic SMA. Small fibres of the same histochemical type fit together like pieces of a jigsaw, suggesting they are split or branching fibres. Close comparison with the H & E serial section confirms this.   ATP-ase pH 9.4 × 300

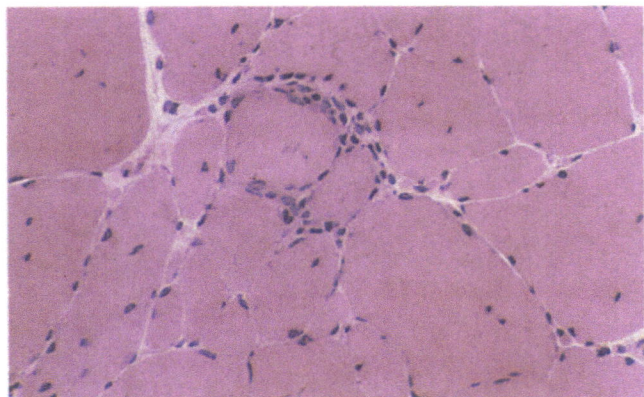

Figure 5.17 Chronic SMA. Focus of chronic inflammatory cells around a split fibre. Such secondary myopathic changes are not uncommon in chronic denervation and relate to the extreme stresses imposed upon innervated fibres.   H & E × 300

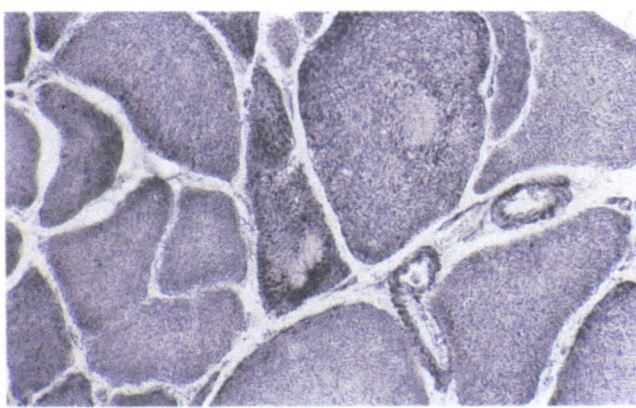

Figure 5.18 Chronic SMA. Targetoid fibre and myofibrillar disarray in a hypertrophied fibre.   NADH-TR × 450

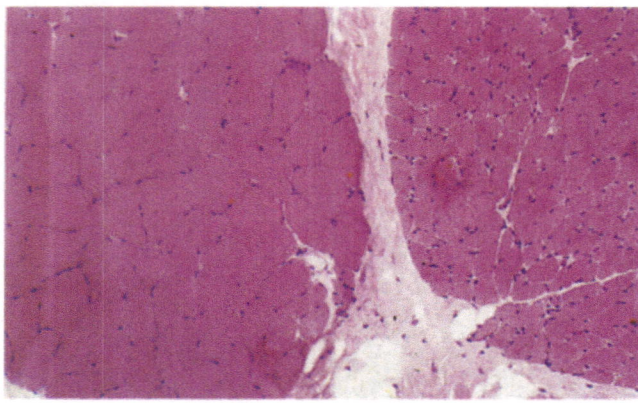

Figure 5.19 Mild chronic SMA (Kugelberg–Welander type). Deltoid muscle of a 14-year-old boy with proximal muscle weakness. Walked at 16 months, but tended to fall a lot. Abnormal gait from early childhood and never able to run well. CPK slightly elevated. Biopsy shows a fascicle of moderately atrophic fibres, which contrasts with the adjacent fascicle containing mildly hypertrophied fibres. (Same case is shown in Figures 5.20–5.24.)   H & E × 75

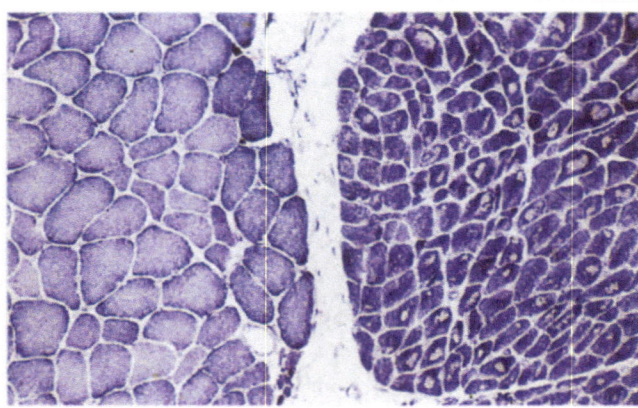

Figure 5.20 Mild chronic SMA. Serial section to Figure 5.1a. The fibres appear to be of uniform histochemical type and there are numerous targets in the smaller fibres. The changes suggest repetitive sequences of denervation and re-innervation.   NADH-TR × 75

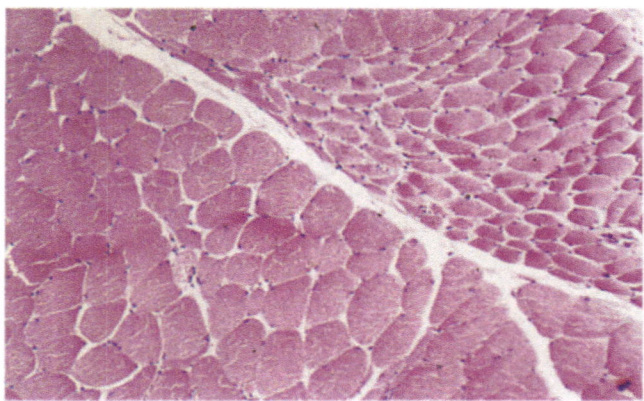

Figure 5.21 Mild chronic SMA. Large group of moderately atrophic angular fibres, contrasting with mildly hypertrophied fibres, which form the majority.   H & E × 75

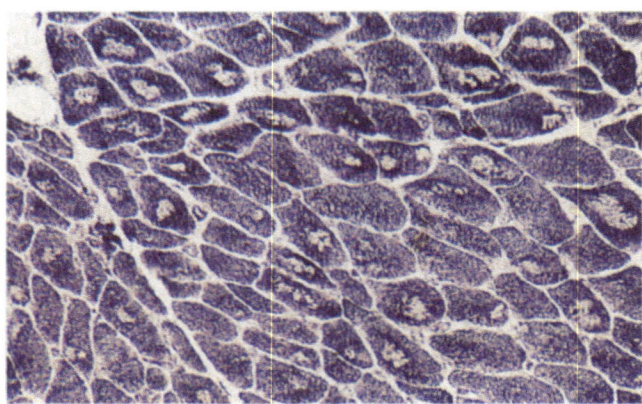

Figure 5.22 Mild chronic SMA. The grouped atrophic fibres contain targets. These may occur in early denervation or during re-innervation.   NADH-TR × 180

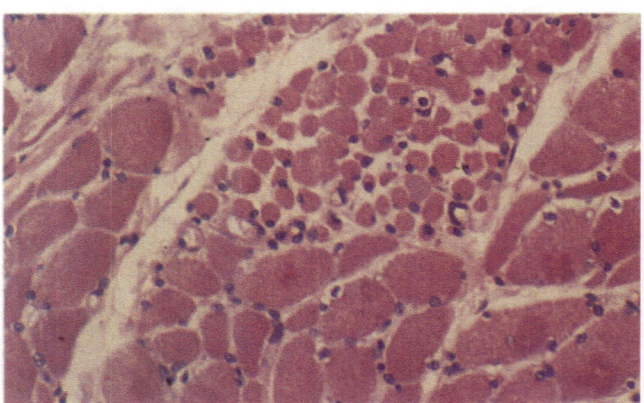

Figure 5.23 Mild chronic SMA. Group of very tiny, rounded, atrophic fibres. Eosinophilic targets can be seen in the larger fibres. Severely atrophic fibres, which suggest long-standing denervation, were comparatively scarce in this biopsy.   H & E × 180

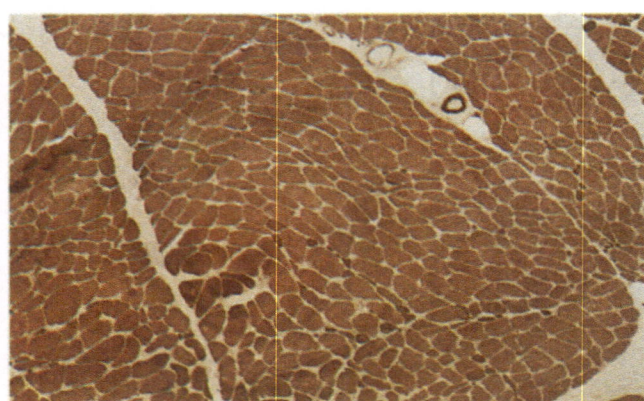

Figure 5.24 Mild chronic SMA. Fascicles of almost uniform fibre type, type 1, are produced by re-innervation.   ATP-ase pH 9.4 × 30

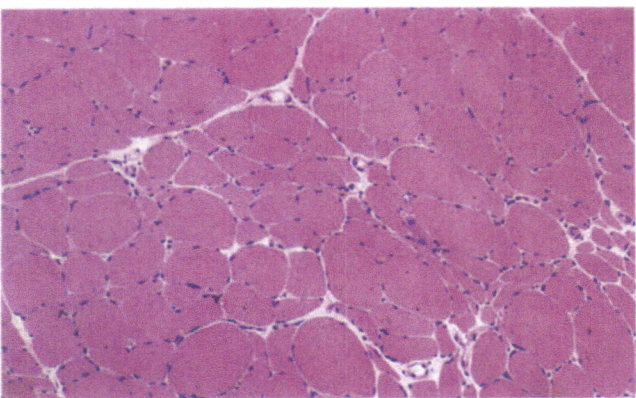

Figure 5.25 Distal SMA. Gastrocnemius muscle of 15-year-old boy observed to have an abnormal gait at 13 years. He showed remarkable wasting of the calves and intrinsic foot muscles, but normal muscle bulk above the knees. There was no upper limb wasting and sensation was normal. No family history. 2 years later his condition is virtually unchanged. Biopsy shows small group atrophy and mild compensatory hypertrophy. (Same case is shown in Figures 5.26–5.30.) H & E × 75

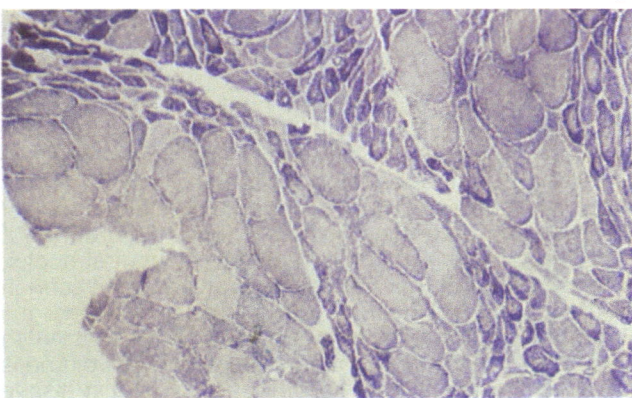

Figure 5.26 Distal SMA. Small groups of atrophic fibres which contain many targets. The hypertrophied fibres, which are mostly type 1 with the myosin ATP-ase reaction, show only a weak oxidative enzyme reaction, suggesting they are re-innervated fibres.   NADH-TR × 75

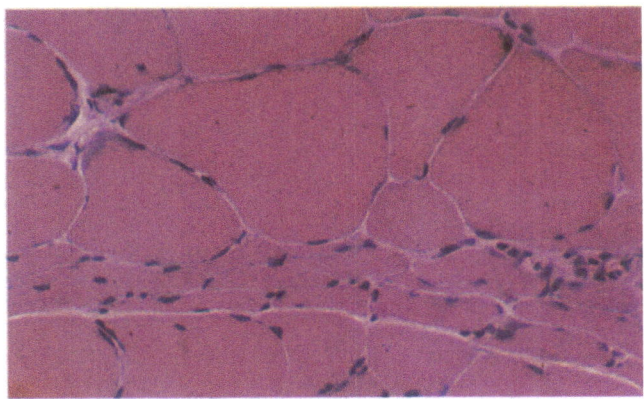

Figure 5.27 Distal SMA. Small group of angular, atrophic, denervated fibres between fibres showing compensatory hypertrophy.   H & E × 300

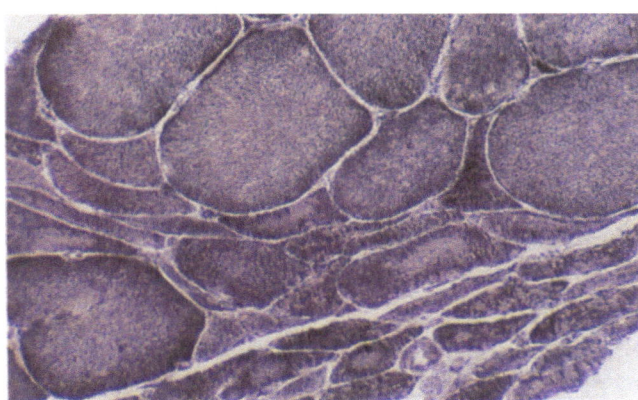

Figure 5.28 Distal SMA. Adjacent section to Figure 5.27. Several atrophic fibres have a targetoid appearance.   NADH-TR × 300

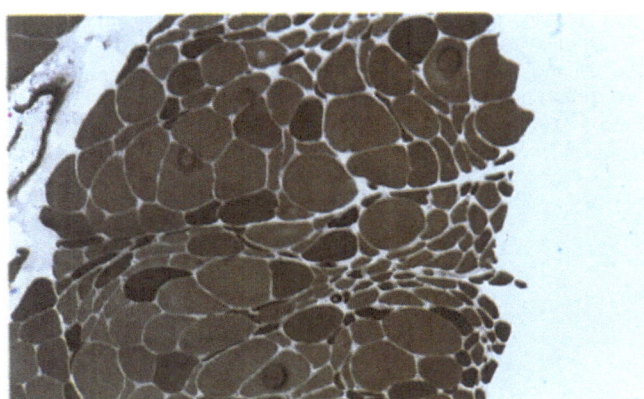

Figure 5.29 Distal SMA. Groups of atrophic fibres at the periphery of hypertrophied fibres.   ATP-ase pH 9.4 × 75

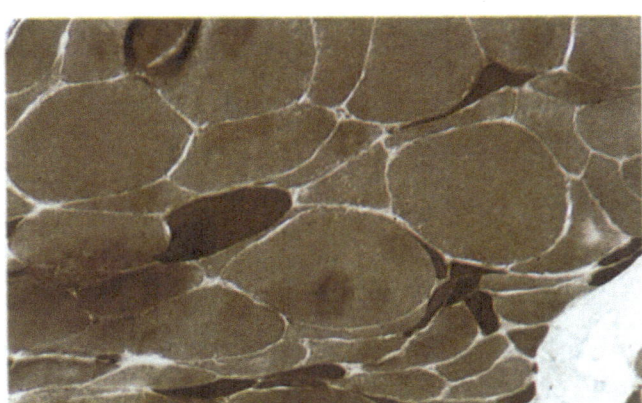

Figure 5.30 Distal SMA. Atrophic fibres are both type 1 and type 2, but hypertrophied fibres are type 1 (light).   ATP-ase pH 9.4 × 300

only represented by pyknotic nuclear clusters at the periphery of grossly hypertrophied fibres. The fibre distribution pattern usually reveals clear evidence of re-innervation of normal sized and hypertrophied fibres, with type groups of both type 1 and type 2 fibres. Target fibres are not uncommon in type 1 fibres (Figure 5.22). Secondary myopathic changes such as central nuclei, fibre splitting and myofibrillar disarray are often seen in the larger fibres[22] (Figure 5.22). Occasional necrotic fibres undergoing phagocytosis may be present. With the passage of time reduction in muscle fibre volume is associated with adipose and fibrous connective tissue replacement.

Differential Diagnosis

In late onset forms of SMA, secondary myopathic changes may dominate the histology, hence the long-standing confusion with dystrophy. This pattern and the differential diagnosis of the limb girdle syndrome is discussed in Chapter 10. Adult onset SMA cannot be distinguished from slowly progressive motor neuron disease by muscle biopsy. Clinical absence of upper motor neuron disease is the most reliable indicator of SMA and has been confirmed at postmortem[23]. Distinction from Becker dystrophy can be difficult and is discussed in Chapter 8.

References

1. Pearn, J. (1980). Classification of spinal muscular atrophies. *Lancet*, **1**, 919–22

2. Walton, J. N. (1983). Changing concepts of neuromuscular disease. *Hosp. Update*, **9**, 949–58

3. Emery, A. E. H., Davie, A. M., Holloway, S. and Skinner, R. (1976). International collaborative study of the spinal muscular atrophies. 2. Analysis of genetic data. *J. Neurol. Sci.*, **30**, 375–84

4. Pearn, J. H., Carter, C. O. and Wilson, J. (1973). The genetic identity of acute infantile spinal muscular atrophy. *Brain*, **96**, 463–70

5. Pearn, J. H. and Wilson, J. (1973). Acute Werdnig–Hoffman disease. *Arch. Dis. Childh.*, **48**, 425–30

6. Pearn, J., Bundey, S., Carter, C. O., Wilson, J., Gardner-Medwin, D. and Walton, J. N. (1978). A genetic study of sub-acute and chronic spinal muscular atrophy in childhood. *J. Neurol. Sci.*, **37**, 227–48

7. Pearn, J., Gardner-Medwin, D. and Wilson, J. (1978). A clinical study of chronic childhood spinal muscular atrophy. *J. Neurol. Sci.*, **38**, 23–37

8. Emery, A. E. H., Hausmanowa-Petrusewicz, I., Davie, A. M., Holloway, S., Skinner, R. and Borkowska, J. (1976). International collaborative study of spinal muscular atrophies. 1. Analysis of clinical and laboratory data. *J. Neurol. Sci.*, **29**, 83–94

9. Pearn, J. H. and Wilson, J. (1973). Chronic generalised spinal muscular atrophy of infancy and childhood. *Arch. Dis. Childh.*, **48**, 768–74

10. Hausmanowa-Petrusewicz, I., Zaremba, J. and Borkowska, J. (1979). Chronic form of spinal muscular atrophy. *J. Neurol. Sci.*, **43**, 313–27

11. Pearn, J. H., Hudgson, P. and Walton, J. N. (1978). A clinical and genetic study of spinal muscular atrophy of adult onset. *Brain*, **101**, 591–606

12. Stefanis, C. *et al.* (1975). X-linked spinal and bulbar muscle atrophy of late onset: a separate type of motor neuron disease? *J. Neurol. Sci.*, **24**, 493–503

13. Harding, A. E., Bradbury, P. G. and Murray, N. M. F. (1983). Chronic asymmetrical spinal muscular atrophy. *J. Neurol. Sci.*, **59**, 69–83

14. Pearn, J. and Hudgson, P. (1978). Anterior horn cell degeneration and gross calf hypertrophy with adolescent onset. A new spinal muscular atrophy syndrome. *Lancet*, **1**, 1059–61

15. Bouwsma, G. and van Wijngaarden, G. K. (1980). Spinal muscular atrophy and hypertrophy of the calves. *J. Neurol. Sci.*, **44**, 275–9

16. Harding, A. E. and Thomas, P. K. (1980). Hereditary distal spinal muscular atrophy. *J. Neurol. Sci.*, **45**, 337–48

17. Young, I. D. and Harper, P. S. (1980). Hereditary distal spinal muscular atrophy with vocal cord paralysis. *J. Neurol. Neurosurg. Psychiatry*, **43**, 413–18

18. DeReuck, J., van den Bossce, H., DeCoster, W. and Hooft, C. (1978). Infantile spinal muscular atrophy. Unusual fibre typing and distribution in a muscle biopsy. *Eur. Neurol.*, **17**, 142–8

19. Hausmanowa-Petrusewicz, I., Fidianska, A., Dobosz, I., Drac, H. and Ryniewsicz, B. (1975). The foetal character of the lesion in the acute form of Werdnig–Hoffman disease. In Bradley, W. G., Gardner-Medwin, D. and Walton, J. N. (eds.) *Recent Advances in Myology, International Congress Series*. pp. 546–56. (Amsterdam: Excerpta Medica)

20. Fitzsimons, R B. and Hoh J. F. Y. (1981). Embryonic and foetal myosins in human skeletal muscle. *J. Neurol Sci.*, **52**, 367–84

21. Dubowitz, V. (1978). The spinal muscular atrophies. In Schaffer, A. J. and Markowitz, M. (eds.) *Muscle Disorders in Childhood. Major Problems in Clinical Paediatrics*. pp. 147–78

22. Mastaglia, F. L. and Walton, J. N. (1971). Histological and histo-chemical changes in skeletal muscle from cases of chronic juvenile and early adult spinal muscular atrophy (the Kugelberg–Welander syndrome). *J. Neurol. Sci.*, **12**, 15–44

23. Huang, K. and Luo, Y. (1983). Adult spinal muscular atrophy. A report of 4 cases. *J. Neurol. Sci.*, **61**, 249–59

Peripheral Neuropathy

Peripheral neuropathy or polyneuropathy is a clinical syndrome characterized by acute or chronic, symmetrical and simultaneous disturbance of function in many peripheral nerves. The causes are legion and include toxic inflammatory, metabolic and genetically determined conditions. There is usually impairment of both sensory and motor function, although one or other may dominate the clinical picture. Distal segments of the limbs are most severely affected. Only disorders with a significant motor nerve component will result in muscle weakness. The peripheral nerve pathology may be segmental demyelination or axonal degeneration. In demyelinating neuropathies nerve conduction is usually markedly slowed, but it may be normal in the neuronal form, provided some large, fast conducting axons remain. Changes in the muscle biopsy are usually most severe when there is axonal degeneration. The pathological spectrum is covered by two categories, the chronic, hereditary peripheral neuropathies and acute acquired postinfective neuropathy.

Hereditary Sensory and Motor Peripheral Neuropathies (Peroneal Muscular Atrophy)

Unravelling the complexities of the hereditary peripheral neuropathies is bedevilled by the numerous eponymous terms in the literature. Charcot–Marie–Tooth disease is, however, the well-established name for a clinical syndrome characterized by peroneal muscular atrophy (PMA), weakness of the hands and mild distal sensory impairment. The syndrome probably represents two or more separate disorders with different pathogenesis, but mostly autosomal dominant inheritance. They can be classified on the basis of peripheral nerve conduction velocity, which correlates with the pathology and also shows concordance within individual families[1]. Low conduction velocity is associated with segmental demyelination and palpable nerves (hypertrophic neuropathy). The thickened nerves are due to 'onion bulb' Schwann cell proliferation, which accompanies remyelination. Normal conduction velocity is associated with axonal degeneration and only minimal demyelination (neuronal form of PMA). The site of the neuronal lesion is uncertain. Intermediate nerve conduction velocity reflects a combination of pathological features. In addition, some neuronal forms may be associated with upper motor neuron lesions or the clinical picture of Friedreich's ataxia. Onset of the hypertrophic neuropathy is usually in the first 10 years, whereas late onset, after 40 years, is quite common in the neuronal form[2]. Peroneal muscular atrophy is often more severe in the neuronal form and patients develop the so-called 'inverted champagne bottle' legs. Other rare, clinically overlapping disorders include infantile, autosomal recessive hypertrophic neuropathy (Dejerine–Sottas disease)[3] and neuropathy due to abnormal lipid metabolism (Refsum's disease). Clinical or electrophysiological evidence of sensory nerve involvement is the only certain means of distinguishing dominantly inherited peripheral neuropathy from autosomal recessive distal spinal muscular atrophy.

Muscle Biopsy

In order to categorize these neuropathies fully it is essential to combine muscle and sural nerve biopsy. Biopsy of a lower limb muscle reveals a variable degree of neurogenic atrophy. Small group atrophy tends to be more marked in the neuronal form of peroneal muscular atrophy[4], where there is also well-developed type grouping and compensatory hypertrophy of remaining fibres (Figures 6.1–6.4). Type groups of large fibres may be of both type 1 and type 2 fibres. In addition, relating to the chronicity of the condition, secondary myopathic changes are often conspicuous. However, early in the course of this disease before all these changes have occurred, mild denervation atrophy can resemble the less severe, demyelinating disorder, hence the need for examination of a peripheral nerve. A predominantly demyelinating neuropathy may induce isolated fibre atrophy and sometimes an almost selective type 1 atrophy, which could be confused with congenital fibre type disproportion if the clinical picture is ignored (Figures 6.5–6.16). Susceptibility of type 1 fibres is due to interruption of the normal continual, low threshold stimulation of type 1 motor units[5].

The Guillain–Barre Syndrome

Acute, postinfective polyneuropathy, the Guillain–Barre syndrome, is probably the commonest, acquired peripheral neuropathy associated with significant muscle weakness. Typically there is an acute febrile illness, followed within days or a few weeks by rapidly spreading weakness of proximal and distal muscles. This may progress to flaccid paralysis and assisted ventilation may be required for weak respiratory muscles. EMG shows slowing or complete block in nerve conduction, which is due to inflammatory, segmental demyelination. The pathological changes are very similar to those of experimental allergic neuritis, suggesting a hypersensitivity mechanism, perhaps initiated by a viral infection[6]. When demyelination is severe it may be accompanied by axonal degeneration. Occasionally if weakness is confined to proximal muscles the clinical picture may resemble polymyositis. In most cases gradual remyelination brings full

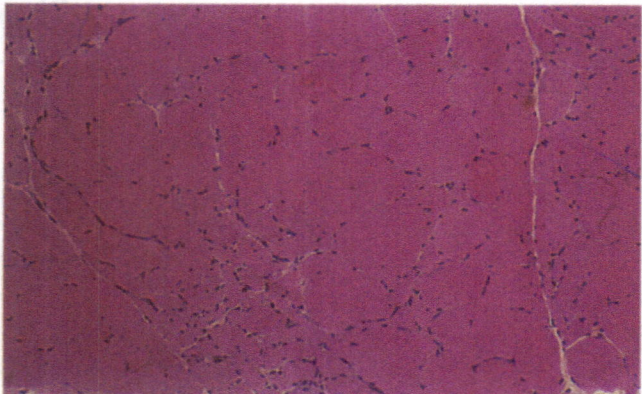

Figure 6.1 Chronic peripheral neuropathy. Quadriceps biopsy from a 41-year-old woman with peroneal muscular atrophy. Onset of symptoms 3 years previously. Muscle wasting has progressed rapidly. She also has reduced nerve conduction velocity in her arms. Peripheral nerves are not palpable. The biopsy shows the typical picture of denervation small group atrophy. The rapid progression and marked wasting suggest this is predominantly a neuronal type of peroneal muscular atrophy, although the altered nerve conduction indicates a demyelinating component. (Same case shown in Figures 6.2–6.4.) H & E × 180

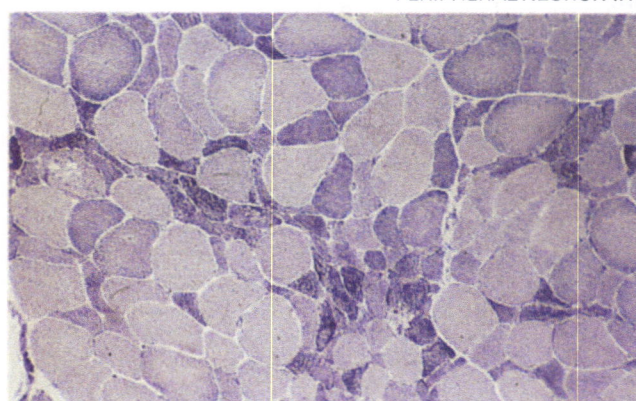

Figure 6.2 Chronic peripheral neuropathy. Small group atrophy and angular darkly staining fibres with the oxidative reaction. NADH-TR × 180

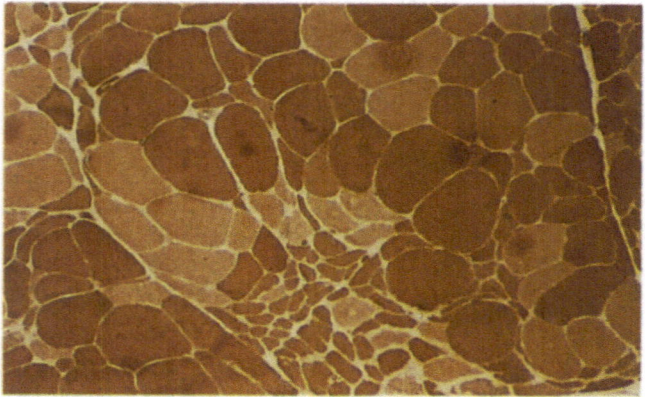

Figure 6.3 Chronic peripheral neuropathy. Grouped atrophy. The atrophic, denervating fibres are both type 1 and type 2. A few type 2 fibres are mildly hypertrophied. ATP-ase pH 9.4 × 180

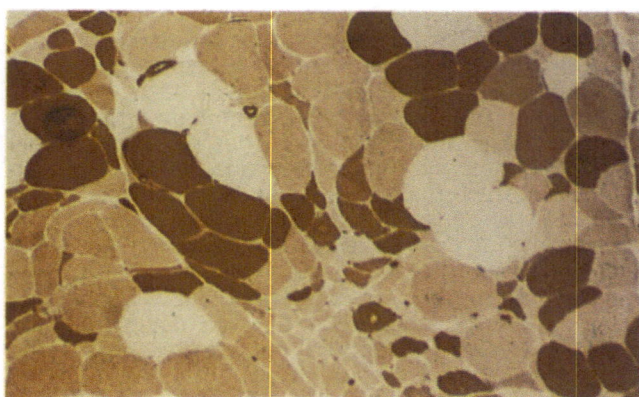

Figure 6.4 Chronic peripheral neuropathy. Serial section to Figure 6.3. Grouped atrophy, involving both type 1 and 2 fibres. This form of chronic peripheral neuropathy, which is largely due to axonal degeneration, shows more severe muscular atrophy than a purely demyelinating disorder. Histology shows the typical picture of denervation atrophy. ATP-ase pH 4.6 × 180

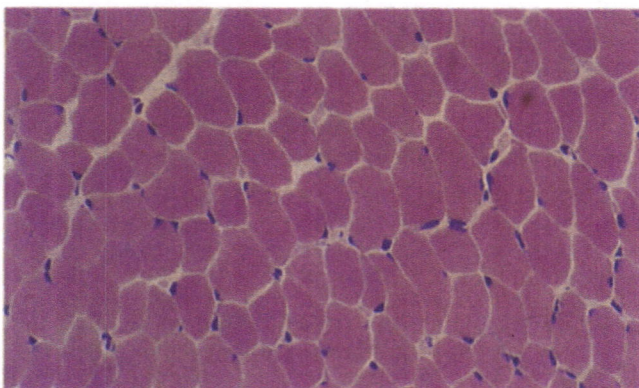

Figure 6.5 Hereditary chronic peripheral neuropathy, with marked reduction in nerve conduction velocity, but without palpable peripheral nerves. Quadriceps biopsy from a 4-year-old boy whose mother and maternal grandmother have the disorder. His grandfather did not show signs of disease until 43 years and lived until 80 years. The disorder was diagnosed in his mother at 5 years and at 23 years she is quite severely incapacitated and barely able to walk unaided. Her son walked at a normal age, but fell frequently. At 4 years he walks unaided, but is unable to run or jump. The biopsy shows some small fibres, but no grouped atrophy. Combined clinical and pathological findings suggest this is an intermediate form of chronic peripheral neuropathy. (Same case is shown in Figures 6.6–6.10.) H & E × 300

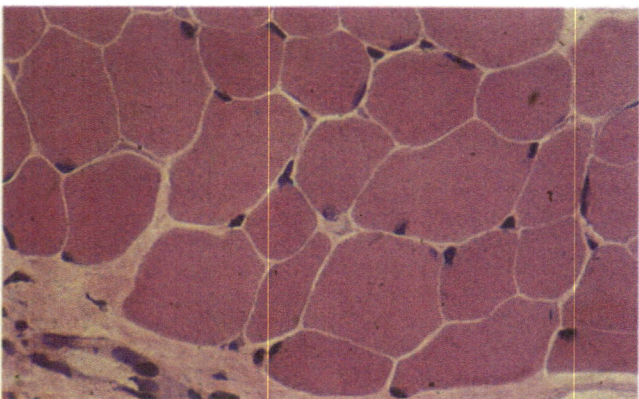

Figure 6.6 Hereditary chronic peripheral neuropathy. Small fibres are rounded and dispersed amongst mildly hypertrophied fibres. There are none of the tiny, angular fibres, typical of denervation atrophy. H & E × 750

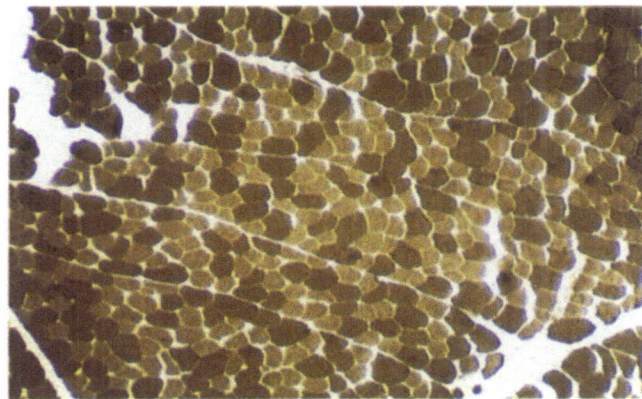

Figure 6.7 Hereditary chronic peripheral neuropathy. A normal mosaic pattern of fibre type distribution. Even at low magnification it is apparent that the larger fibres are type 2 fibres (dark). ATP-ase pH 9.4 × 180

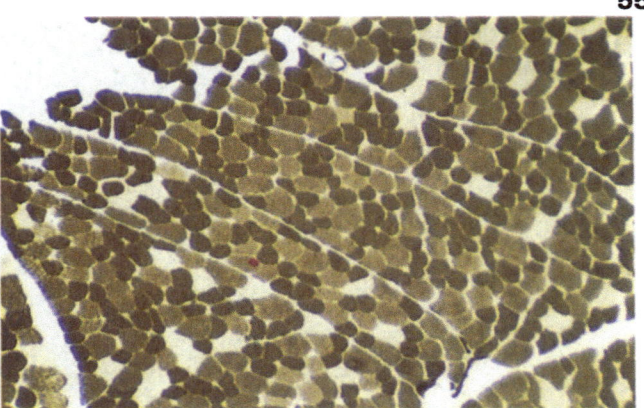

Figure 6.8 Hereditary chronic peripheral neuropathy. Serial section to Figure 6.7. The larger fibres are type 2 fibres, but there is a predominance of 2B fibres (intermediate staining) over 2A fibres (light). ATP-ase pH 4.6 × 180

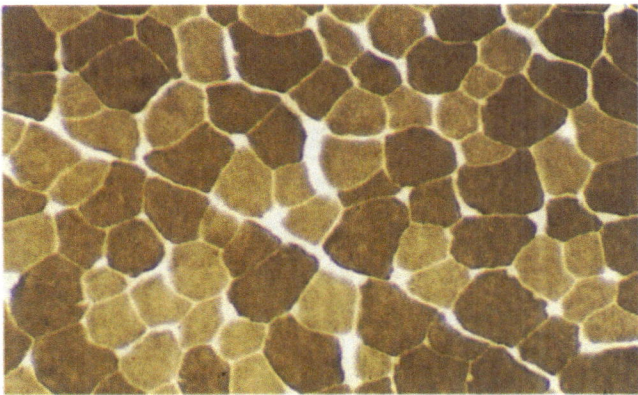

Figure 6.9 Hereditary chronic peripheral neuropathy. There is a dual fibre population. Almost all the small fibres are type 1. Type 1 fibres are mildly atrophic, whereas some type 2 fibres (dark) are slightly enlarged. ATP-ase pH 9.4 × 300

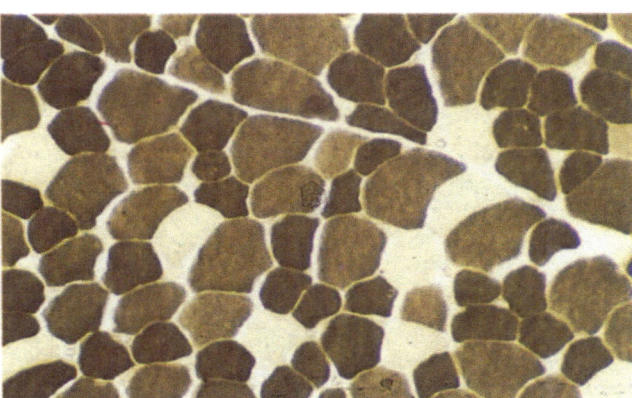

Figure 6.10 Hereditary chronic peripheral neuropathy. The small fibres (dark) are mostly type 1 (dark). Some 2B fibres (intermediate) are slightly enlarged, whereas type A (light) are normal size. This disparity in fibre sizes which accompanies demyelinating peripheral neuropathy may reflect the normal dependence of type 1 fibres upon continual low threshold neuronal stimulation. ATP-ase pH 4.6 × 300

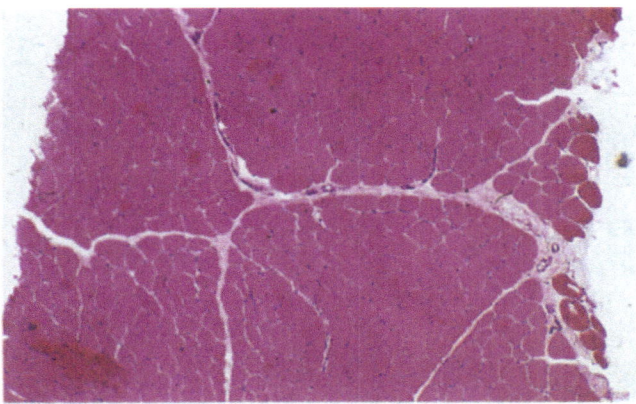

Figure 6.11 Hypertrophic chronic peripheral neuropathy. Quadriceps biopsy from a 31-year-old man with mild peroneal muscular atrophy and pes cavus, apparent for several years. Palpable peripheral nerves and greatly reduced nerve conduction velocity. At low magnification, some variation in fibre size is evident, but not the grouped atrophy of denervation. (Same case shown in Figures 6.12–6.14 and biopsy of a son in Figures 6.15 and 6.16.) H & E × 30

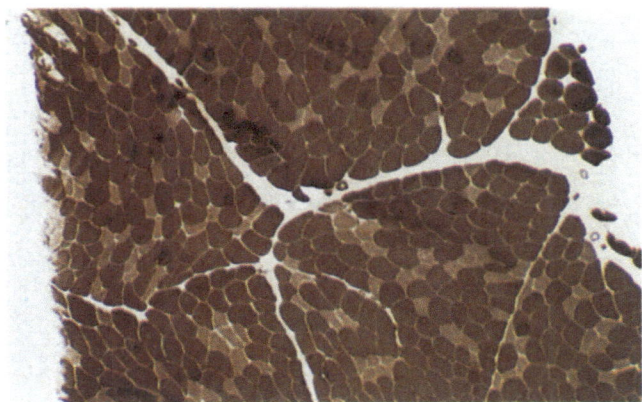

Figure 6.12 Hypertrophic peripheral neuropathy. There is mild type 2 predominance. The small fibres (light) are type 1 fibres. ATP-ase pH 9.4 × 30

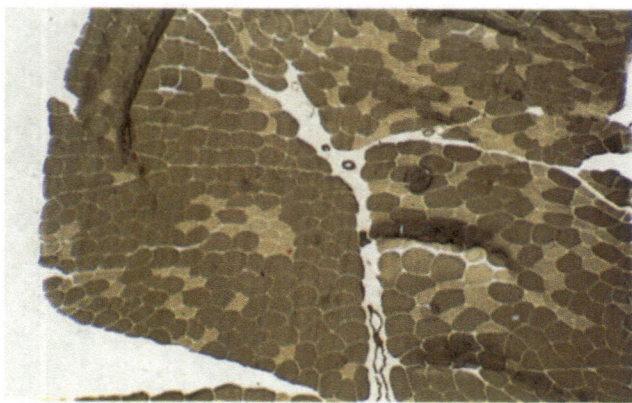

Figure 6.13 Hypertrophic peripheral neuropathy. Type 2 predominance and small (atrophic) type 1 fibres.   ATP-ase pH 9.4 × 30

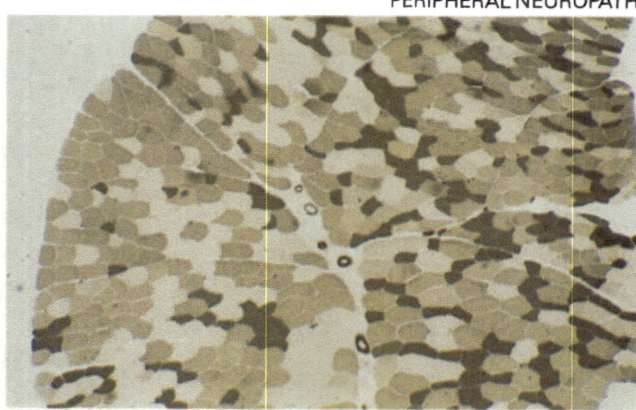

Figure 6.14 Hypertrophic peripheral neuropathy. Serial section to Figure 6.13. The atrophic type 1 fibres (dark) are best demonstrated by this reaction. Although there is type 2 predominance, it is not the type grouping of re-innervation. The type 2 fibres are a mixture of 2A and 2B. The quadriceps muscle was not demonstrably weakened in this man, but the biopsy has revealed clear evidence of the effects of a demyelinating, chronic peripheral neuropathy.   ATP-ase pH 4.6 × 30

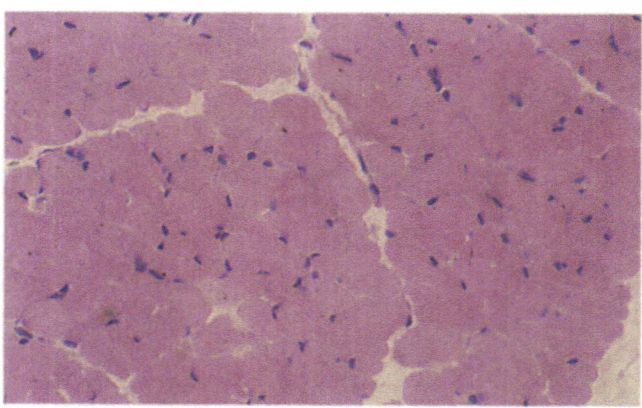

Figure 6.15 Hereditary chronic peripheral neuropathy. Quadriceps biopsy from the 18-month-old son of the patient shown in Figures 6.11–6.14. He showed delay in reaching motor milestones. He was able to sit unsupported, but was not crawling, and unable to pull himself up into a standing position. His legs, particularly distal muscles were hypotonic in comparison with his arms. At this age he had not developed palpable nerves. The biopsy shows variation in fibre size, but this is quite difficult to detect with only an H & E stain. (Same case shown in Figure 6.16.)   H & E × 300

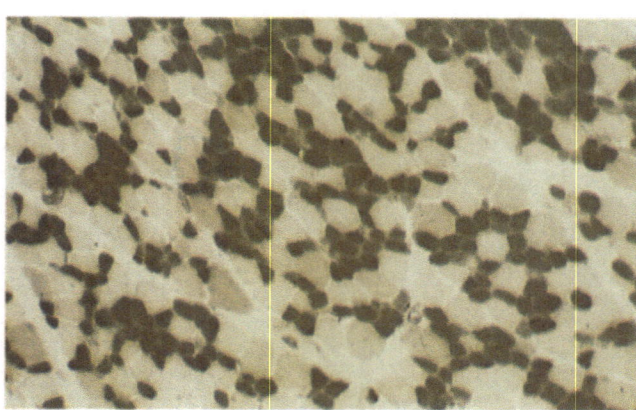

Figure 6.16 Hereditary chronic peripheral neuropathy. The myosin ATP-ase reaction shows very clearly that this child has the same histochemical pattern of type 1 atrophy as seen in his father's muscle.   Myosin ATP-ase pH 4.6 × 300

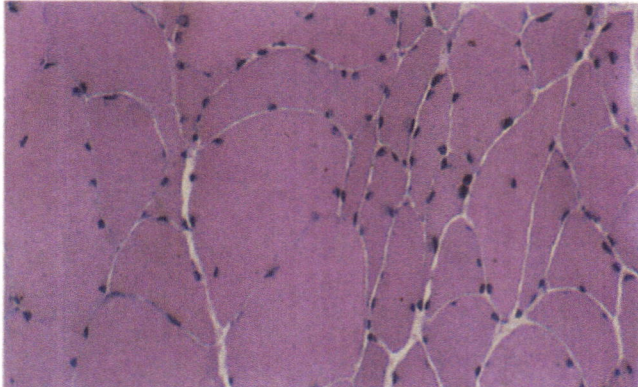

Figure 6.17 Guillain–Barre syndrome. Quadriceps from a 61-year-old man with severe proximal muscle weakness, of recent onset. Clinical picture and EMG suggested Guillain–Barre syndrome. He also had multiple myeloma with chronic renal failure. The biopsy contains some groups of small angular fibres, suggesting denervation atrophy. (Same case shown in Figure 6.18.)   H & E × 300

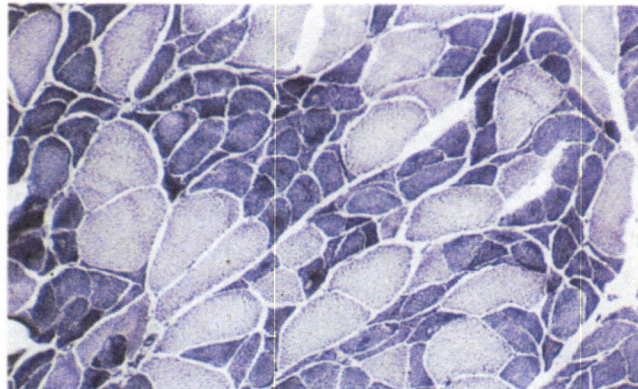

Figure 6.18 Guillain–Barre syndrome. Small groups of angular atrophic fibres, which stain darkly with the oxidative enzyme reaction, suggesting denervation atrophy.   NADH-TR × 180

recovery. A few patients fail to respond to steroid therapy and others have extensive neuronal degeneration that leaves a neurological deficit. Occasional patients relapse, increasing the likelihood of residual weakness.

Muscle Biopsy

Changes in the muscle biopsy will depend upon the timing of the biopsy and the severity of axonal degeneration. Early in the acute phase, mild atrophy of both fibre types may be seen, without the characteristic angular fibres and grouping of established denervation. Small group atrophy develops within a few weeks in severe cases and probably indicates neuronal degeneration (Figures 6.17 and 6.18). Target fibres may appear in the recovery phase. Permanent weakness will be associated with mild chronic denervation atrophy.

References

1. Madrid, R., Bradley, W.G. and Davis, C.J.F. (1977). The peroneal muscular atrophy syndrome. Clinical, genetic, electrophysiological and nerve biopsy studies. *J. Neurol. Sci.*, **32**, 91–122 and 123–6

2. Buchthal, F. and Behse, F. (1977). Peroneal muscular atrophy and related disorders. *Brain*, **100**, 41–66

3. Guzzetta, F., Ferrière, G. and Lyon, G. (1982). Congenital hypomyelination polyneuropathy. Pathological findings compared with polyneuropathies starting later in life. *Brain*, **105**, 395–416

4. Nukada, H., Pollock, M. and Haas, L.F. (1982). The clinical spectrum and morphology of type II hereditary sensory neuropathy. *Brain*, **105**, 647–65

5. Gale, A.N., Gomez, S. and Duchen, L.W. (1982). Changes produced by a hypomyelinating neuropathy in muscle and its innervation. Morphological and physiological studies in the trembler mouse. *Brain*, **105**, 373–93

6. Weller, R.O. and Cervos-Navarro, J. (1977). Inflammatory disorders of peripheral nerves. In *Pathology of Peripheral Nerves*. pp. 128–30. (London: Butterworth and Co.)

MYASTHENIA GRAVIS

Myasthenia gravis (MG) is now well established as an autoimmune disease mediated by antibodies to acetylcholine receptors which initiate structural damage to the motor end plate. Simplification of the normally complex junctional folds of the end plate correlates with defective neuromuscular transmission (Figures 7.1–7.3, Diagrams 7.1 and 7.2). There is a distinctive clinical picture of increased fatiguability and temporary muscle weakness. Initial symptoms are often ptosis, diplopia or blurring of vision, due to involvement of the extra-ocular muscles. In the majority of patients the disease soon becomes generalized, affecting speech and swallowing as well as limb muscles[1]. Sometimes there is severe bulbar weakness with sparing of limb muscles. The most severe generalized disease involves the respiratory muscles, increasing susceptibility to chest infection. In approximately 20% of patients, clinical manifestations remain limited to the extra-ocular muscles, although EMG investigation will reveal more widespread abnormalities. It is suggested that if the disease has been localized for a year, further progression is unlikely[1]. In chronic disease temporary muscle weakness may give way to persistent weakness, accompanied by atrophy. In all patients symptoms tend to fluctuate.

There is a female preponderance, and clinical presentation is most often between 20 and 40 years. Onset may occur in childhood or adolescence and some of these early-onset slowly progressive cases prove to have a familial basis. Late onset, i.e. over 50 years, is more common in men. MG may appear temporarily in the neonate, whose mother has generalized disease. Rare, persistent congenital forms also occur, but have a different, non-immune pathogenesis from the classical disease[2]. The thymus is enlarged in the majority of patients. Some 60% have a hyperplastic thymus and 15% a thymoma[3]. In those with a thymic neoplasm prognosis is determined by the invasive properties of the tumour and by other associated autoimmune disorders, such as polymyositis or red cell aplasia. Myasthenia itself tends to be more severe in patients with a thymoma. Drug-induced MG is also reported. This is one of the several immunologic disorders that can be induced by penicillamine therapy[4].

Pathogenesis

Antibodies to acetylcholine receptors (AChR) of IgG class can be detected in the great majority of patients. The effector role of these antibodies has been amply demonstrated by experimental autoimmune MG in animals, induced by inoculation of purified AChR combined with an adjuvant and by the natural, passive transfer of antibodies in neonatal MG[5,6]. In both experimental and naturally occurring diseases antibody is bound to the postsynaptic membrane[7]. In normal neuromuscular transmission the arrival of the action potential at the nerve terminal causes fusion of numerous synaptic vesicles with the presynaptic membrane and release of many quanta of acetyl choline (ACh). ACh diffuses across the synaptic cleft, binds to the specific receptors located on the tips of junctional folds and thereby induces a change in membrane permeability. AChR antibody may interfere with this action by more than one mechanism.

Antibody can compete with ACh for the binding site, thus preventing depolarization. However the majority of antibodies have been shown to react with an immunogenic region of the receptor molecule that is distinct from the binding site[8]. In normal muscle cells there is a continual turnover of AChR, which become internalized and taken up by the lysosomal system[9]. This process is accelerated in MG as a result of cross-linkage of divalent antibody on the cell membrane[10]. Normally, increased degradation is compensated for by increased synthesis. This happens to a certain extent and may explain the stable state of many chronic myasthenics[9]. Nevertheless compensation is not complete and one reason is the concurrent disorganization of junctional folds. Degeneration of junctional folds and simplification of the postsynaptic membrane is probably the major cause of AChR reduction and impaired neuromuscular transmission. This end plate destruction is attributed to focal lysis via the complement pathway. Complement components C3 and C9 have been demonstrated on the postsynaptic membrane[7].

Despite the pathogenetic role of AChR antibody the levels of serum antibody do not show close correlation with clinical severity. This discrepancy may be explained by antibodies of different specificities and ability to fix complement. Therapeutic measures that reduce the level of antibody are nevertheless generally beneficial.

Identification of the effector mechanism does not explain why it occurs. Antibody production is T-cell dependent and in many young female patients a wide variety of autoantibodies are produced[8]. A strong association with HLA-B8 implies a genetic disposition. A unifying concept of pathogenesis suggests the thymus itself is the initial site of antibody production[11]. Non-lymphoid stromal cells of the thymus, referred to as myoid cells, have been shown to develop AChR on the cell membrane. In the younger patient there is frequently a hyperplastic thymus, which is the site of germinal centre formation and B-cell production. It is suggested that altered AChR within the thymus provide the stimulus for an autoimmune response. The

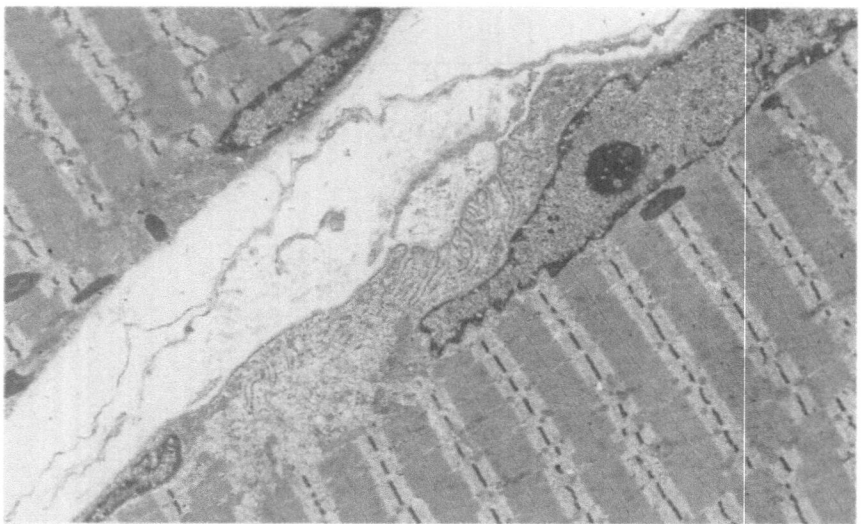

Figure 7.1 Normal motor end plate showing an axonal terminal lying in a groove in the surface of the muscle cell membrane. The sarcolemma adjacent to the axon shows complex infolding, the junctional folds. Electron micrograph × 2000

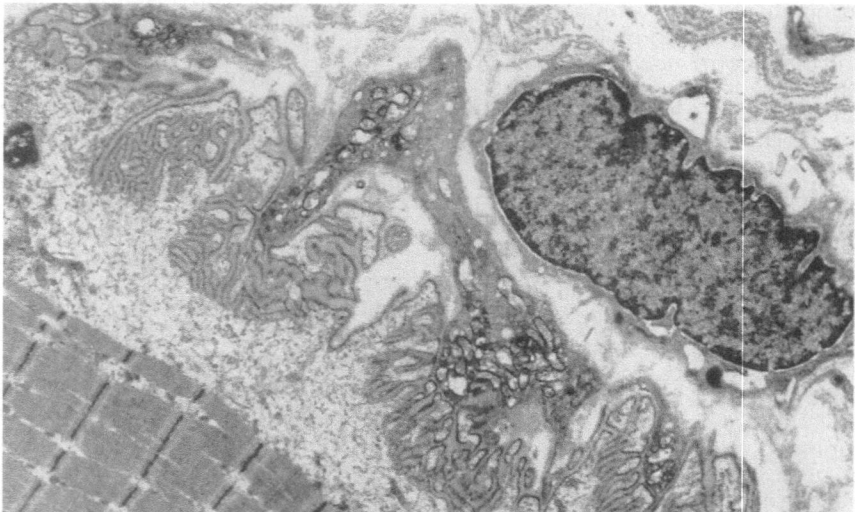

Figure 7.2 Normal motor end plate showing four axon terminals and greater detail of the junctional folds. Electron micrograph × 4000

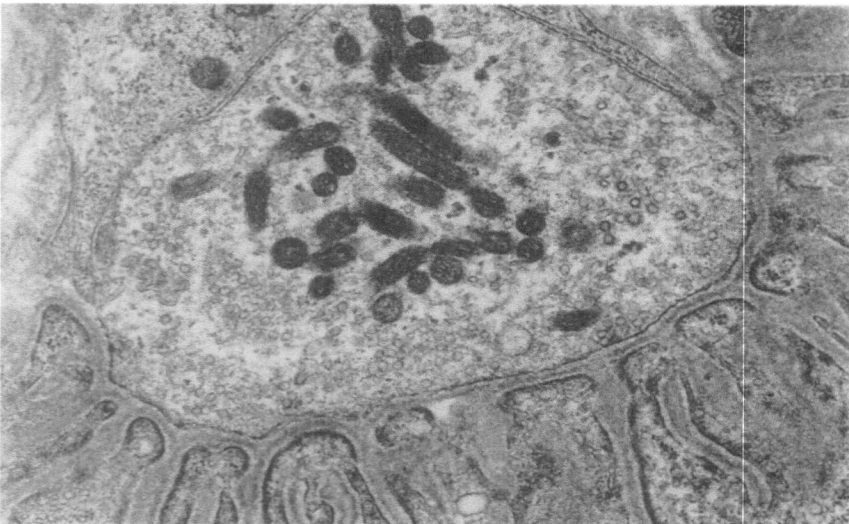

Figure 7.3 Normal axon terminal containing synaptic vesicles and mitochondria. Schwann cell cytoplasm extends up to the junction but not into the synaptic cleft. A basement membrane separates muscle sarcolemma from the axolemma. Electron micrograph × 15 200

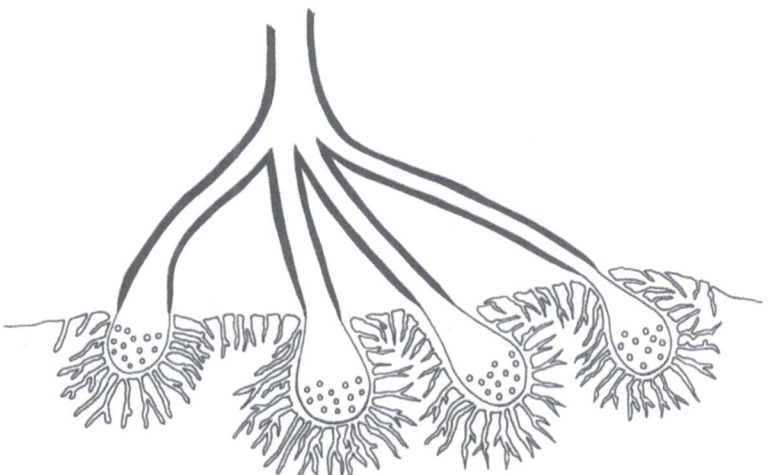

Diagram 7.1 Diagram of a normal motor end plate. Several axon terminals lie within shallow grooves in the muscle cell surface, surrounded by deep, complex invaginations of the sarcolemma

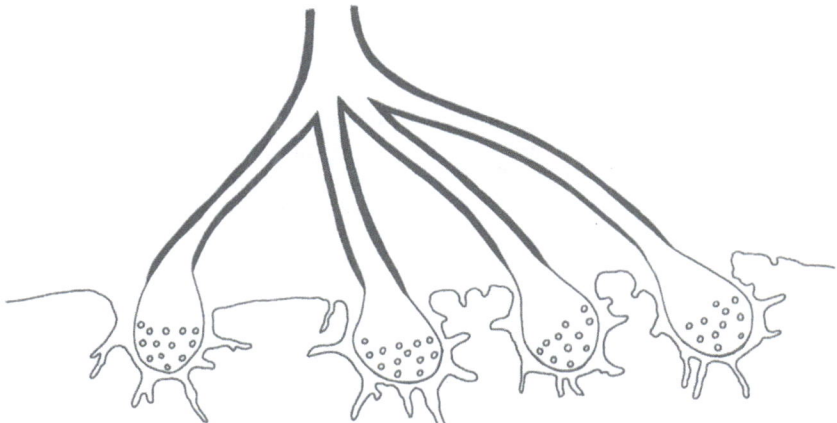

Diagram 7.2 Diagram of the motor end plate in myasthenia gravis. There is gross simplification of the junctional folds, which are shallower, broader and less complex than normal

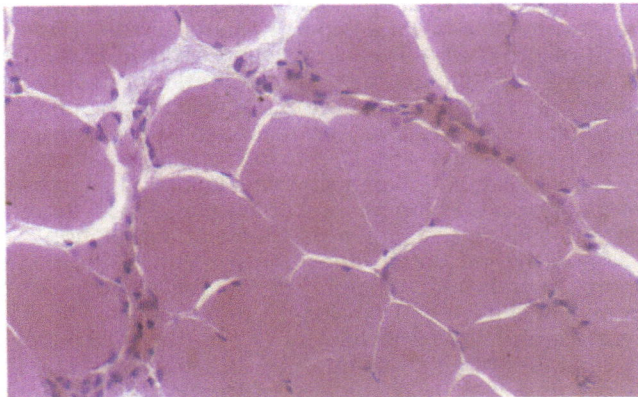

Figure 7.4 Chronic myasthenia gravis Deltoid biopsy from a 40-year-old woman with chronic, generalized myasthenia gravis. There is small group atrophy, consistent with established denervation atrophy. The denervated fibres are minute and easily overlooked in this biopsy in which the majority of fibres are of normal size.   H & E × 180

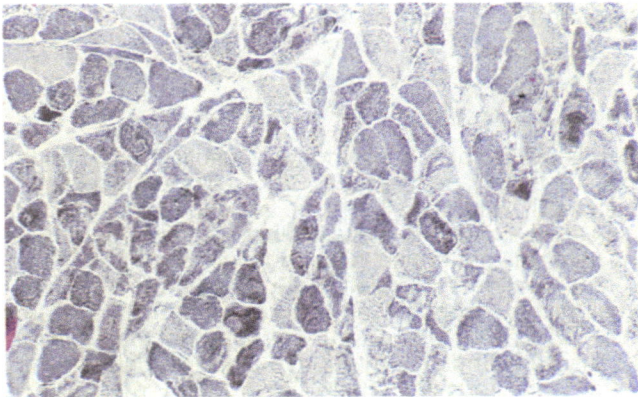

Figure 7.5 Chronic myasthenia gravis. Deltoid biopsy from a 72-year-old man with chronic generalized myasthenia gravis, showing global limb weakness and moderate wasting of the shoulder girdle muscles. CPK normal. The biopsy shows moderate atrophy, with scattered angular fibres and a moth-eaten appearance of the cytoplasm with the oxidative enzyme reaction. Co-existent polymyositis was considered but there was no firm evidence and the patient responded well to neostigmine. (Same case shown in Figures 7.6 and 7.7.)   NADH-TR × 75

receptors are conceivably altered by viral infection of these cells. The production of antibody is dependent upon a clone of T-cells capable of responding to AChR antigens and co-operating with B cells. The success of thymectomy is explained by elimination of the source of primed immunocompetent cells, which not only respond to intrathymic antigens, but to the AChR of skeletal muscle cells. Thymic neoplasms may have a similar effect on self tolerance, by disrupting normal architecture of the residual thymus.

The rare congenital forms of MG (as opposed to maternally transmitted neonatal disease) have a completely different pathogenesis. These appear to be the result of various biochemical defects operating at the neuromuscular junction. Probable mechanisms include end plate acetylcholine esterase deficiency, defective AChR-induced ion channels and defective AChR resynthesis[2]. Autoantibodies are not present in these disorders.

Diagnosis

In almost all patients with a suggestive clinical picture the diagnosis can be confirmed or refuted by response to anticholinesterase drugs, such as intravenous edrophonium. An unequivocal increase in strength occurs in MG but not in other neuromuscular disorders. However, in a few with predominantly ocular manifestations, the response is too small to be quantitated and in others a negative result may be confused by a subjective response. In these cases electrodiagnosis can provide a definitive diagnosis. Repetitive stimulation of a motor nerve confirms the diagnosis when the successive muscle potentials exhibit clear decrement in size[12]. This is a less sensitive method, but easier to perform and interpret, than single fibre EMG. The latter provides a sensitive detector for MG by measuring the jitter, i.e. the variation in latency from nerve impulse to action potential following successive impulses to individual fibres[13]. Reduced end plate sensitivity in MG increases jitter. Thus it is apparent that muscle biopsy has a relatively small part to play in the routine clinical diagnosis of MG. There is overlap with other immunological disorders including polymyositis in a small proportion of myasthenics[14]. Biopsy is probably only required for these and other atypical cases.

Muscle Biopsy

The diagnosis of MG will not be established by routine muscle biopsy techniques. When limb muscles are examined histologically in the absence of permanent clinical weakness no abnormalities may be found with the usual histochemical techniques. In chronic MG, persistent weakness correlates with single fibre atrophy or small group atrophy in the more severe case (Figures 7.4–7.7). Occasional foci of lymphocytes are an inconsistent finding. They have been described in the extra-ocular muscles where fibre atrophy may also be more severe[15]. The significance of lymphoid infiltrates is uncertain because experimental evidence and fine structural observations suggest that direct cell-mediated destruction of motor end plates does not occur.

The only consistent morphological abnormalities in MG are found at the motor end plate (Diagrams 7.1 and 7.2). Their detection requires a motor end point biopsy,

methylene vital staining or silver staining of the terminal innervation and possibly an exhaustive EM search. In man, as a research procedure, rather than a diagnostic technique, it may be possible to obtain the innervation zone from intercostal muscle during a thymectomy operation. Intercostal muscle is also an ideal muscle to study at autopsy, because the innervation zone is easily located in short muscle fibres. The Schofield's silver technique gives excellent results in postmortem material. In MG the nerve terminals appear elongated and fine terminal sprouts may be found. These abnormalities are particularly striking in the extra-ocular muscles[15].

Electron microscopy of motor end plates in early MG reveals alterations in junctional folds; some are missing and synaptic clefts may be widened. In chronic MG these changes are more severe. Destruction of junction folds leads to simplification of the normally complex end plate folds[16,17] (Diagrams 7.1 and 7.2). Large gaps appear between the pre- and postsynaptic membranes and there is vesicular debris on the postsynaptic surface. Electron-dense fuzzy material has been observed on the tips of junctional folds where the AChR are situated[17].

Myasthenic Syndrome – Eaton–Lambert Syndrome

Clinically the myasthenic, or Eaton–Lambert syndrome can resemble generalized myasthenia gravis, but it is a motor end plate disorder with a completely different pathogenesis. The disorder is a rare, non-metastatic manifestation of malignancy, usually oat cell carcinoma of the bronchus and thus most patients are men over 40 years. It has occasionally been described in association with autoimmune diseases in younger patients without malignancy[18]. The main clinical features are weakness and excess fatiguability of the proximal limb and girdle muscles, particularly the leg muscles. In some cases this is combined with ptosis, blurring of vision, speech and swallowing difficulties. Tendon reflexes, which are usually preserved in MG, are depressed or absent. In contrast to MG, whilst prolonged effort exacerbates weakness, there is often a temporary improvement after a few attempts at voluntary contraction. There is no significant response to anticholinesterases, but a definite improvement with guanidine. Patients usually have at least mild proximal muscle wasting and the EMG may reveal myopathic changes. The true nature of this disorder may be overlooked without specific tests of neuromuscular transmission. The response to a single peripheral nerve stimulus is an abnormally small action potential, stimulation at a slow rate leads to progressive reduction in amplitude, but characteristically there is paradoxical potentiation at fast rates of stimulation[12].

Abnormal neuromuscular transmission in the myasthenic syndrome is due to defective release of acetylcholine (ACh) from the nerve terminals. The ACh content and synthetic activity of the nerve terminal is normal, but reduced quanta of ACh are released by the nerve impulse[19]. The defect in neuromuscular transmission has been transferred to mice by repeated injections of the IgG fraction of patient serum[20]. Clinical and experimental evidence suggest that in the myasthenic syndrome antibody bound to the presynaptic membrane interferes with ACh release[21].

As in myasthenia gravis, muscle biopsy is not the way to establish the diagnosis, but may help to exclude other disorders.

Biopsy

By light microscopy, changes are quite non-specific. There may be scattered angular atrophic fibres or a suggestion of small group atrophy (Figures 7.8–7.10). Motor end plates appear normal by light microscopy (Figure 7.11). Electron microscopy has revealed abnormalities of end plate morphology quite different from MG. The postsynaptic membrane is not simplified, but unduly complex, with increased folds and sometimes the axon terminals are completely filled with synaptic vesicles (Figures 7.12 and 7.13)[22]. Changes in the nerve terminal have been detected by the freeze fracture technique. In the presynaptic membrane the regions associated with synaptic vesicle release are referred to as active zones. Large intramembranous particles in these zones represent voltage-sensitive calcium channels that control transmitter release. In the myasthenic syndrome these active zones have been found to be disorganized or absent, suggesting they are the target of autoantibody attack[23].

Muscle Disorders Associated with Malignancy

The Eaton–Lambert syndrome is a well-defined, but extremely rare, complication of malignancy; however patients with malignant tumours frequently exhibit some degree of muscle weakness. Most commonly this is due to the combined effects of cachexia, immobility and disuse atrophy. Protein synthesis in muscle is depressed in patients with cancerous cachexia[24]. The association between dermatomyositis and malignancy in adults is described in Chapter 13. Widely disseminated tumour with haematogenous spread to muscle is another unusual cause (see Chapter 18). A rare, focal, flitting myopathy of embolic origin has been reported as a terminal event in patients with carcinoma[25]. The systemic emboli produced arteriolar occlusion and small muscle infarcts, chiefly in the lower legs, and were thought to originate from non-bacterial thrombotic endocarditis. A sensorimotor neuropathy due to combined axon loss and segmental demyelination has been described in association with malignancy and, like the myasthenic syndrome and dermatomyositis, it is probably a paraneoplastic syndrome with an immunological basis[26]. Motor neuron disease has also been reported in patients with carcinoma[27]. Malignant neoplasia and motor neuron disease both have a peak incidence in the elderly. Thus it is not surprising that the two disorders sometimes coincide. A causal relationship can only be proposed for the very few cases where motor neuron disease has apparently remitted on resection of the tumour[28]. In the majority of patients there is no such association and exhaustive tumour-seeking investigations in patients with motor neuron disease are quite unwarranted.

Muscle Biopsy

There is no specific histological picture that can be labelled as carcinomatous myopathy. Patients with associated motor neuron disease or peripheral neuropathy will show varying degrees of neurogenic atrophy. The histology of dermatomyositis associated with malignancy is indistinguishable from uncomplicated dermatomyositis or polymyositis. Cachexia and disuse atrophy are likely to produce atrophy of all fibre types, but type 2 fibres are most severely affected.

References

1. Grob, D. (1983). Clinical manifestations of myasthenia gravis. In Albuquerque, E. X. and Eldefrawi, A. T. (eds.) *Myasthenia Gravis*. (London: Chapman & Hall), pp. 319–45

2. Engel, A. G. *et al.* (1981). Recently recognised congenital myasthenic syndromes. *Ann. NY Acad. Sci.*, **377**, 614–39

3. Tindall, R. S. A. (1980). Humoral immunity in myasthenia gravis: effect of steroids and thymectomy. *Neurology*, **30**, 554–7

4. Burres, S. A., Kanter, M. E., Richman, D. P. and Amason, B. G. W. (1981). Studies on the pathophysiology of chronic D-penicillamine-induced myasthenia. *Ann. NY Acad. Sci.*, **377**, 640–51

5. Lennon, V. A. (1978). The immunopathology of myasthenia gravis. *Human Pathol.*, **9**, 541–51

6. Engel, A. G. (1984). Myasthenia gravis and myasthenic syndromes. *Ann. Neurol.*, **16**, 519–34

7. Engel, A. G., Sahashi, K. and Fumagalli, G. (1981). The immunopathology of acquired myasthenia gravis. *Ann. NY Acad. Sci.*, **377**, 159–74

8. Biesecker, G. and Koffler, D. (1983). Immunology of myasthenia gravis. *Human Pathol.*, **14**, 419–23

9. Fumagalli, G., Engel, A. G. and Lindstrom, J. (1982). Ultrastructural aspects of acetyl choline receptor turnover at the normal end plate and in auto-immune myasthenia gravis. *J. Neuropathol. Exp. Neurol.*, **41**, 567–79

10. Drachman, D. B. *et al.* (1981). Antibody-mediated mechanisms of ACh receptor loss in myasthenia gravis: clinical relevance. *Ann. NY Acad. Sci.*, **377**, 175–88

11. Wekerle, H. *et al.* (1981). Thymic myogenesis, T lymphocytes and the pathogenesis of myasthenia gravis. *Ann. NY Acad. Sci.*, **377**, 455–76

12. Desmedt, J. E. (1983). Electrophysiological validation of myasthenia gravis. In Albuquerque, E. X. and Eldefrawi, A. T. (eds.) *Myasthenia Gravis*. (London: Chapman & Hall), pp. 249–74

13. Sanders, D. B. (1983). Electrodiagnosis of myasthenia gravis: recent techniques. In Albuquerque, E. X. and Eldefrawi, A. T. (eds.) *Myasthenia Gravis*. (London: Chapman & Hall), pp. 275–96

14. Behan, W. M. H., Behan, P. O. and Doyle, D. (1982). Association of myasthenia gravis and polymyositis with neoplasia, infection and autoimmune disorders. *Acta Neuropathol. (Berl.)*, **57**, 221–9

15. Duchen, L. W. (1975). Pathology of the innervation of skeletal muscle. In Harrison, C. V. and Weinbren, K. (eds.) *Recent Advances in Pathology*. (Edinburgh: Churchill Livingstone), pp. 215–48

16. Engel, A. G., Tsujihata, M., Lindstrom, J. M. and Lennon, V. A. (1976). The motor end plate in myasthenia gravis and in experimental autoimmune myasthenia gravis. A quantitative ultrastructural study. *Ann. NY Acad. Sci.*, **274**, 60–79

17. Nash, J. E. (1983). Ultrastructure of normal and myasthenic end plates. In Albuquerque, E. X. and Eldefrawi, A. T. (eds.) *Myasthenia Gravis*. (London: Chapman & Hall), pp. 391–422

18. Gutmann, L., Crosby, T. W., Takamori, M. and Martin, J. D. (1972). The Eaton–Lambert syndrome and auto-immune disorders. *Am. J. Med.*, **53**, 354–6

19. Molenaar, P. C., Newsom-Davis, J., Polak, R. L. and Vincent, A. (1982). Eaton–Lambert syndrome: acetyl choline and choline acetyl transferase in skeletal muscle. *Neurology*, **32**, 1061–5

20. Lang, B., Newsom-Davis, J. M., Wray, D., Vincent, A. and Murray, N. (1981). Auto-immune aetiology for myasthenic (Eaton–Lambert) syndrome. *Lancet*, **2**, 224–6

21. Vincent, A. (1983). Humoral immunity in myasthenia gravis and the Eaton–Lambert syndrome. In Albuquerque, E. X. and Eldefrawi, A. T. (eds.) *Myasthenia Gravis*. (London: Chapman & Hall), pp. 311–16

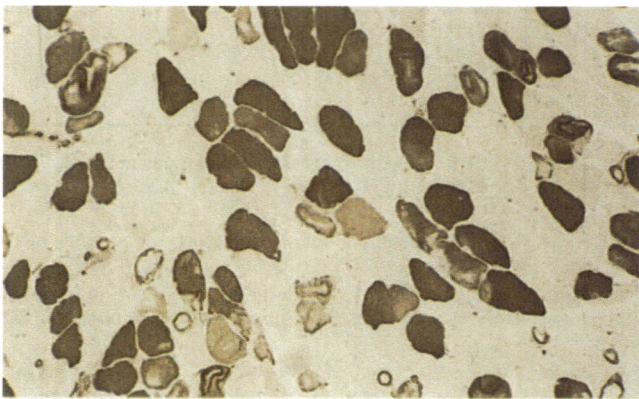

Figure 7.6 Chronic myasthenia gravis. Irregularly distributed atrophic fibres of both types and patchy staining with the myosin ATP-ase reaction. Some fibres show loss of enzyme activity in the centre. Myosin ATP-ase pH 4.5 × 75

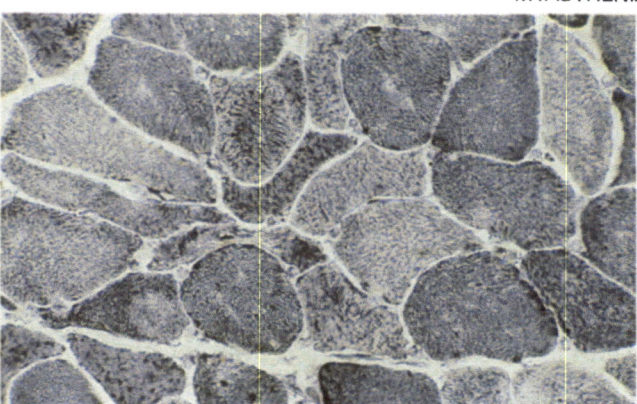

Figure 7.7 Chronic myasthenia gravis. Small angular fibres suggesting denervation atrophy. There is patchy disruption of the cytoplasmic architecture. NADH-TR × 180

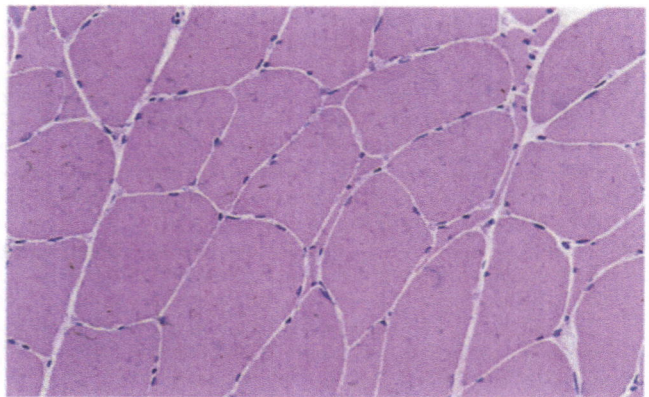

Figure 7.8 Eaton–Lambert syndrome. Quadriceps biopsy from a 70-year-old man with known carcinoma of the bronchus and recent onset of proximal muscle weakness. EMG findings characteristic of the myasthenic syndrome. The biopsy contains angular atrophic fibres and there is a suggestion of small group atrophy. (Same case shown in Figures 7.9–7.13.) H & E × 180

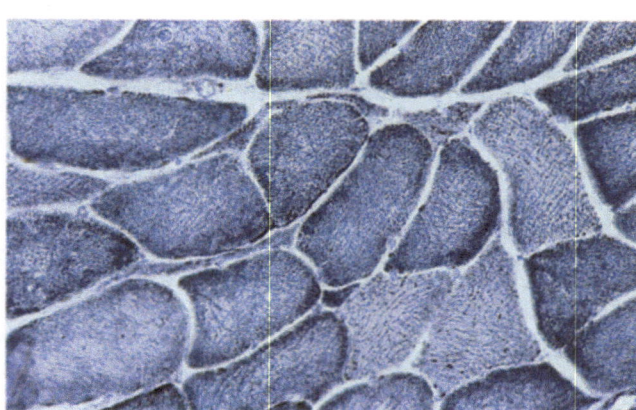

Figure 7.9 Myasthenic syndrome. Angular atrophic fibres amongst normal sized fibres. NADH-TR × 180

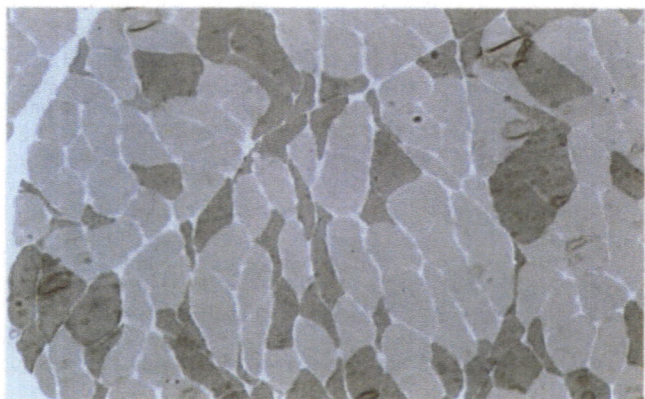

Figure 7.10 Myasthenic syndrome. The atrophic fibres are of both types, but are predominantly type 2 fibres. Myosin ATP-ase pH 9.4 × 75

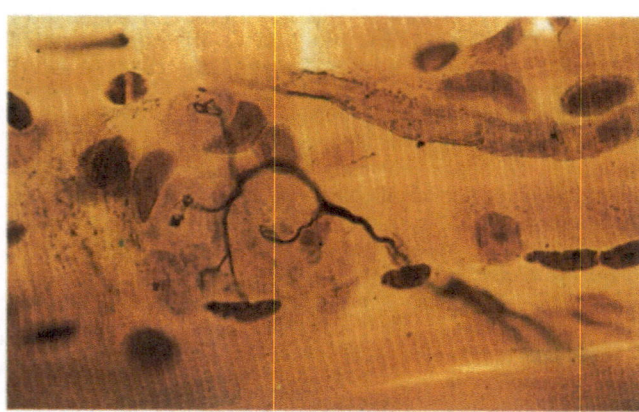

Figure 7.11 Myasthenic syndrome. A motor end plate appears normal by light microscopy. Schofield's silver staining technique × 300

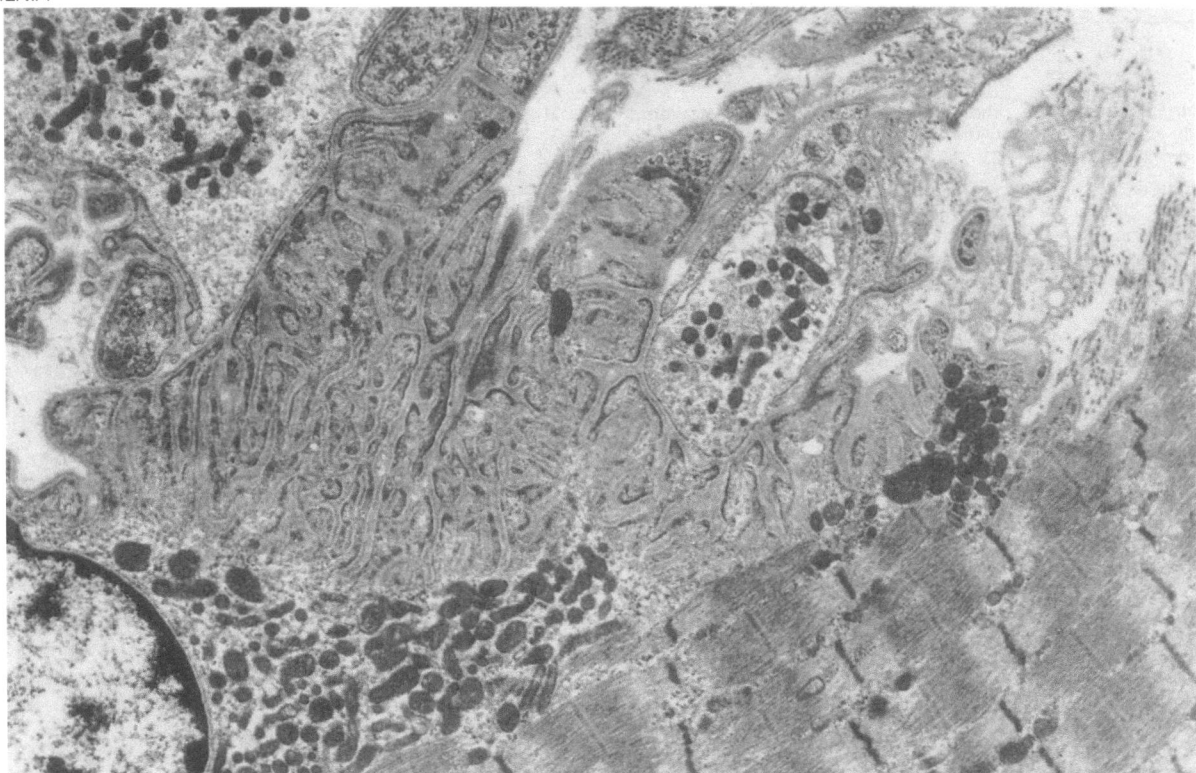

Figure 7.12 Myasthenic syndrome. A motor end plate with two axon terminals. Detailed measurements have shown that there is more complex infolding and thus a greater area of the postsynaptic membrane in the myasthenic syndrome. The numerous branching clefts in this end plate quite possibly represent an increase, but this can only be determined with certainty by accurate measurement of many end plates and many sections. There is considerable normal variation and the appearance also varies with the plane of section.   Electron micrograph × 7100

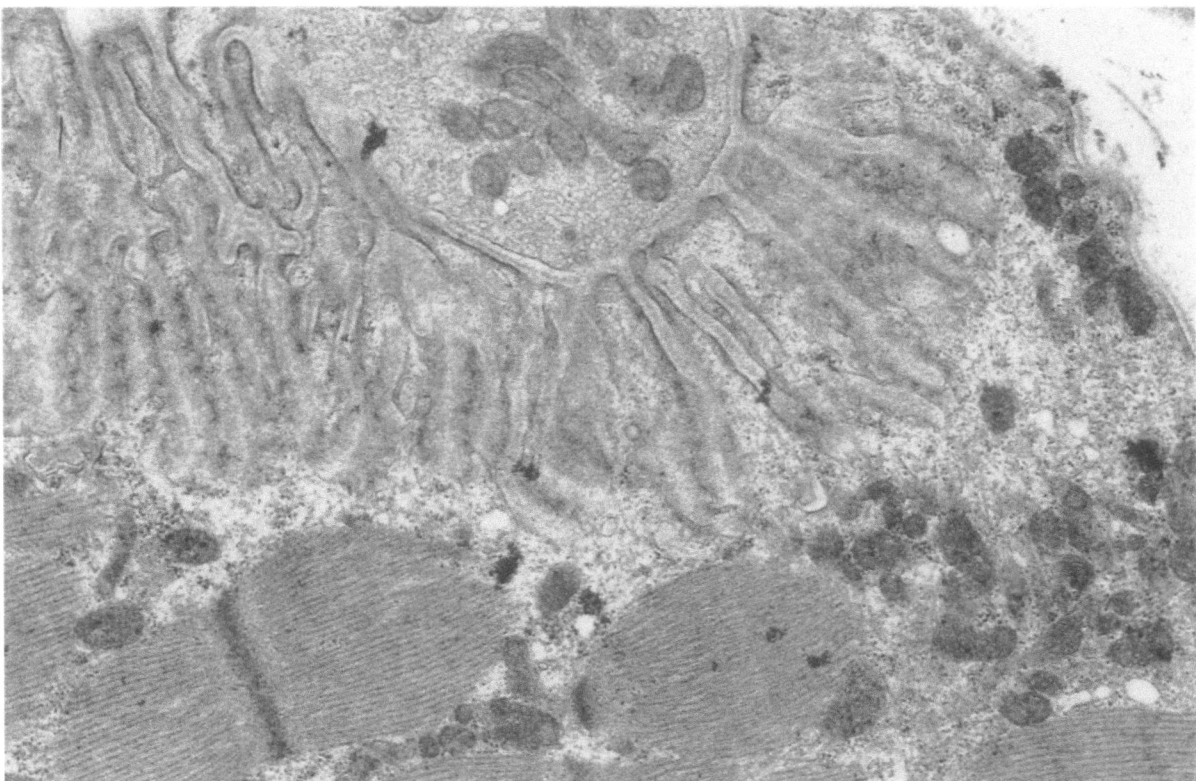

Figure 7.13 Myasthenic syndrome. Detail of an axon terminal which appears to be completely filled with synaptic vesicles.   Electron micrograph × 19 000

22. Santa, T., Engel, A. G. and Lambert, E. G. (1972). Histometric study of neuromuscular junction ultrastructure. II: Myasthenic syndrome. *Neurology*, **22**, 370–6

23. Fukunaga, H., Engel, A. G., Osame, M. and Lambert, E. H. (1982). Deficiency of presynaptic membrane active zones and active zone associated intramembrane particles in the Lambert–Eaton myasthenic syndrome. In Abstracts of the Fifth International Congress on Neuromuscular Diseases, Marseilles, France

24. Emery, P. W., Edwards, R.H.T., Rennie, M. J. and Halliday, D. (1984). Protein synthesis in muscle measured in vivo in cachetic patients with cancer. *Br. Med. J.*, **289**, 584–6

25. Heffner, R. R. (1971). Myopathy of embolic origin in patients with carcinoma. *Neurology*, **21**, 840–6

26. Weller, R. O. and Cervos-Navarro, J. (1977). Neuropathy in malignant disease. In *Pathology of Peripheral Nerves*. (London: Butterworths), pp. 135–6

27. Gritzman, M. C. D., Fritz, V. U., Perkins, S. and Kaplan, C. L. (1983). Motor neuron disease associated with carcinoma. *S. African Med. J.*, **63**, 288–91

28. Mitchell, D. M. and Olczak, S. A. (1979). Remission of a syndrome indistinguishable from motor neurone disease after resection of bronchial carcinoma. *Br. Med. J.*, **2**, 176–7

Muscular Dystrophy

Introduction

Muscular dystrophies are, by definition, inherited, progressive, wasting diseases of muscle. Duchenne dystrophy is the commonest, the most severe and inexorably progressive condition. Other forms, largely distinguished by selective muscle involvement, e.g. oculopharyngeal and facioscapulohumeral dystrophy, are more variable in their rate of progression. Many theories of causation have at some time held sway, including vascular and neural hypotheses, but current lines of research suggest cell membrane defects underlie the progressive muscle breakdown[1]. Biopsy has an essential role in early diagnosis and accurate classification of muscular dystrophy. A vague or probable diagnosis of dystrophy gives no guide to prognosis and cannot be a basis for genetic counselling.

Duchenne Muscular Dystrophy

This is a sex-linked recessive disorder with an incidence of approximately 1 in 3000 live male births[2]. Clumsy movements usually attract attention between 3 and 5 years of age, but when there is a family history and heightened awareness, the parents may identify an affected son at an early age. About one-third of cases are sporadic, due to new mutations[2] and in these children diagnosis is often delayed until school age and comparison with their peers. Young boys have a waddling gait, they fall easily and have difficulty in rising from the floor. There is a steadily progressive muscle weakness, with initial selective involvement of proximal muscles and gradual distal extension[3]. In the early years calf hypertrophy may be conspicuous. At first this is probably a genuine compensatory hypertrophy, progressing to pseudohypertrophy due to fibro-fatty replacement and eventually to diminution of muscle bulk. There is a fairly constant downhill clinical course. The boy is likely to be wheelchair-bound by 10–12 years and severely disabled by contractures and spinal deformities in the teens. Survival beyond the early twenties is exceptional, most succumbing to pneumonia. ECG abnormalities are usually present[4] and occasional patients may die of cardiac arrhythmia. Mental retardation is also a common association of Duchenne dystrophy[3] and may initially be held responsible for the physical clumsiness.

When Duchenne dystrophy becomes clinically evident, biopsy will always be diagnostic. Histological abnormalities have also been demonstrated in the preclinical phase and earlier diagnosis is possible in at-risk male infants. Bradley et al., who examined a small series, suggested that biopsy should not be performed before 2 months of age because very early changes may be quite minor and non-specific[5].

Pathogenesis

Fine structural and freeze fracture studies have revealed focal defects in the sarcolemma which are considered to be the basis of an increased permeability[6-9]. It is postulated that an abnormally permeable cell membrane permits focal influxes of calcium ions which both trigger hypercontraction and activate endogenous proteases, leading to segmental necrosis[10]. An increased calcium content has been demonstrated in muscle fibres in Duchenne dystrophy[11]. The question of whether or not the membrane defect is restricted to muscle has not been resolved[12]. Red cell membrane abnormalities are described, but these may be epiphenomena due to changes in serum enzymes. There is no recognized morphological basis for the mental retardation.

Biochemistry

The serum creatine kinase is greatly elevated in Duchenne dystrophy. In the early years it may be 200 times the normal upper limit and then gradually declines[13]. In advanced disease, when the muscle mass is severely reduced, the level approaches normal. The peak serum enzyme concentration probably occurs around 2 years and precedes obvious clinical manifestations[13]. This early rise supports the concept that increased cell membrane permeability precedes necrosis. It also provides a valuable screening test for at-risk male infants.

Duchenne Dystrophy in Females and Carrier Detection

Typical Duchenne dystrophy only occurs in boys and very rarely in females with Turner's syndrome and an XO chromosome constitution. Detection of female carriers is important for genetic counselling. A minority (approximately one-tenth) of carriers show some calf hypertrophy and/or proximal muscle weakness. A very few are quite severely affected with a progressive weakness that must be differentiated from an autosomal recessive, limb girdle dystrophy as the genetic counselling is quite different. The majority, however, have no clinical manifestations[2]. The serum creatine kinase is raised in about two-thirds of carriers, but it is not an infallible guide. The level falls in early pregnancy, with increasing age and, most importantly, a normal value does not exclude carrier status[2]. Biopsy sometimes reveals definite although often very minor abnormalities, but in other cases there is normal histology[14,15]. It has been suggested that electron microscopy may reveal subtle abnormalities undetected by light microscopy[16] but artifacts are easily produced

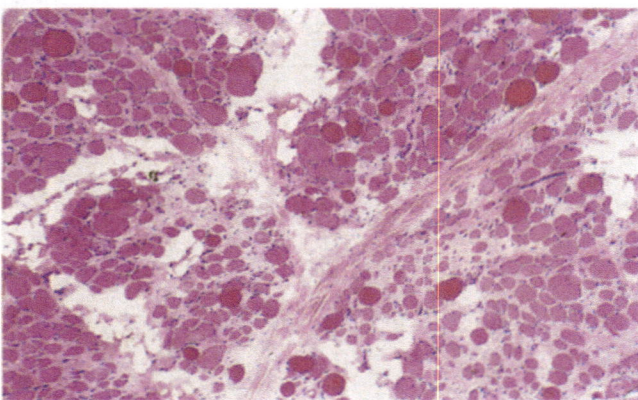

Figure 8.1 Duchenne dystrophy in a 7-year-old boy. He was late in walking and had frequent falls. He showed generalized, but predominantly proximal muscle weakness, with a positive Gower's manouevre. CPK – very high. Quadriceps muscle biopsy shows variation in fibre size and moderate perimysial and endomysial fibrosis. Even at low magnification some large rounded, eosinophilic fibres stand out. (Same case is shown in Figures 8.2–8.9.)   H & E × 75

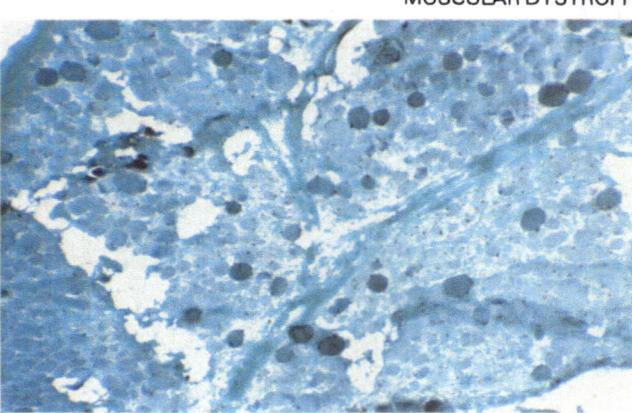

Figure 8.2   Duchenne dystrophy. The large hyaline fibres stain darkly with the trichrome method.   Gomori's trichrome × 75

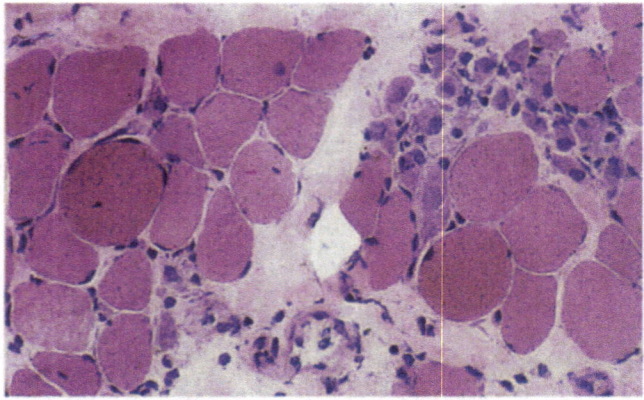

Figure 8.3   Duchenne dystrophy. A cluster of small basophilic regenerating myotubes. This field contains two of the large, rounded eosinophilic, hyaline fibres, which result from hypercontraction. In addition, there is a moderate increase in the interstitial fibrous connective tissue. (Serial sections are shown in Figures 8.4–8.6 and Figure 8.9.)   H & E × 180

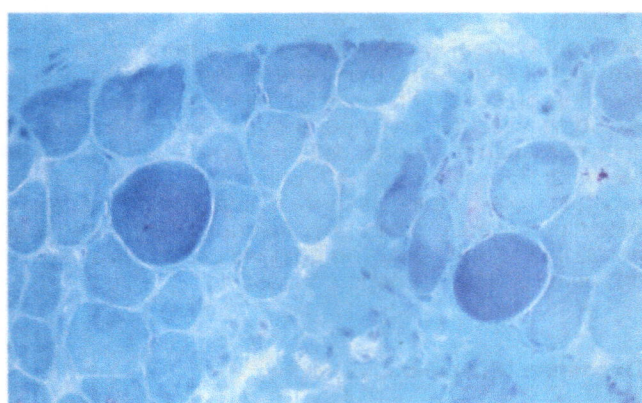

Figure 8.4   Duchenne dystrophy. The hyaline fibres stain deeply with the trichrome reaction, which also emphasizes the interstitial fibrosis.   Gomori's trichrome × 180

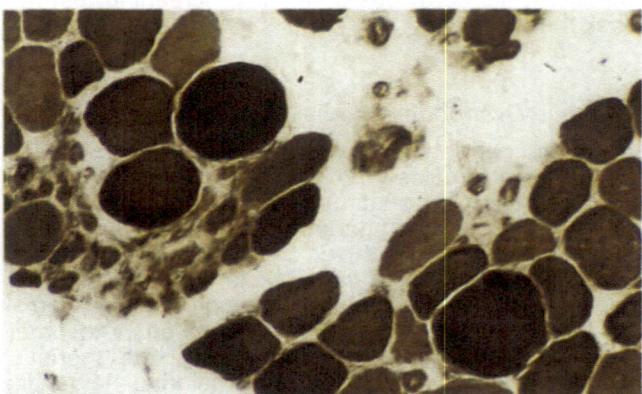

Figure 8.5   Duchenne dystrophy. The two hyaline fibres are intensely positive with myosin ATP-ase at all pHs. There is a cluster of tiny, regenerating 2C fibres.   ATP-ase pH 9.4 × 180

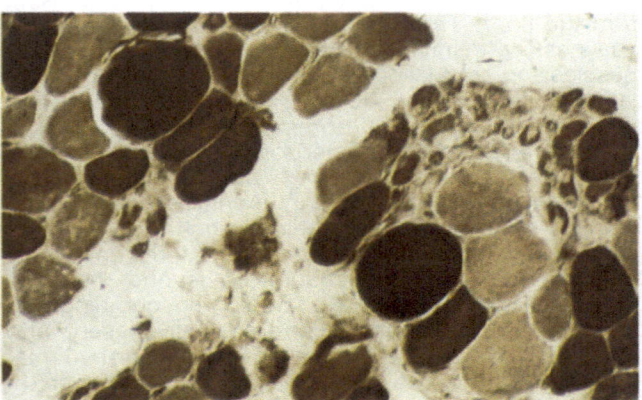

Figure 8.6   Duchenne dystrophy. The hyaline fibres show an equally positive reaction with myosin ATP-ase at acid pH.   ATP-ase pH 4.5 × 180

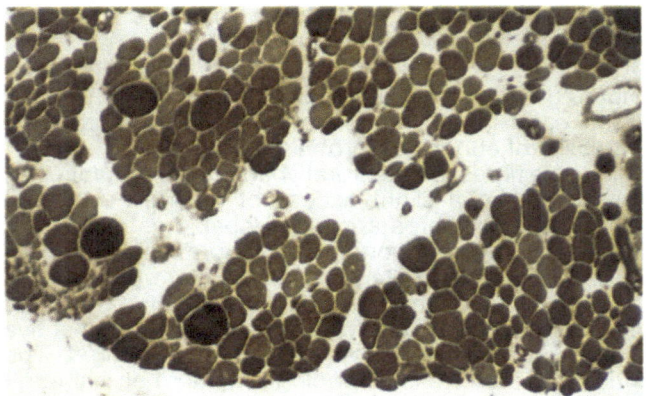

Figure 8.7 Duchenne dystrophy. Fibre type differentiation is poor with the routine myosin ATP-ase reaction. This is partly accounted for by the many hyaline fibres, which stain very darkly.   ATP-ase pH 9.4 × 75

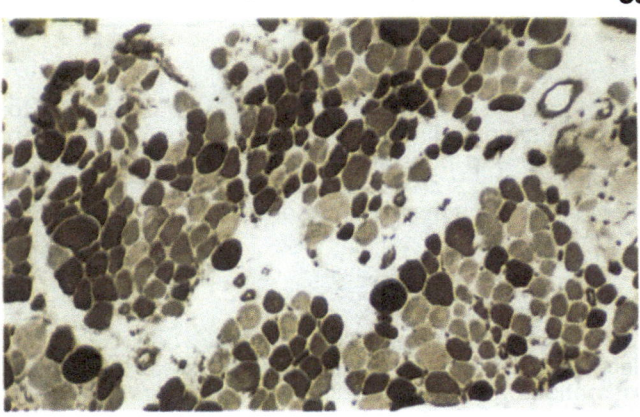

Figure 8.8 Duchenne dystrophy. Serial section of Figure 8.7. Fibre type differentiation is clearer, although most of the hyaline fibres are still darkly stained. Fibres with an intermediate reaction are probably mostly 2C.   ATP-ase pH × 4.6

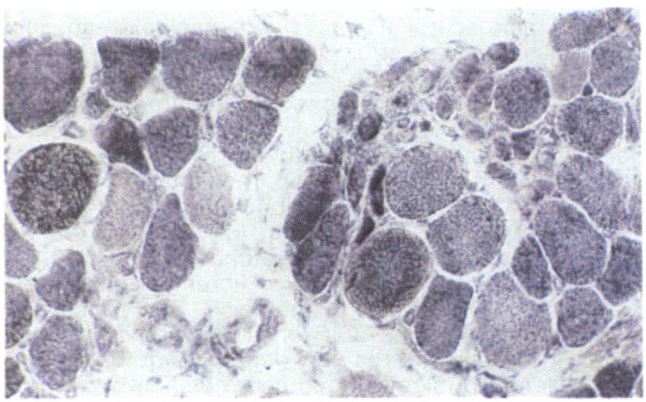

Figure 8.9 Duchenne dystrophy. Marked abnormalities of myofibrillar architecture are unusual in Duchenne dystrophy, possibly because longstanding fibre hypertrophy does not occur in rapidly progressive disease. This biopsy shows essentially normal fibre architecture, except in the two hyaline fibres, where myofibrils appear clumped.   NADH-TR × 180

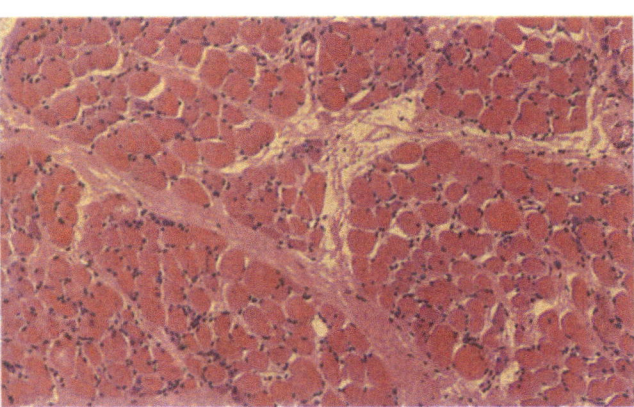

Figure 8.10 Duchenne dystrophy in a 3-year-old boy. He was noted to have an awkward gait and found difficulty in climbing stairs. CPK is extremely high. Quadriceps biopsy shows characteristic histology, with variation in fibre size. Moderate perimysial fibrosis is already clearly visible. (Same case is shown in Figures 8.11 and 8.12.)   H & E × 75

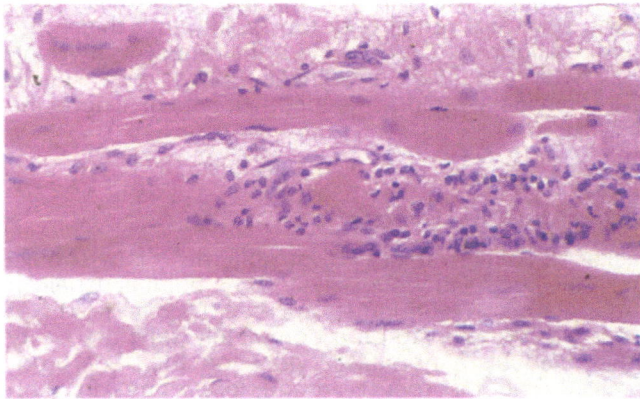

Figure 8.11 Duchenne dystrophy. Longitudinal section showing segmental necrosis. Amorphous pink cytoplasm in necrotic muscle.   H & E × 300

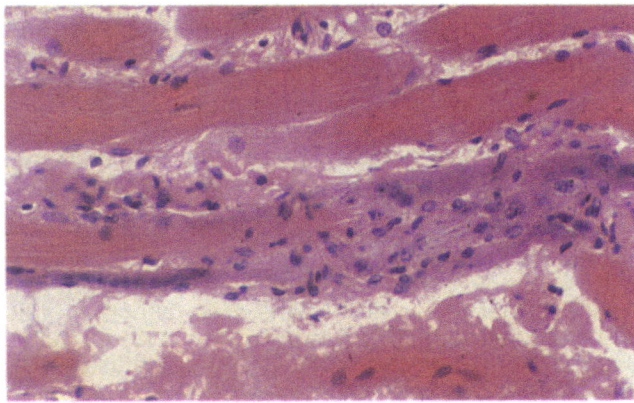

Figure 8.12 Duchenne dystrophy. Basophilic regenerating myotubes growing along the scaffold of a necrotic fibre, in biopsy of a 3-year-old patient.   H & E × 300

and it would seem to be highly dangerous practice to base the serious diagnosis of a Duchenne carrier upon such scant and possibly misleading evidence. For the future, specific X chromosome DNA probes promise to provide a more sensitive method[17].

Antenatal Detection

Until recently Duchenne dystrophy could not be detected *in utero*. Fetal serum creatine kinase estimations do not give reliable results[2] and fetal myoglobin estimation is equally unsatisfactory[18]. Although pathological abnormalities have been reported in muscle of at-risk male abortuses[19], their specificity is highly questionable, as similar changes are sometimes found in other fetuses. However, as with carrier detection, hopefully the problem is about to be solved by methods of X chromosome analysis[16].

Biopsy

In childhood the major pathological features of Duchenne dystrophy are hyaline fibres, necrotic and regenerating fibres (Figures 8.1–8.18). The sequence of necrosis and regeneration produces wide variation in fibre size. Progressive breakdown of muscle fibres leads to fibro-fatty replacement, which dominates the histology in later years. Hyaline fibres are a conspicuous, almost diagnostic finding in the early clinical phase. These are large, rounded deeply eosinophilic fibres, scattered throughout the biopsy (Figures 8.1, 8.2, 8.15–8.18). They result from segmental hypertraction, which probably precedes or is associated with fibre necrosis[20]. Hyaline fibres have been shown to have a high calcium content[21], and are particularly well demonstrated by the Gomori's trichrome method (Figures 8.4 and 8.17). The ATP-ase reaction may distinguish them as type 1 or type 2 fibres, but more often they stain darkly at all pHs. Necrotic fibres, identified by pale staining amorphous cytoplasm and invasion by phagocytes, are numerous in the early clinical years. These are often present in small clusters and in longitudinal section it is apparent that the change is segmental (Figure 8.11). Necrosis is followed by regeneration from satellite cells (Figure 8.12). In transverse section small, basophilic, regenerating fibres are usually arranged in groups, sometimes up to 10–20 fibres (Figures 8.3 and 8.14). The grouping of necrotic and regenerating fibres has suggested that additional neural or vascular factors must operate, but these have not been identified[22]. The ATP-ase reaction may show mild type 1 predominance. Distinction between fibre types is sometimes poor at pH 9.4, but clearer at acid pH. Many 2C fibres correlating with the regenerating clusters are present (Figures 8.5 and 8.6). Dubowitz claims a complete absence of 2B fibres[23], but I am not convinced that this is always the case, although they can be difficult to distinguish from 2C fibres. All these abnormalities are present in the preclinical phase and a pathognomonic biopsy can be obtained after the first few months of life[24].

Active regeneration is particularly prevalent in the early stages, but it is sometimes abortive and clearly fails to keep pace with the fibre breakdown. Progression of the disease is marked by loss of muscle fibres and a great increase in fibro-fatty connective tissue. Around 3 years of age there is already separation of fascicles by fibrous tissue and considerable endomysial fibrosis

(Figure 8.10). The abundance of interstitial connective tissue early in the course of the disease raises the possibility of abnormal fibroblastic activity[22].

In viable fibres architectural changes are insignificant. There may be a slight excess of central nuclei and occasional split fibres appear, probably as a result of incomplete regeneration[25], but abnormalities of myofibrillar arrangement are infrequent (Figure 8.9).

Study of the terminal innervation has revealed unemployed axons ramifying blindly within connective tissue, but no evidence of collateral sprouting[26]. The end plates are often morphologically normal, although sole plate retraction and immature end plates are sometimes described[27]. The end plates tend to be scattered outside the normal narrow innervation zone. The changes can all be attributed to loss of muscle fibres and re-innervation of some regenerating fibres. There is nothing to suggest a primary neural defect.

Electron Microscopy

Electron microscopy has revealed many non-specific abnormalities of fine structure, including the details of necrosis and regeneration. Satellite cells are numerous in the early years. Hypercontracted segments appear electron dense, with thick wavy Z lines bunched together[20], whereas in completely necrotic segments the cytoplasm is granular and myofibrils cannot be recognized. The plasma membrane is absent over a necrotic segment. In addition to these advanced changes, tiny, focal defects have been identified in the sarcolemma of non-necrotic fibres[6], sometimes associated with very superficial and localized degenerative changes[7]. It is suggested that tiny membrane breaks are not only genuine, but the earliest detectable morphological change preceding hypercontraction and necrosis[6,22].

Differential Diagnosis

Although other disorders may be considered clinically, on biopsy the only possible differential diagnosis is Becker dystrophy. The histology can be similar, but Becker dystrophy is much rarer. When the biopsy fits with Duchenne dystrophy, sadly the great majority of young boys will prove only too rapidly that this is the correct diagnosis. Conversely, if the biopsy of a young boy with muscle weakness does not show characteristic histology he does not have Duchenne dystrophy.

Becker Muscular Dystrophy

Becker, X-linked muscular dystrophy has many clinical similarities with Duchenne dystrophy, but it is usually a milder condition with longer survival. Despite points of overlap it is known to be a completely separate entity determined by a non-allelic gene on the X-chromosomes[3]. The disorder is much less common than Duchenne dystrophy. The average age of onset is later in Becker dystrophy, usually after 7 years and sometimes not until late 'teens. However, there is a wide range and considerable overlap with Duchenne dystrophy[28]. Clumsiness has been noticed at 2 years of age and, of course like Duchenne dystrophy, the disorder is generally recognized earlier when there is a family history[29]. The distribution of weakness is similar with initial pelvic girdle weakness and progression to involve the upper limbs. Pseudohypertrophy of the calves is present in the majority. The rate of progression is usually much slower than in Duchenne dystrophy, so that patients are still ambulant in their 'teens and usually until the twenties. A few continue walking until the 4th and 5th decades. The mean age at death is much later, around 40 years. Patients with Becker dystrophy are usually of normal intelligence. In the early stages the serum creatine kinase is very high and gives no distinction from Duchenne dystrophy. The main differences from Duchenne dystrophy are the slower progression and greater longevity. Therefore in the young child it may be impossible to distinguish the two disorders unless there is a family history. There may be subtle differences in the biopsy, referred to below, but not all studies have revealed these. Emery considers the age of becoming chairbound as the best criterion[28]. The ECG may also be helpful, because the early ECG changes that are common in Duchenne dystrophy are usually absent in Becker dystrophy. Within a single kindred the clinical course is usually similar[29], although occasionally siblings have shown marked clinical differences[30].

Biopsy

All the histological changes described in Duchenne dystrophy, including opaque, hyaline fibres, necrosis and regeneration, can be found in Becker dystrophy and histological distinction may be impossible. However, in parallel with the protracted clinical course, the changes tend to be milder in Becker dystrophy at comparable ages (Figures 8.19–8.24). The extent of fibre loss and fibrosis in the older child or teenager is far less than in Duchenne dystrophy. Fibre type differentiation with the ATP-ase reaction at pH 9.4 is sometimes poor in Duchenne dystrophy, but there is generally a clear distinction in Becker dystrophy. Type 1 predominance is quite common and Dubowitz has described type 2B fibre deficiency[31]. Internal nuclei and split fibres may be quite numerous in Becker dystrophy[29], but they are relatively infrequent in Duchenne dystrophy. A recent histopathological report of Becker dystrophy confirmed these myopathic changes, but also described group atrophy and type grouping, suggesting that a neurogenic component may play a part in the pathogenesis of this disease[32].

Differential Diagnosis

Sporadic Becker dystrophy must be distinguished from chronic spinal muscular atrophy (the limb girdle syndrome) with autosomal recessive inheritance, because very different genetic counselling is required. Definite type grouping and small group atrophy point to SMA. SMA also tends to show more hypertrophied fibres with abnormalities of internal architecture, whilst frequent hyaline fibres suggest the dystrophy. However, groups of small fibres, perhaps derived from regeneration or splitting can be found in Becker dystrophy and distinction may not be easy[33]. It would seem appropriate to check the serum CPK levels of close female relatives whenever possible, as levels are likely to be elevated in most carriers of dystrophy, but not in heterozygotes with SMA.

When there is a family history of affected male relatives the clinical diagnosis of Becker dystrophy may

be unchallenged. However, there are other rare X-linked muscle disorders which cannot be reliably distinguished without full investigation and biopsy. In particular, there is an X-linked form of chronic SMA which also gives calf hypertrophy in adolescence[34]. The EMG and biopsy in this condition are clearly neurogenic and distinction is worthwhile because the prognosis is usually better.

Severe Muscular Dystrophy in Girls

Female carriers of the Duchenne gene who have clinical symptoms are rarely as severely affected as boys[35]. Genuine severe muscular dystrophy is an exceptional rarity in girls. Only a few cases with probable autosomal inheritance have been reported. There is considerable clinical similarity with Duchenne dystrophy and the serum CPK is very high. However the ability to walk is maintained slightly longer.

Muscle biopsy shows fibre necrosis and regeneration and hyaline fibres similar to Duchenne dystrophy. However muscle destruction is less severe in early childhood and tends to have a focal pattern.

References

1. Rowland, L. P. (1976). Pathogenesis of muscular dystrophies. *Arch. Neurol.*, **33**, 315–21

2. Emery, A. E. H. (1980). Duchenne muscular dystrophy: genetic aspects, carrier detection and antenatal diagnosis. *Br. Med. Bull.*, **36**, 117–22

3. Gardner-Medwin, D. (1980). Clinical features and classification of the muscular dystrophies. *Br. Med. Bull.*, **36**, 109–15

4. Hunter, S. (1980). The heart in muscular dystrophy. *Br. Med. Bull.*, **36**, 133–4

5. Bradley, W. G., Hudgson, P., Larkson, P. F., Papapetropoulos, T. A. and Jenkinson, M. (1972). Structural changes in the early stages of Duchenne muscular dystrophy. *J. Neurol. Neurosurg. Psychiatry.*, **35**, 451–5

6. Carpenter, S. and Karpati, G. (1979). Duchenne muscular dystrophy. Plasma membrane loss initiates muscle cell necrosis unless it is repaired. *Brain*, **102**, 147–61

7. Bahram, M. and Engel, A. G. (1975). Duchenne dystrophy: electron microscopic findings pointing to a basic or early abnormality in the plasma membrane of the muscle fibre. *Neurology*, **25**, 1111–20

8. Shotton, D. M. (1982). Quantitative freeze-fracture electron microscopy of dystrophic muscle membranes. *J. Neurol. Sci.*, **57**, 161–90

9. Wakayama, Y., Okayasu, H., Shibuya, S. and Kumagai, T. (1984). Duchenne dystrophy: Reduced density of orthogonal array subunit particles in muscle plasma membrane. *Neurology*, **34**, 1313–17

10. Duncan, C. J. (1978). Role of intracellular calcium in promoting muscle damage: a strategy for controlling the dystrophic condition. *Experientia*, **34**, 1531–5

11. Maunder, C. A., Yarom, R. and Dubowitz, V. (1977). Electron microscopic X-ray microanalysis of normal and diseased human muscle. *J. Neurol. Sci.*, **33**, 323–34

12. Lucy, J. A. (1980). Is there a membrane defect in muscle and other cells? *Br. Med. Bull.*, **36**, 187–92

13. Pennington, R. J. T. (1980). Clinical biochemistry of muscular dystrophy. *Br. Med. Bull.*, **36**, 123–6

14. Morris, C. J. and Raybould, J. A. (1971). Histochemically demonstrable fibre abnormalities in normal skeletal muscle and muscle from carriers of Duchenne muscular dystrophy. *J. Neurol. Neurosurg. Psychiatry.*, **34**, 348–56

15. Dubowitz, V. (1975). Carrier detection and genetic counselling in Duchenne dystrophy. *Develop. Med. Child. Neurol.*, **17**, 352–56

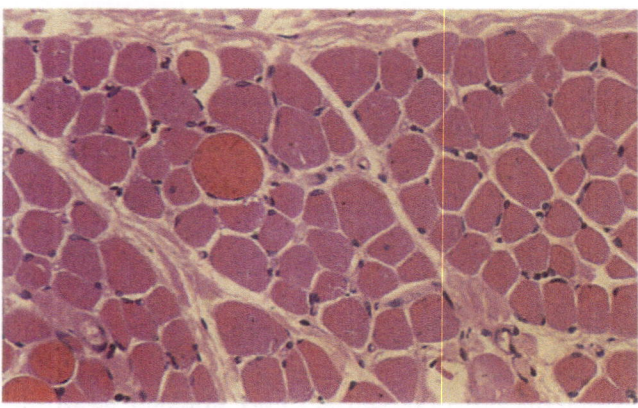

Figure 8.13 Duchenne dystrophy in a 6-year-old boy, with the typical clinical picture and greatly elevated CPK. Quadriceps biopsy shows variation in fibre size and occasional large, hyaline fibres.   H & E × 180

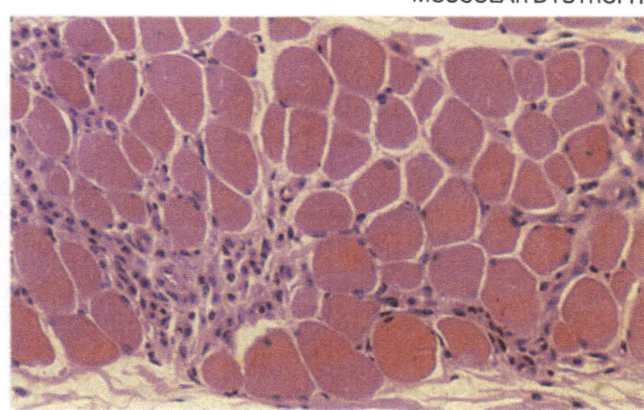

Figure 8.14 Duchenne dystrophy. Cluster of tiny, regenerating myotubes.   H & E × 180

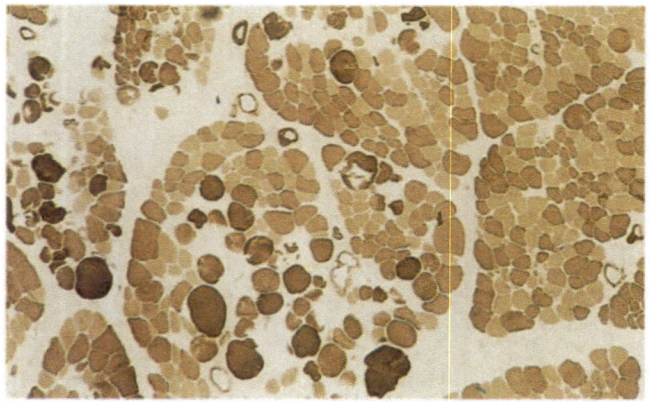

Figure 8.15 Duchenne dystrophy. Hyaline fibres show a positive reaction with the routine myosin ATP-ase reaction. (Serial sections shown in Figures 8.17 and 8.18.)   ATP-ase × 75

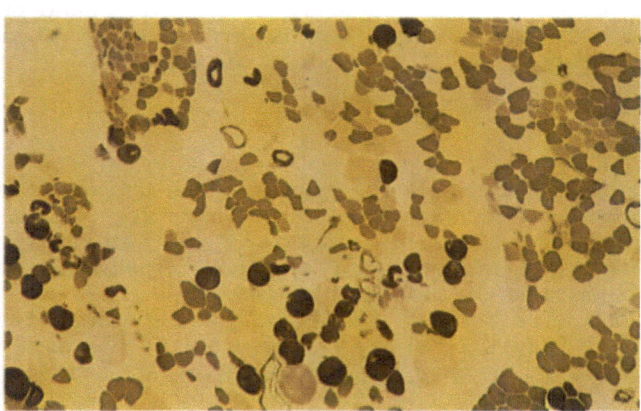

Figure 8.16 Duchenne dystrophy. Some appararently hyaline fibres retain fibre differentiation with myosin ATP-ase at this pH.   ATP-ase pH 4.6 × 75

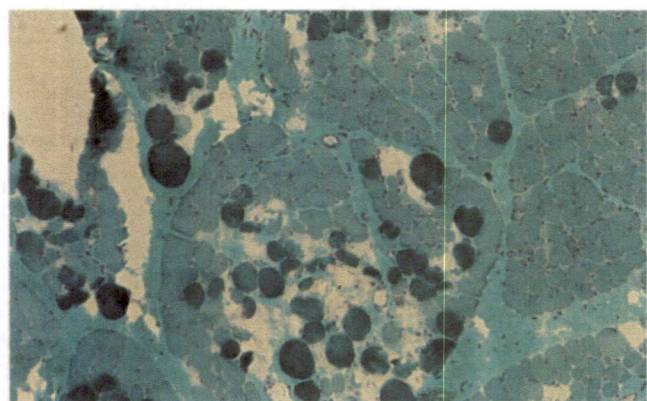

Figure 8.17 Duchenne dystrophy. Many, irregularly scattered hyaline fibres are revealed by this stain.   Gomori's trichrome × 75

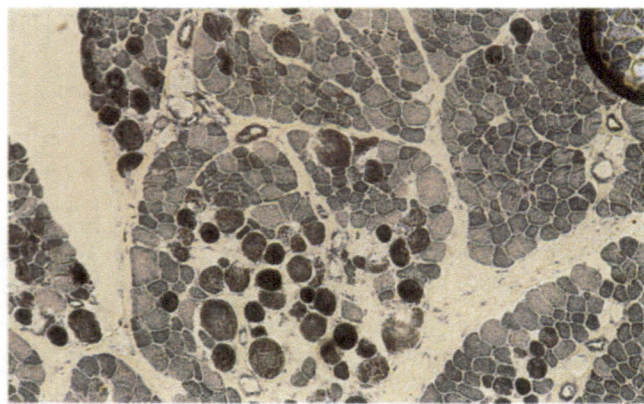

Figure 8.18 Duchenne dystrophy. Most hyaline fibres show a strongly positive oxidative enzyme reaction, irrespective of fibre type.   NADH-TR × 75

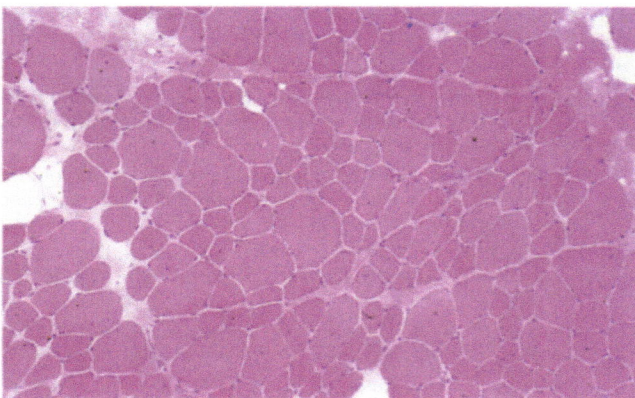

Figure 8.19 Becker dystrophy. 7-year-old boy with difficulty in walking since age 3 years. He had a slightly waddling gait and walked on the balls of his feet. Leg muscles mildly hypertrophied. Normal tone and muscle power. The biopsy shows variation in fibre size, but not the degree of fibrosis expected in Duchenne dystrophy and there are no obvious hyaline fibres. (Same case shown in Figures 8.20–8.24) H & E × 180

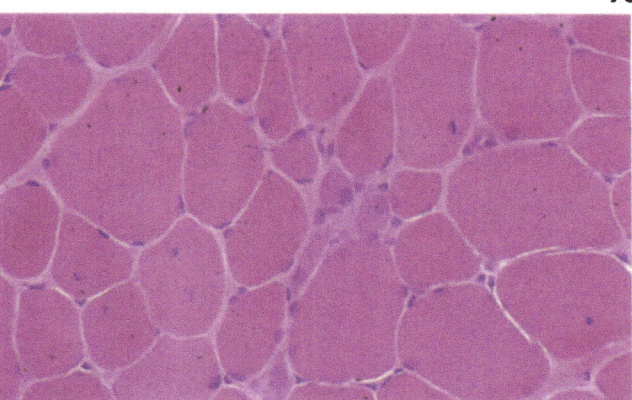

Figure 8.20 Becker dystrophy. There is variation in fibre size with some greatly hypertrophied fibres, a slight increase in endomysial fibrous connective tissue and a few regenerating fibres. These features would be unusual in a congenital myopathy and suggest a dystrophic process. H & E × 300

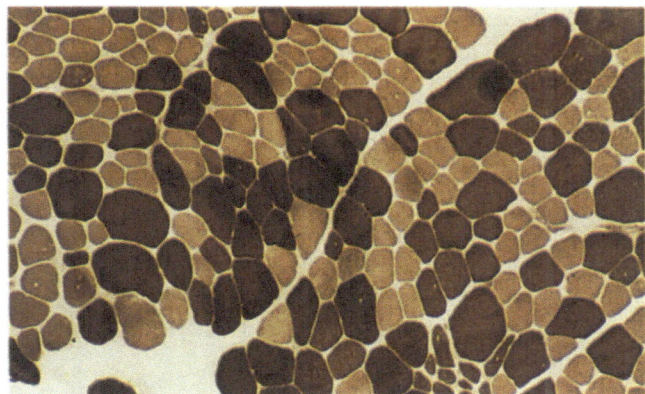

Figure 8.21 Becker dystrophy. The large fibres are mainly type 2, whereas the small fibres are mainly type 1. However, there are scattered small type 2 fibres, unlike the picture of congenital fibre type disproportion. ATP-ase pH 9.4 × 180

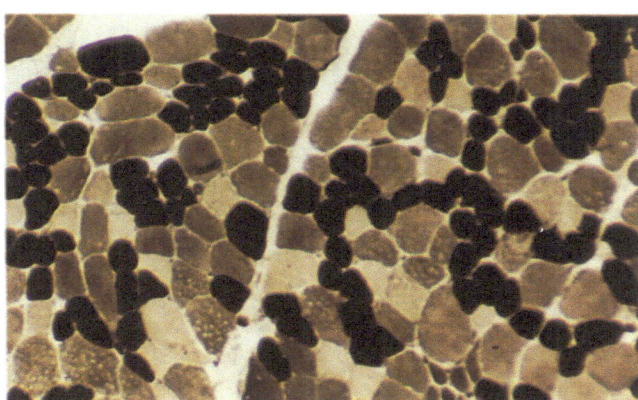

Figure 8.22 Becker dystrophy. There is clear fibre type differentiation and a normal mosaic distribution pattern. ATP-ase pH 4.3 × 180

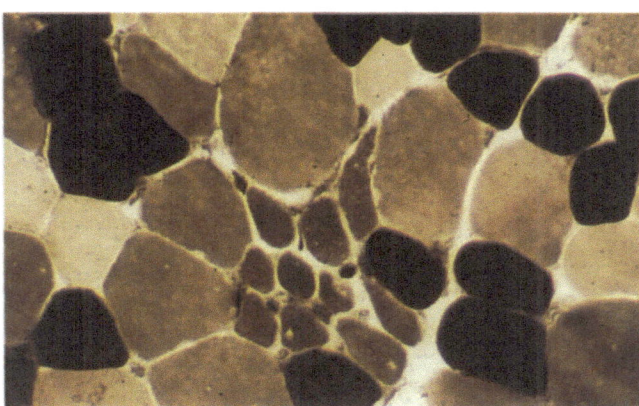

Figure 8.23 Becker dystrophy. A small group of type 2C fibres, which probably correspond with regenerating fibres. ATP-ase pH 4.3 × 300

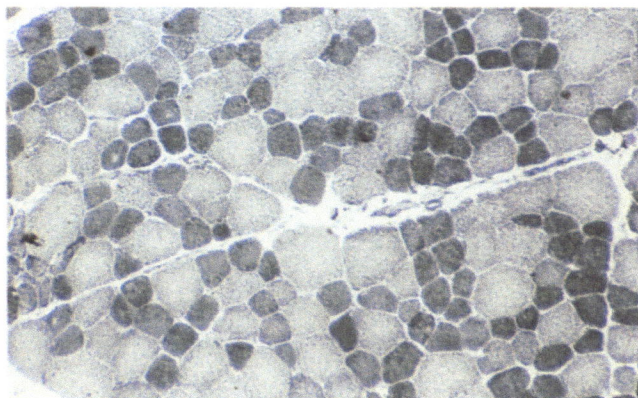

Figure 8.24 Becker dystrophy. There are no obvious fibre architectural abnormalities. The changes in this biopsy are mild in comparison with Duchenne dystrophy. Although the picture bears some resemblance to congenital fibre type disproportion, the presence of regenerating fibres and endomysial fibrosis indicate there is some tissue destruction. This is more in keeping with the slowly progressive Becker dystrophy. NADH-TR × 180

16. Afifi, A. K., Bergman, R. A. and Zellweger, H. (1973). A possible role for electron microscopy in detection of carriers of Duchenne type dystrophy. *J. Neurol. Neurosurg. Psychiatry*, **36**, 643–50

17. Murray, J. M. *et al.* (1982). Linkage relationships of a cloned DNA sequence on the short arm of the X chromosome to Duchenne muscular dystrophy. *Nature (London)*, **300**, 69–71

18. Edwards, R. J., Rodeck, C. H. and Watts, D. C. (1984). The diagnostic value of plasma myoglobin levels in the adult and fetus at risk for Duchenne muscular dystrophy. *J. Neurol. Sci.*, **63**, 173–82

19. Emery, A. E. H. and Burt, D. (1980). Intracellular calcium and pathogenesis and antenatal diagnosis of Duchenne muscular dystrophy. *Br. Med. J.*, **280**, 355–7

20. Cullen, M. J. and Fulthorpe, J. J. (1975). Stages in fibre breakdown in Duchenne muscular dystrophy. An electron microscopic study. *J. Neurol. Sci.*, **24**, 179–200

21. Bodensteiner, J. B. and Engel, A. G. (1978). Intracellular calcium accumulation in Duchenne dystrophy and other myopathies. A study of 567 000 muscle fibres in 114 biopsies. *Neurology*, **28**, 439–46

22. Cullen, M. J. and Mastaglia, F. L. (1980). Morphological changes in dystrophic muscle. *Br. Med. Bull.*, **36**, 145–52

23. Dubowitz, V. and Brooke, M. H. (1973). The muscular dystrophies. In Walton, J. N. (ed.) *Muscle biopsy: A Modern Approach*. pp. 168–81. (Philadelphia: W. B. Saunders)

24. Hudgson, P., Pearce, G. W. and Walton, J. N. (1967). Preclinical muscular dystrophy. Histopathological changes observed on muscle biopsy. *Brain*, **90**, 565–76

25. Schmalbruch, H. (1984). Regenerated muscle fibres in Duchenne muscular dystrophy: A serial section study. *Neurology*, **34**, 60–5

26. Coers, C. and Telerman-Toppett, N. (1977). Morphological changes of motor units in Duchenne's muscular dystrophy. *Arch. Neurol.*, **34**, 396–402

27. Harriman, D. G. F. (1976). A comparison of the fine structure of motor end-plates in Duchenne dystrophy and in human neurogenic diseases. *J. Neurol. Sci.*, **28**, 233–47

28. Emery, A. E. H. and Skinner, R. (1976). Clinical studies in benign (Becker type) X-linked muscular dystrophy. *Clin. Genet.*, **10**, 189–201

29. Ringel, S. P. *et al.* (1977). The spectrum of mild X-linked recessive muscular dystrophy. *Arch. Neurol.*, **34**, 408–16

30. Furukawa, T. and Peter, J. B. (1977). X-linked muscular dystrophy. *Ann. Neurol.*, **2**, 414–16

31. Dubowitz, V. and Brooke, M. H. (1973). Becker's muscular dystrophy. In Walton, J. N. (ed.) *Major Problems in Neurology*. Vol. 2. pp. 182–8. (Philadelphia: W. B. Saunders)

32. ten Houten, R. and De Visser, M. (1984). Histopathological findings in Becker-type muscular dystrophy. *Arch. Neurol.*, **41**, 729–33

33. Goebel, H. H. *et al.* (1979). Becker's X-linked muscular dystrophy: histological, enzyme-histochemical, and ultrastructural studies of two cases, originally reported by Becker. *Acta Neuropathol. (Berl.)*, **46**, 69–77

34. Pearn, J. and Hudgson, P. (1978). Anterior horn cell degeneration and gross calf hypertrophy with adolescent onset. A new spinal muscular atrophy syndrome. *Lancet*, **1**, 1059–61

35. Gardner-Medwin, D. and Johnston, H. M. (1984). Severe muscular dystrophy in girls. *J. Neurol. Sci.*, **64**, 79–87

Congenital Muscular Dystrophy

Congenital muscular dystrophy (CMD) is a controversial condition which encompasses more than one entity. The label is derived from muscle histology which shows changes of dystrophic nature very early in life. One distinctive type appears almost exclusive to the Japanese and seems to be one of the commonest causes of the floppy infant syndrome in Japan[1].

In contrast, a completely separate and comparatively rare form of CMD exists in the West[2]. This disorder frequently presents at birth with hypotonia, often associated with contractures and congenital dislocation of the hips[3]. Milder cases are recognized from the delay in reaching motor milestones. Congenital contractures usually progress and others may develop early in childhood. Limb muscle weakness is most severe proximally and mild facial weakness is common. The respiratory muscles may become involved later in childhood. In early childhood the degree of weakness is extremely variable. Some patients are severely incapacitated. Many do manage to walk, but often need the help of calipers. A slowly progressive course is common and respiratory insufficiency may cause death in late childhood[2]. However, Jones et al. provide a more optimistic outlook[3]. They stress that regular physiotherapy from an early age may delay or prevent contractures and improve mobility. With this treatment many patients in their series of 27 cases actually improved or at least remained static. The serum creatine phosphokinase is usually moderately elevated in early life and may decline later. Affected siblings suggest autosomal recessive inheritance in some cases[2]. The severity of this disorder does not correlate well with either serum enzyme levels or muscle histology and it is impossible to predict the clinical course from these parameters.

The nature of CMD is quite unknown. Loss of muscle fibres early in life supports an intrauterine disturbance in myogenesis, but there is probably more than one cause. A programmed biochemical defect may operate in some cases. A disorder of collagen formation has been queried[4]. In non-progressive cases a single environmental insult could be responsible.

The Japanese type of CMD, originally described by Fukuyama, is an inherited, wasting disease. Clinically and pathologically the muscle disorder is similar to the Western condition[5]. However, in Japanese children a constant association with severe central nervous system abnormalities, particularly micropolygria, cerebral and cerebellar cortical disorganization, indicates an entirely separate disease[6]. Only a handful of apparently similar cases have been described in children of other races[7].

Biopsy

The histology is quite unlike that of congenital myopathies (Figures 9.1–9.6). There is marked variation in fibre size with both large and small fibres. There is usually evidence of necrosis and regeneration particularly at an early age. Even in the very young infant there is an increase in endomysial and perimysial connective tissue and sometimes fatty replacement[8] (Figures 9.1 and 9.2). Scattered foci of chronic inflammatory cells may be found, especially in relation to necrotic muscle fibres (Figure 9.2). The ATP-ase reaction may reveal normal fibre type distribution or sometimes type 1 predominance. There are various non-specific architectural abnormalities, including an increase in central nuclei and a moth-eaten pattern with the oxidative enzyme reaction. Although changes in an early biopsy do not always correlate with clinical status, second biopsies in patients with progressive disease have shown increased severity with marked atrophy and extensive fibrosis[2]. Electron microscopy has not revealed any convincing specific abnormalities. The many tiny fibres have an immature appearance[4]. Abundant collagen fibrils are present in the interstitium and one study described many interstitial myofibroblasts.

Differential Diagnosis

Although the early clinical picture may suggest a congenital myopathy the histology is quite different. The wide variations in fibre size and fibrosis are not found in any of the congenital myopathies. Similarly, spinal muscular atrophy in the very young infant does not show such variability in fibre size, nor the moth-eaten fibres or fibrosis. However, in a slightly older child, chronic spinal muscular atrophy and, in a boy, Duchenne dystrophy may enter the differential diagnosis. Small angular fibres, grouped atrophy and fibre type grouping are all important features that indicate SMA. Obviously, clinical differences that distinguish Duchenne dystrophy will be sought. Pseudohypertrophy is not a feature of CMD and early contractures are not seen in Duchenne dystrophy. The CPK is usually much higher in Duchenne dystrophy. In the biopsy the degree of fibrosis and fatty infiltration seen in a young child with CMD is likely to be greater than in the very young boy with Duchenne dystrophy. However, hyaline fibres are the most important difference. Some necrotic fibres are usual in CMD, but not the numerous large hyaline fibres that are so characteristic of both preclinical and early clinical stages of Duchenne dystrophy.

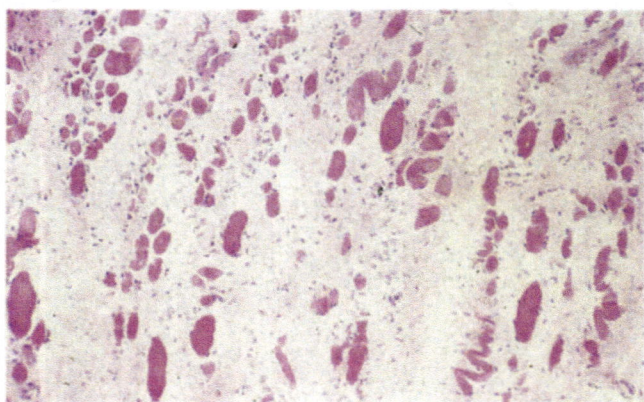

Figure 9.1 Congenital muscular dystrophy. Seven-month-old female infant with retarded motor milestones and generalized hypotonia. The biopsy shows a great paucity of muscle fibres with extensive fibrous replacement. (Same case shown in Figure 9.2.)   H & E × 180

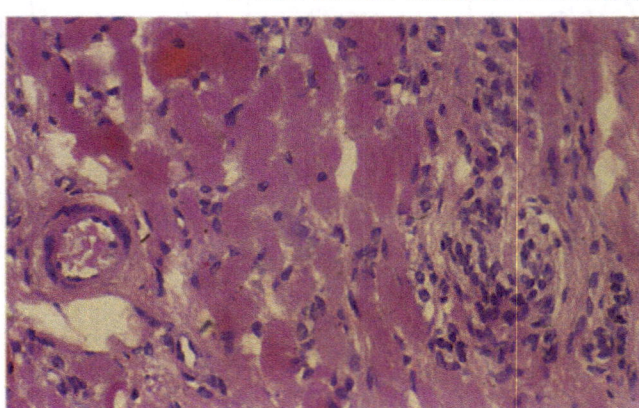

Figure 9.2 Congenital muscular dystrophy. The biopsy shows interstitial, endomysial fibrosis and a focus of chronic inflammatory cells.   H & E × 300

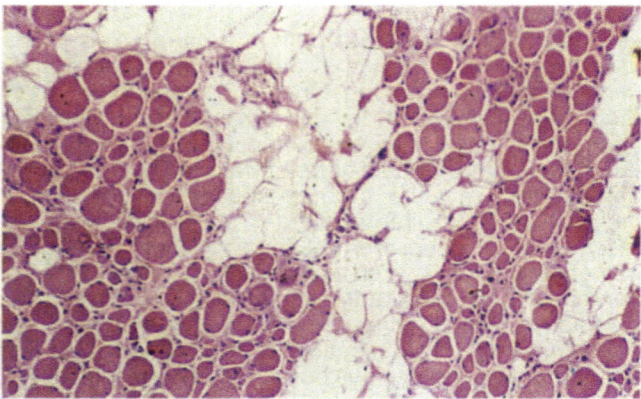

Figure 9.3 Congenital muscular dystrophy. Biopsy from a child of 3½ years. There is variation in fibre size and considerable fibro-fatty replacement of muscle. (Same case shown in Figures 9.4–9.6.)   H & E × 180

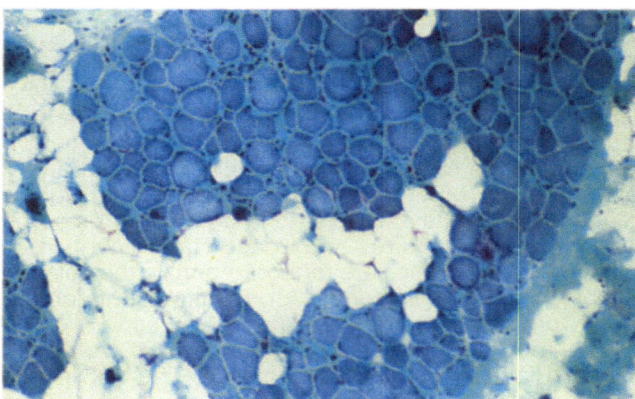

Figure 9.4 Congenital muscular dystrophy. The biopsy shows endomysial fibrosis and fatty replacement of muscle, but it does not show the numerous hyaline fibres that occur in Duchenne dystrophy in the young child.   Gomori's trichrome × 180

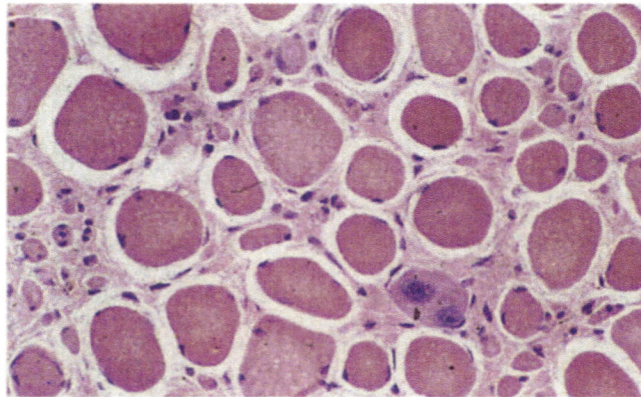

Figure 9.5 Congenital muscular dystrophy. There is variation in fibre size, with an occasional regenerating fibre and a great excess of endomysial collagenous connective tissue.   H & E × 300

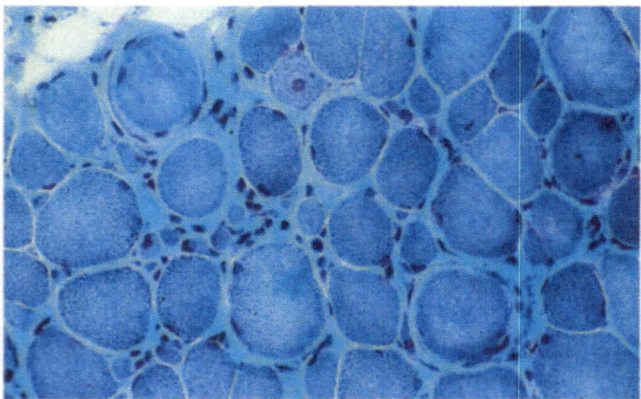

Figure 9.6 Congenital muscular dystrophy. The trichrome stain highlights the conspicuous endomysial fibrosis. The degree of fibrosis and fibro-fatty replacement in this 3-year-old child is considerably greater than in Duchenne dystrophy at this age.   Gomori's trichrome × 300

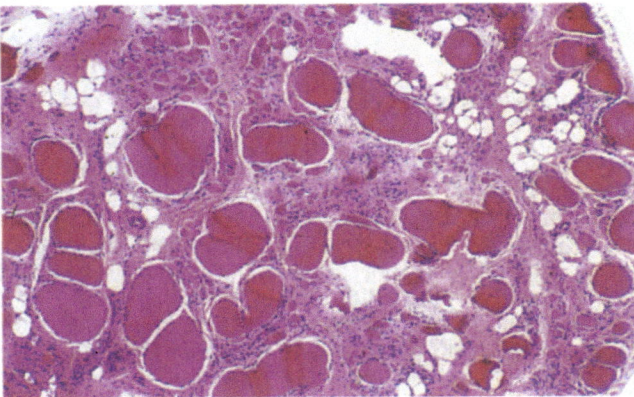

Figure 9.7 Childhood facioscapulohumeral dystrophy. six-year-old boy with the typical clinical picture of facial weakness and winging of the scapulae. The biopsy shows marked variation in fibre size, with both grossly hypertrophied fibres and severely atrophic fibres. There is also considerable interstitial fibrosis. The picture is readily acceptable as a muscular dystrophy, but this interpretation can be challenged. Chronic denervation could produce the same changes, with the hypertrophied fibres representing surviving motor units. In cases such as this, invariably, there is no absolute proof for either aetiology. (Same case shown in Figures 9.8–9.10.)   H & E × 180

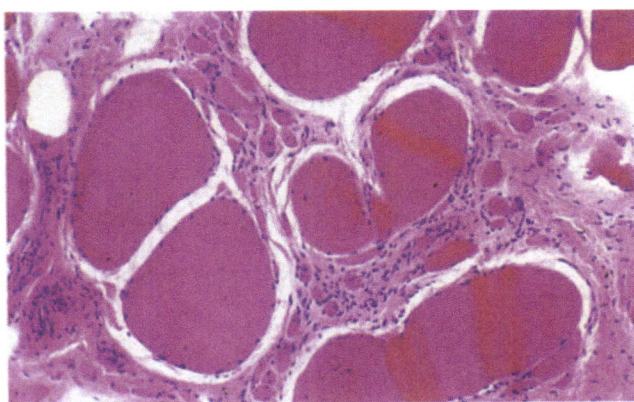

Figure 9.8 Childhood facioscapulohumeral dystrophy. Grossly hypertrophied fibres contrast with intervening groups of very tiny fibres. There is also marked endomysial fibrosis.   H & E × 300

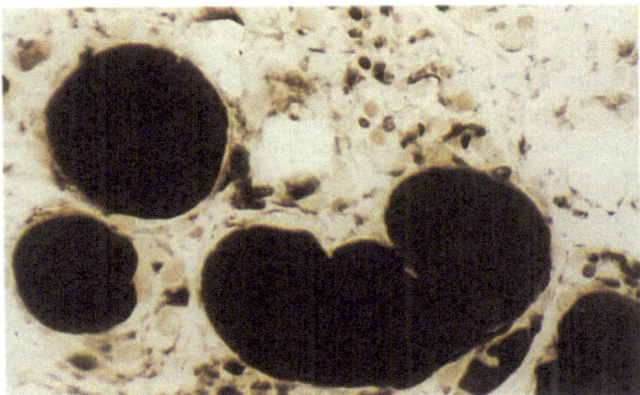

Figure 9.9 Childhood facioscapulohumeral dystrophy. The hypertrophied fibres throughout this biopsy are uniformly type 1 fibres, with the myosin ATP-ase reaction. Atrophic fibres are both type 1 and type 2.   ATP-ase pH 4.3 × 300

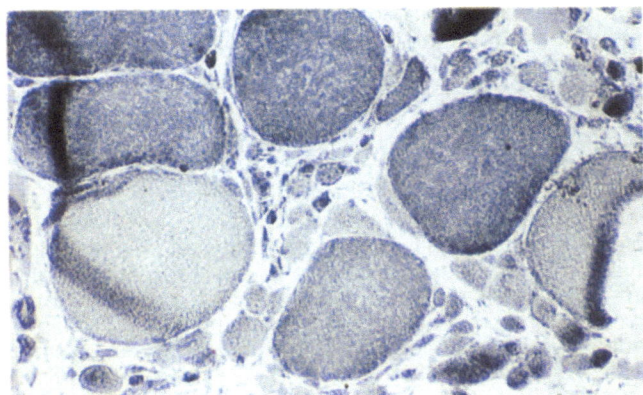

Figure 9.10 Childhood facioscapulohumeral dystrophy. Although the large fibres are uniformly type 1 with myosin ATP-ase, some show only a weak oxidative enzyme reaction. This mixed histochemical pattern is known to occur with re-innervation. Thus chronic spinal muscular atrophy should be considered as a differential diagnosis.   NADH-TR × 300

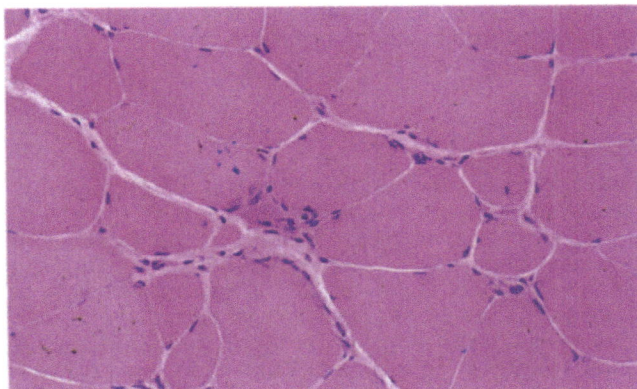

Figure 9.11 Facioscapulohumeral dystrophy. Deltoid biopsy from a 20-year-old man whose clinical picture is quite characteristic of that generally accepted as facioscapulohumeral dystrophy. He has always been round shouldered and finds difficulty in lifting things above his shoulders. He has slight facial weakness, wasting of shoulder girdle muscles with winging of the scapulae. Reflexes are absent in his arms. His legs are normal. CPK is normal. EMG shows myopathic changes. His father has a longstanding diagnosis of muscular dystrophy, with weakness involving shoulder and pelvic girdle, but is still able to walk. A younger brother also has the same round shouldered appearance. The biopsy shows scattered atrophic fibres, with a suggestion of a slight increase in endomysial fibrous connective tissue. (Same case shown in Figures 9.12–9.14.)   H & E × 180

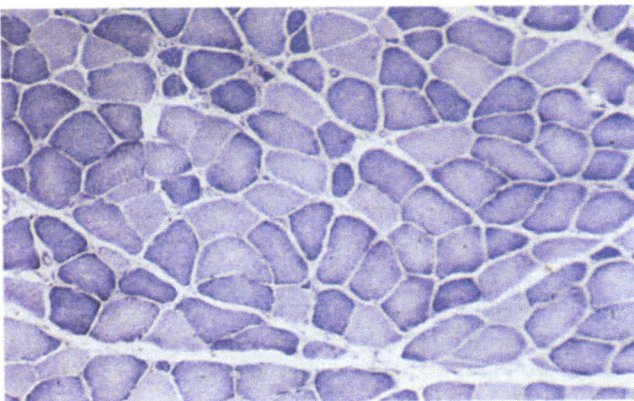

Figure 9.12 Facioscapulohumeral dystrophy. There are scattered small rounded fibres, but not the grouped atrophy or darkly stained angular fibres characteristic of denervation and no coarsely granular fibres to suggest abnormal mitochondria.   NADH-TR × 75

Facioscapulohumeral (FSH) Dystrophy

Facioscapulohumeral dystrophy has been well known as a dominantly inherited disorder for many years. However, identification of this disorder is not as straight-forward as some early studies suggested. Some patients with a facioscapulohumeral distribution of weakness have been shown by muscle biopsy to have different conditions, e.g. polymyositis or mitochondrial myopathy[9]. In addition, a neurogenic form exists, probably related to the spinal muscular atrophies. Clinical overlap exists between FSH and scapulo-peroneal syndromes. The latter seems to encompass both neurogenic and myopathic disorders. Because of this clearly 'mixed bag' it is very difficult to establish indisputable criteria of FSH dystrophy. The sceptic wonders if it really exists. Many reports have failed to exclude neurogenic disease. Suffice it to say that a facioscapulohumeral distribution of weakness cannot be accepted at 'face' value as dystrophy; only further careful clinicopathological correlation, EMG studies and, where possible, examination of terminal inner-vation will distinguish clinically similar disorders, with different prognostic and genetic implications.

The disorder, currently regarded as genuine FSH dystrophy, is uncommon and shows wide variation in clinical expression, even within the same family[10]. Shoulder girdle and facial weakness are usually detected in the 2nd and 3rd decade, although a few patients present in childhood[11] (Figures 9.7–9.10), and in others the condition is not recognized until late middle age. Generally weakness is only slowly progres-sive. The neck flexors, biceps and triceps are usually affected, but deltoids may be preserved, a point to note, because this muscle is often chosen for upper limb muscle biopsy. Obvious asymmetrical weakness should arouse suspicion of neurogenic disease. The CPK is usually mildly but not greatly elevated and sometimes it is normal.

Biopsy

The histopathological picture is not as clearly defined as that of Duchenne dystrophy. A few necrotic or regener-ating fibres may be found, but they are rarely numerous and often completely absent. In fact, the biopsy may show only minimal abnormalities (Figures 9.11–9.18). Variation in fibre size is generally mild. Isolated, very tiny, angular fibres are sometimes seen, but not grouped atrophy. The ATP-ase reaction shows clear fibre type differentiation and usually normal distribution. The NADH-TR reaction sometimes reveals a spotty or lobulate pattern in small type 1 fibres, shown by electron microscopy to be due to accumulations of mitochondria and sarcoplasmic reticulum[12]. There are no particularly characteristic fine structural abnorm-alities. Interstitial inflammatory cell infiltrates may be present between fibres or between fascicles. These may be quite large, mimicking polymyositis. Munsat described two patients with a facioscapulohumeral syndrome and a clear pattern of dominant inheritance, but the histology was indistinguishable from polymyo-sitis[13]. In this disorder and others unrelated to poly-myositis, chronic inflammatory cells may be a response to muscle cell death rather than a cause. Eventual progression to fibro-fatty replacement has been described and a rare association with Coat's syndrome (exudative telangiectasia of the retina)[14].

Differential Diagnosis

Polymyositis, chronic SMA and mitochondrial myopathy have all been reported as causes of facio-scapulohumeral syndrome. Biopsy should readily eliminate mitochondrial myopathy by demonstration of ragged red fibres. Small group atrophy suggests chronic spinal muscular atrophy and should stimulate an EMG search for denervation. A facioscapulohumeral syndrome is an unusual manifestation of polymyositis but it is obviously important to recognize this treatable disorder. Inflammation, necrosis and regeneration suggest polymyositis. Even though FSH dystrophy can be identical this picture probably justifies a proper trial of steroids. Two patients described by Munsat, who appear to have had genuine inherited myopathies, actually showed some improvement on steroids, but this experience is not universal. Failure to maintain improvement with adequate dosage will challenge the original diagnosis and a second biopsy may be indicated. Definite progression and fibro-fatty replace-ment will favour the dystrophy.

Oculopharyngeal Dystrophy

This appears to be a separate, clearly defined, disorder of late onset, showing autosomal dominant inheritance with complete penetrance. The clinical picture is usually very similar in each generation. Ptosis, ophthalmoplegia and dysphagia are the major clinical problems which appear in the 4th and 5th decade and progress slowly[15]. Proximal limb muscles are also involved and suitable for biopsy, but the weakness is relatively mild. Extreme weakness of palatal and pharyngeal muscles may cause severe dysphagia, resulting in malnutrition and sometimes death from aspiration pneumonia. The disease is largely confined to Europeans, the majority, but not all, being of French-Canadian descent[16]. The EMG is usually myopathic and the CPK is often normal. Increased serum immunoglobulins are frequently found, although the significance is unknown[17]. On the basis of EMG and histology, oculopharyngeal dystrophy has been generally accepted as a purely myopathic disorder. However, recently even in this disorder the concept has been challenged. In an autopsy report Probst et al. describe a diminution of large fibres and thinning of myelin sheaths in the cranial nerves suggesting chronic axonal atrophy[17].

Biopsy

The most severe changes are found in the extraocular, pharyngeal and diaphragmatic muscles[15]. However, the lesser abnormalities present in proximal limb muscles generally provide sufficient diagnostic evidence (Figures 9.19–9.24). These muscles show marked variation in size and increased central nuclei. Small angular fibres may be found between hyper-trophic fibres (Figure 9.22), but there is no well-developed grouped atrophy (Figures 9.23 and 9.24). The fibre type distribution is usually normal. The NADH-TR reaction may show moth-eaten fibres, occasional whorled or target fibres. Cytoplasmic vacuoles, variously referred to as 'rimmed' or 'lined' vacuoles are a particularly characteristic, although not specific feature (Figures 9.19–9.21). These vacuoles are only found in a small percentage of fibres, usually atrophic type 1 fibres[15]. They have a rounded, somewhat irregular outline and measure up to 20 μm diameter. Usually only one vacuole, occasionally two, is seen in each fibre in transverse section. H & E shows a basophilic rim and in the centre there is granular, basophilic debris, which is sometimes dislodged on sectioning (Figure 9.20). These structures are demonstrated well by Gomori's trichrome, as the rim is stained red and the granular contents are purplish-red. Although the vacuoles are probably associated with cell degeneration, completely necrotic or regenerating fibres are unusual. Increased endomysial fibrous connective tissue accompanies atrophy and at postmortem the extraocular pharyngeal and diaphragmatic muscles show very extensive fibro-fatty replacement.

Electron Microscopy

The cytoplasmic vacuoles are generally considered to be autophagic and formed from the end products of lysosomes. The granular debris is composed of membranous whorls, dense bodies, glycogen granules and sometimes filamentous material. This aggregate is not always membrane bound[18]. There are several reports of filamentous inclusions in the sarcolemmal nuclei[19].

Differential Diagnosis

The vacuoles are a helpful feature, but not essential to diagnosis. Myopathic changes in the appropriate clinical context are sufficient. Vacuoles are not specific and are occasionally seen in very different disorders including chronic spinal muscular atrophy, polymyositis and myotonic dystrophy[18]. They are particularly common in inclusion body myositis[20], which also shows intranuclear filaments.

The clinical picture on its own may have considerable overlap with disorders in the so-called 'ophthalmoplegia plus' group. Besides ophthalmoplegia and ptosis, many of these patients show an excessive tendency to fatigue and the age of onset is often earlier[21,22]. The distinguishing biopsy feature is numerous abnormal mitochondria, suggesting an underlying metabolic defect. Thus, despite clinical similarity, the pathogenesis is probably quite different from oculopharyngeal dystrophy.

Distal Myopathy

This is a slowly progressive disorder, characterized by late onset distal muscle weakness, in which there is no firm evidence of denervation and investigations generally suggest a myopathy. It is a well-recognized, dominantly inherited disorder in Sweden[23], but only a few familial and sporadic cases have been identified in other countries. Onset is between the 3rd and 5th decades. Clinically the slowly progressive distal wasting may suggest distal SMA or peroneal muscular atrophy, but the EMG is myopathic and nerve conduction studies are normal[24]. Histology reveals a wide variety of nonspecific myopathic changes: increased variability in fibre size, increased central nuclei, fibre necrosis and phagocytosis. However, the most distinctive abnormalities, which suggest the diagnosis in the appropriate setting, are prominent rimmed vacuoles. These may be very numerous, present in up to 10% of fibres, including both type 1 and type 2 fibres. The edge of

these irregular vacuoles is deeply basophilic with H & E and stains red with Gomori's trichrome. Acid phosphatase activity may be demonstrable in the vacuoles[11]. EMG shows membrane bound vacuoles containing lamellar structures and other cell debris[24,25]. The vacuoles are essentially similar to those found in oculopharyngeal dystrophy and inclusion body myositis and are presumed to be lysosomal in origin[18]. Inclusion body myositis would seem to be a very similar sporadic disorder.

References

1. McMenamin, J. B., Becker, L. E. and Murphy, E. G. (1982). Fukuyama-type congenital muscular dystrophy. *J. Pediatr.*, **101**, 580–2

2. McMenamin, J. B., Becker, L. E. and Murphy, E. G. (1982). Congenital muscular dystrophy: clinicopathologic report of 24 cases. *J. Pediatr.*, **100**, 692–7

3. Jones, R. *et al.* (1979). Congenital muscular dystrophy. The importance of early diagnosis and orthopaedic management in the long term prognosis. *J. Bone Jt. Surg.*, **61B**, 13–17

4. Fidzianska, A. *et al.* (1982). Congenital muscular dystrophy (CMD) – a collagen formative disease. *J. Neurol. Sci.*, **55**, 79–90

5. Nonaka, I., Sugita, H., Takada, K. and Kumagai, K. (1982). Muscle histochemistry in congenital muscular dystrophy with central nervous system involvement. *Muscle Nerve*, **5**, 102–6

6. Kamoshita, S., Konishi, Y., Segawa, M. and Fukuyama, Y. (1976). Congenital muscular dystrophy as a disease of the central nervous system. *Arch. Neurol.*, **33**, 513–16

7. Krijgsman, J. B. *et al.* (1980). Congenital muscular dystrophy and cerebral dysgenesis in a Dutch family. *Neuropaediatrie*, **11**, 108–20

8. Dubowitz, V. (1978). *Muscle Disorders in Childhood*. pp. 59–64. (London: W. B. Saunders)

9. Bradley, W. G., Tomlinson, B. E. and Hardy, M. (1978). Further studies of mitochondrial and lipid storage myopathies. *J. Neurol. Sci.*, **35**, 201–10

10. Brooke, M. H. (1977). Facioscapulohumeral dystrophy. In *A Clinician's View of Neuromuscular Diseases*. pp. 109–15. (Baltimore: Williams and Wilkins)

11. Dubowitz, V. (1978). Facioscapulohumeral muscular dystrophy. In Schaffer, A. J. and Markowitz, M. (eds.) *Muscle Disorders in Childhood. Major Problems in Clinical Paediatrics Series*. pp. 54–8. (London: W. B. Saunders)

12. Harriman, D. G. F. (1976). Facioscapulohumeral muscular dystrophy. In Blackwood, W. and Corsellis, J. A. N. (eds.) *Greenfield's Neuropathy*, 3rd Edn., pp. 875–6. (London: Edward Arnold)

13. Munsat, T. L., Piper, D., Cancilla, P. and Mednick, J. (1972). Inflammatory myopathy with facioscapulohumeral distribution. *Neurology*, **22**, 335–47

14. Wuff, J. D., Lin, J. T. and Kepes, J. J. (1982). Inflammatory facioscapulohumeral muscular dystrophy and Coat's syndrome. *Ann. Neurol.*, **12**, 398–401

15. Little, B. W. and Perl, D. P. (1982). Oculopharyngeal muscular dystrophy, an autopsied case from the French-Canadian kindred. *J. Neurol. Sci.*, **53**, 145–58

16. Gardner-Medwin, D. (1980). Clinical features and classification of the muscular dystrophies. *Br. Med. Bull.*, **36**, 109–15

17. Probst, A. *et al.* (1982). Evidence for a chronic axonal atrophy in oculopharyngeal 'muscular dystrophy'. *Acta Neuropathol. (Berl.)*, **57**, 209–16

18. Fukuhara, N. *et al.* (1980). Rimmed vacuoles. *Acta Neuropathol. (Berl.)*, **51**, 229–35

19. Coquet, M. *et al.* (1983). Nuclear inclusions in oculopharyngeal dystrophy. *J. Neurol. Sci.*, **60**, 151–6

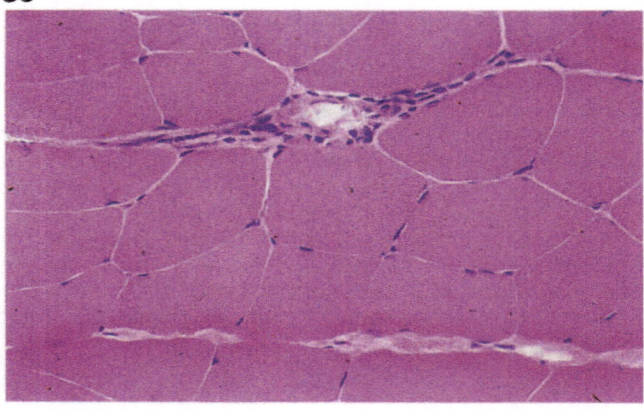

Figure 9.13 Facioscapulohumeral dystrophy. A tiny focus of chronic inflammatory cells around a small blood vessel. H & E × 300

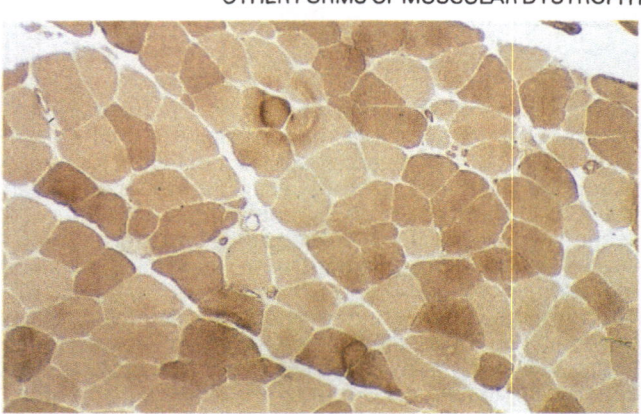

Figure 9.14 Facioscapulohumeral dystrophy. There is essentially normal fibre type distribution and the small rounded fibres include both type 1 and type 2 fibres. It is the association of relatively minor histological abnormalities with the appropriate muscle involvement that support diagnosis of facioscapulohumeral dystrophy. ATP-ase pH 9.4 × 180

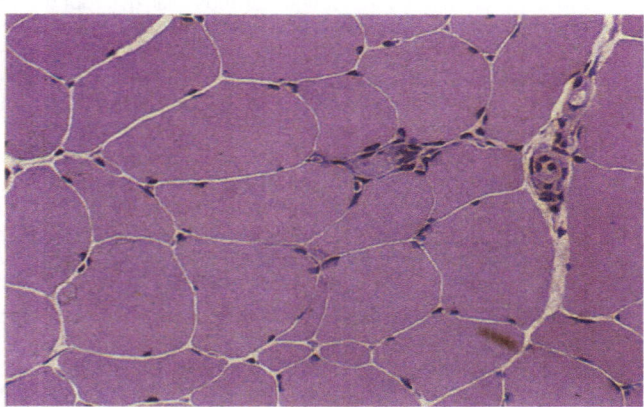

Figure 9.15 Facioscapulohumeral dystrophy. Quadriceps biopsy from a 36-year-old woman with no family history who first became aware of shoulder weakness when playing tennis in her 'teens. In the last few years she had become less mobile and finds difficulty in rising from a low chair. She has facial weakness and gross but asymmetrical wasting of shoulder muscles with normal distal arm muscles. She also has mild weakness of the pelvic girdle and distal leg muscles. CPK is slightly elevated. EMG shows myopathic changes. The biopsy shows scattered atrophic fibres. (Same case shown in Figures 9.16–9.18.) H & E × 300

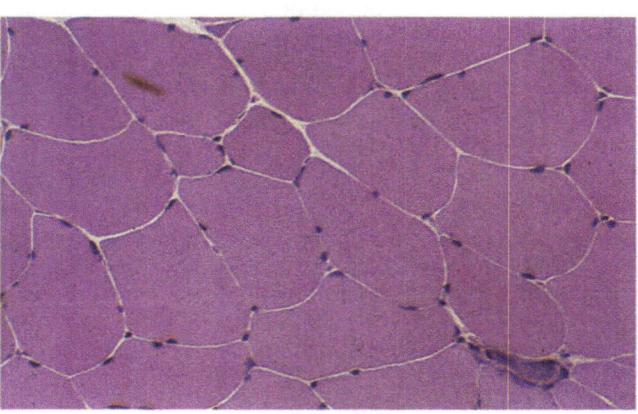

Figure 9.16 Facioscapulohumeral dystrophy. A few small rounded fibres and an isolated, basophilic, regenerating fibre. H & E × 300

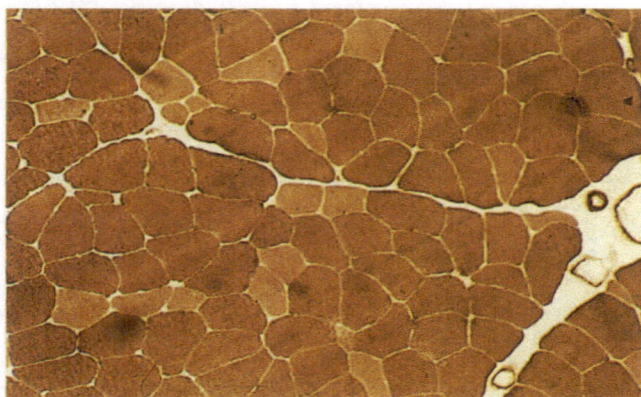

Figure 9.17 Facioscapulohumeral dystrophy. There is essentially normal fibre type distribution, but atrophic fibres are chiefly type 1. ATP-ase pH 9.4 × 180

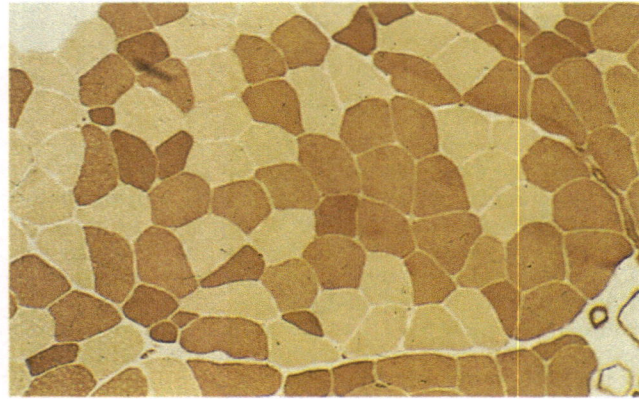

Figure 9.18 Facioscapulohumeral dystrophy. The scattered, small fibres are mostly type 1 fibres. There is no grouped atrophy. These minor abnormalities and the clinical pattern support the conventional diagnosis of facioscapulohumeral dystrophy and dominant inheritance must be anticipated. Nevertheless, this patient does have asymmetry and in the present state of knowledge it is impossible to exclude the possibility that the disorder is really a neural defect. ATP-ase pH 4.5 × 180

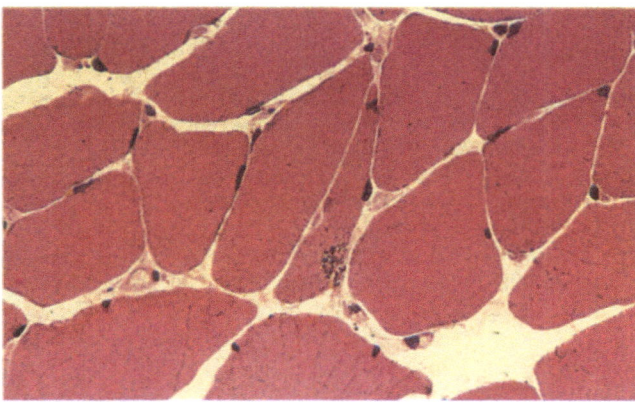

Figure 9.19 Oculopharyngeal dystrophy? Deltoid biopsy from a 67-year-old woman, with no family history, who developed ptosis 4 years previously. A tensilon test was negative. She had no convincing limb weakness, but the biopsy is abnormal. At the time she had no symptoms of dysphagia, but as histology is typical of that described in ocular pharyngeal dystrophy, this is the tentative diagnosis. There are occasional small angular fibres which contain lysosomal vacuoles. (Same case shown in Figures 9.20–9.24.)   H & E × 300

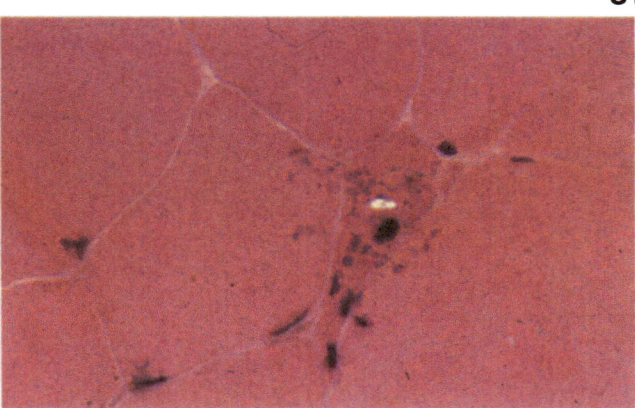

Figure 9.20 Oculopharnygeal dystrophy? A small angular fibre containing a vacuole filled with basophilic debris, which has been partly dislodged by sectioning.   H & E × 450

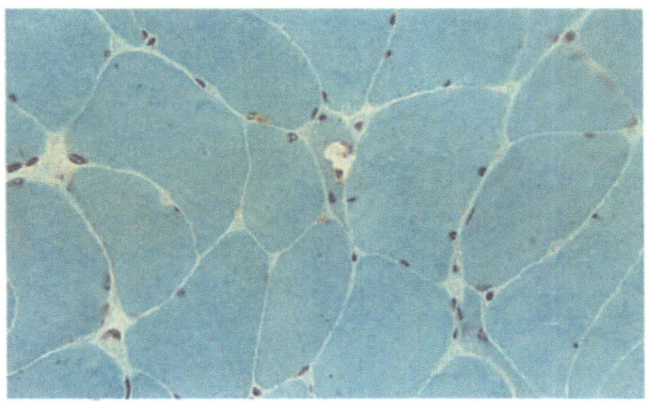

Figure 9.21 Vacuolated, atrophic fibre. The trichrome frequently reveals a red stain rim or reddish contents, but not when the debris is dislodged by sectioning. There were no ragged red fibres to suggest a mitochondrial disorder and no abnormal mitochondria or unusually large collections of mitochondria were found by electron microscopy.   Gomori's trichrome × 300

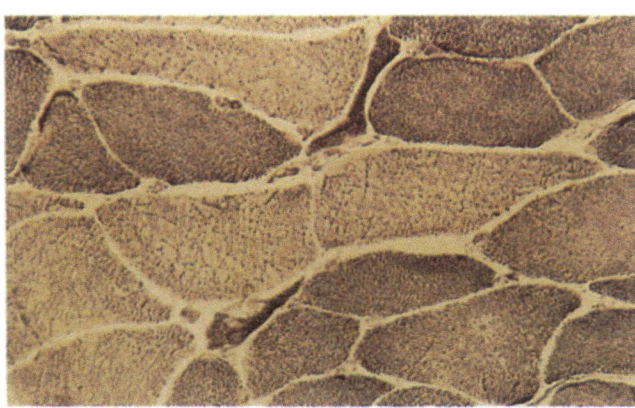

Figure 9.22 Small angular fibres. A few small angular fibres appear compressed between the normal sized fibres. There was no grouped atrophy.   NADH-TR × 300

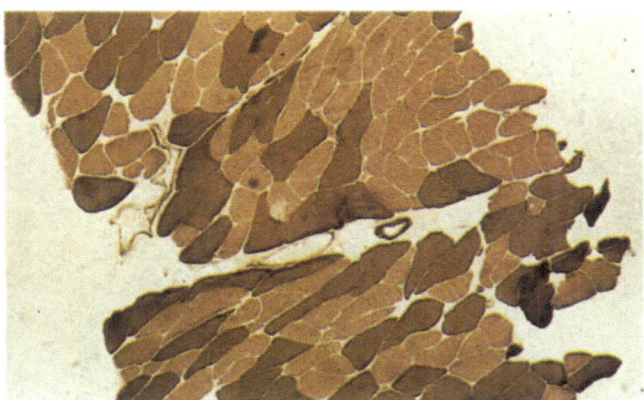

Figure 9.23 Oculopharyngeal dystrophy? The fibre distribution is not entirely normal. There is a suggestion of type grouping of type 1 fibres.   ATP-ase pH 9.4 × 75

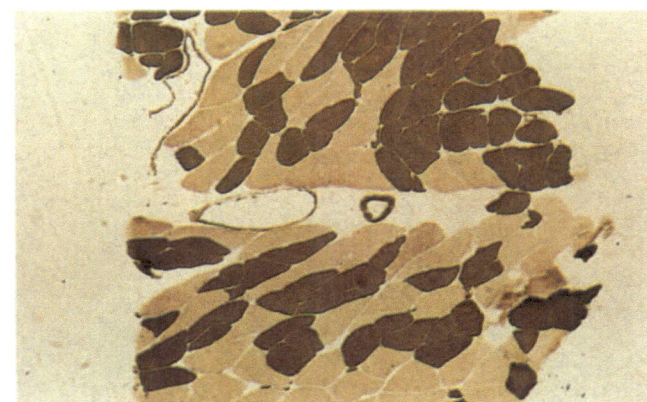

Figure 9.24 Oculopharyngeal dystrophy? Serial section to Figure 9.23 shows a group of type 1 fibres. There is a paucity of 2B fibres.   ATP-ase pH 4.5 × 75

20. Mikol, J. *et al*. (1982). Inclusion-body myositis: clinicopathological studies and isolation of an adenovirus type 2 from muscle biopsy specimen. *Ann. Neurol.*, **11**, 576–81

21. Morgan-Hughes, J. A. and Mair, W. G. P. (1973). Atypical muscle mitochondria in oculoskeletal myopathy. *Brain*, **96**, 215–24

22. Julien, J. *et al*. (1974). Oculopharyngeal muscular dystrophy. A case with abnormal mitochondria and 'fingerprint' inclusions. *J. Neurol. Sci.*, **21**, 165–9

23. Edstrom, L. (1975). Histochemical and histopathological changes in skeletal muscle in late onset hereditary distal myopathy (Welander). *J. Neurol. Sci.*, **26**, 147–57

24. Markesbery, W. R. *et al*. (1977). Distal myopathy: electron microscopic and histochemical studies. *Neurology*, **27**, 727–35

25. Kumamoto, T. *et al*. (1982). Distal myopathy. Histochemical and ultrastructural studies. *Arch. Neurol.*, **39**, 367–71

Introduction

These syndromes are discussed with the dystrophies for historical reasons. Many patients, still living, bear the label of limb girdle dystrophy, although recent studies suggest this diagnosis and likewise that of many cases of scapuloperoneal dystrophy is frequently erroneous[1]. Nevertheless, rare dystrophies with these clinical patterns may exist[2].

General Account

The onset of these syndromes is often in the second decade, but can be earlier or much later. Distinct entities are not easy to pinpoint, even when biopsy and EMG investigations are available. For many years progressive weakness of proximal limb muscles, with apparently myopathic histology and usually autosomal recessive inheritance has been labelled as limb girdle dystrophy. However, it has become very clear that this is a heterogeneous group, including some cases of Becker dystrophy, some female carriers of Duchenne dystrophy and a large majority who do not have a dystrophy at all, but chronic spinal muscular atrophy, with florid, secondary myopathic changes masking the evidence of denervation[1]. A genuine autosomal recessive limb girdle (scapulohumeral) dystrophy may exist, but it is very rare and the upper limbs are affected many years before the pelvic girdle muscles[2].

The scapuloperoneal syndrome describes disorders in which weakness initially appears in the proximal arm muscles and distal leg muscles, sparing the pelvic girdle until later. Clinical overlap with the limb girdle syndrome does occur[3]. Family studies have shown that autosomal dominant[3,4] and recessive[5] and sex-linked recessive disorders[6] all exist and some cases are sporadic. Association with cardiomyopathy is described with both neurogenic and presumed myopathic forms[5,6] and sudden death at a young age has been attributed to cardiac arrhythmia. EMG findings are often inconclusive, showing features of both denervation and myopathy[3,5]. Not infrequently there is apparent discrepancy between the EMG and histology, the one suggesting denervation, the other myopathy. These problems arise because, as with the limb girdle syndrome, myopathic changes are superimposed upon chronic denervation atrophy. The surviving fibres are effectively overloaded and the stresses of attempted muscular activity themselves cause damage, which mimics a primary degenerative disorder. In many families detailed investigations have now established a denervating condition. These are probably further examples of chronic spinal muscular atrophy. However, there are still some families where there is no hint of denervation, although the final proof of autopsy examination is lacking[4,6]. These may be examples of genuine dystrophy, but it must be stressed that compared to Duchenne dystrophy they are exceptionally rare.

Whilst the physician and pathologist must seek to understand these disorders fully, what really matters to the patient is prognosis and pattern of inheritance. Muscle biopsy serves to eliminate the completely different diseases, such as metabolic myopathies and polymyositis, or to confirm one of these chronic neurogenic/myopathic syndromes. Even though histology may fail to separate the neurogenic and myopathic categories, the uncertainty does not matter, as a slowly progressive course can reasonably be predicted. Members of the same family often follow a similar pattern. Patients with a neurogenic limb girdle syndrome may eventually become wheelchair-bound, but many with scapuloperoneal syndromes remain ambulant[2]. Genetic counselling is harder. The limb girdle type of SMA is usually autosomal recessive, but other types of inheritance occur. The variable inheritance of scapuloperoneal syndromes present greater difficulties. A detailed family history, together with examination of the parents and any available relative provides the best hope of accurate counselling.

Biopsy

Histologically it is the plethora of pathological changes that identifies these disorders, rather than any single pathognomonic feature. H & E generally shows great variability in fibre size and shape, including both very large, rounded fibres and tiny atrophic fibres (Figures 10.1–10.12). Atrophic fibres are sometimes angular and if small group atrophy is present it is a pointer to denervation (Figures 10.4, 10.12 and 10.24). Other small fibres are rounded and may represent fibre splitting or regeneration (Figure 10.21). Central nuclei are often quite numerous, particularly in the hypertrophied fibres and often associated with clefts and all degrees of fibre splitting. The ATP-ase reaction may show atrophy of hypertrophy of all fibres types (Figures 10.8 and 10.23). An almost selective type 1 atrophy can be a very early change (Figures 10.13 and 10.14). A type 1 predominance is not uncommon (Figure 10.2), less often type 2A predominance and both may be due to re-innervation. Type 2B deficiency is sometimes found. The NADH-TR reaction reveals a wide variety of abnormal myofibrillar patterns particularly in the larger fibres (Figures 10.19 and 10.20). Thus whorled fibres, ring fibres, moth-eaten or spotty fibres and sarcoplasmic masses all appear. There may be scattered necrotic or regenerating fibres and occasional hyaline fibres (Figures 10.1, 10.11 and

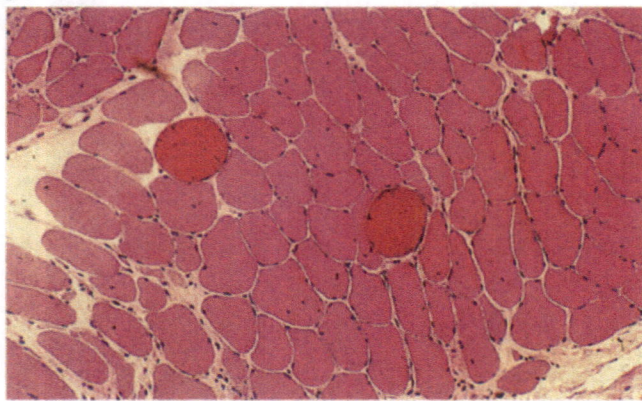

Figure 10.1 Limb girdle syndrome in a 20-year-old woman. Age of onset uncertain, but she showed progressive proximal muscle weakness in her 'teens and became wheelchair-bound by 18 years. No family history of muscle disease. EMG – myopathic. Deltoid biopsy shows variation in fibre size, with a few very tiny fibres. There are also two eosinophilic hyaline fibres. (Same case is shown in Figures 10.2–10.4.) H & E × 75

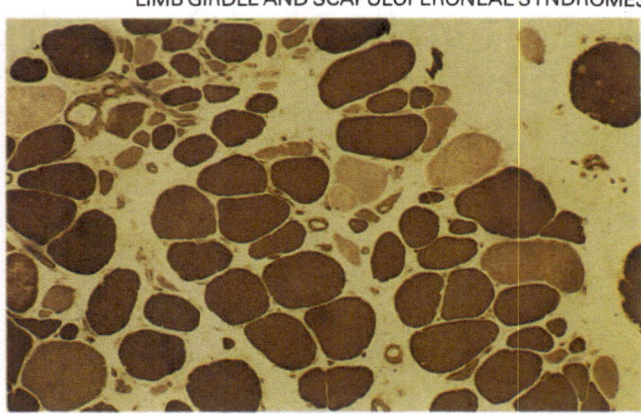

Figure 10.2 Limb girdle syndrome. Variation in fibre size with a type 1 predominance. The atrophic fibres are both type 1 and type 2. ATP-ase pH 4.5 × 75

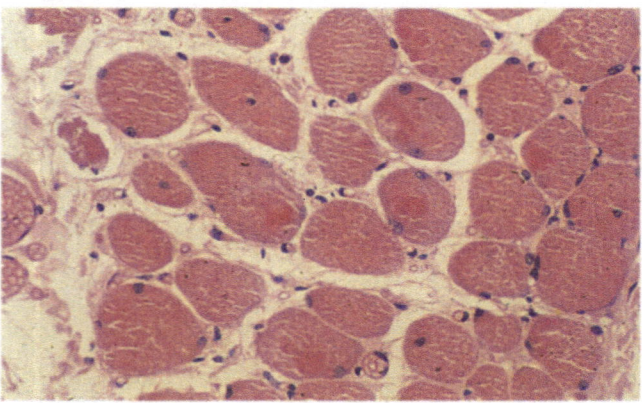

Figure 10.3 Limb girdle syndrome. A group of fibres containing eosinophilic targets, suggestive of denervation. H & E × 180

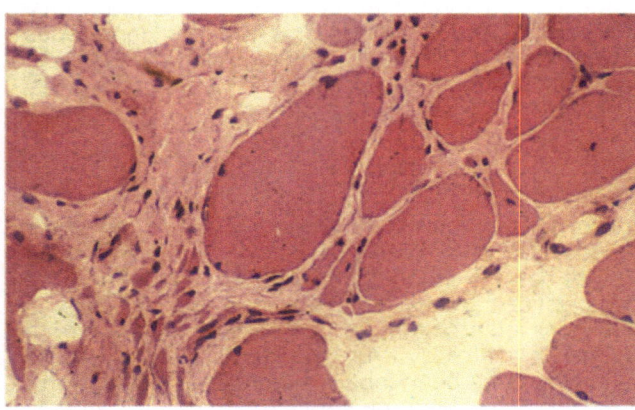

Figure 10.4 Limb girdle syndrome. A group of severely atrophic angular fibres. There is also interstitial fibrosis. The combination of grouped atrophy, targets and type 1 predominance suggest this is a denervating condition, probably chronic spinal muscular atrophy. H & E × 180

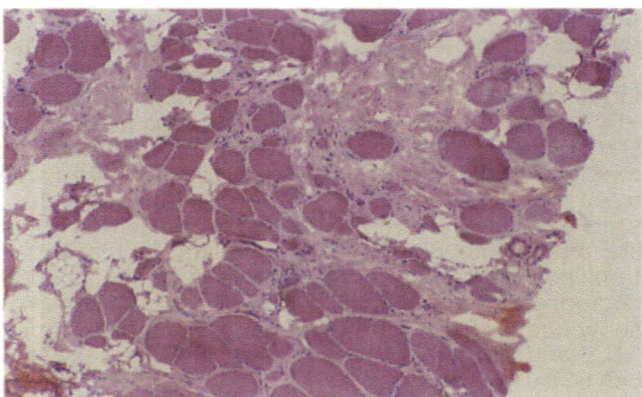

Figure 10.5 Limb girdle syndrome in a 24-year-old man, who had first become aware of weakness in his arms 1 year previously. On examination he showed winging of the scapulae and marked weakness and wasting in biceps and triceps. Weakness of the legs was asymmetrical, but most severe in proximal muscles. There was no calf hypertrophy. He also showed mild facial weakness. CPK was slightly elevated. EMG was myopathic. Deltoid biopsy shows great variation in fibre size and moderate interstitial fibrosis. (Same case is shown in Figures 10.6–10.12. H & E × 30

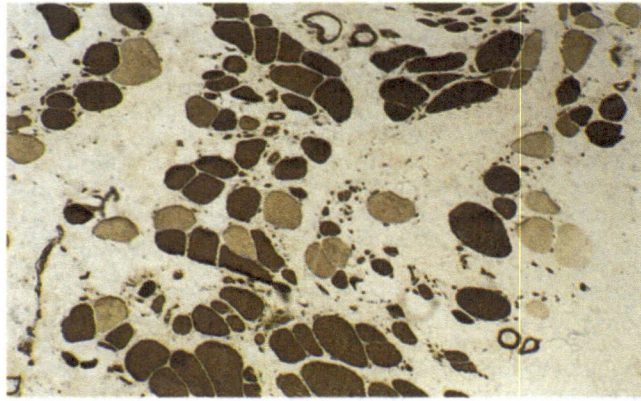

Figure 10.6 Limb girdle syndrome. Serial section to Figure 10.5. A slight type 1 predominance with some hypertrophied type 1 fibres (dark). ATP-ase pH 4.6 × 30

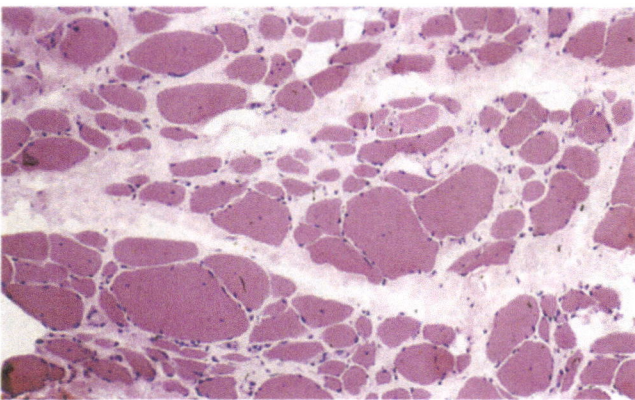

Figure 10.7 Limb girdle syndrome. Variation in fibre size with some greatly hypertrophied fibres. H & E × 75

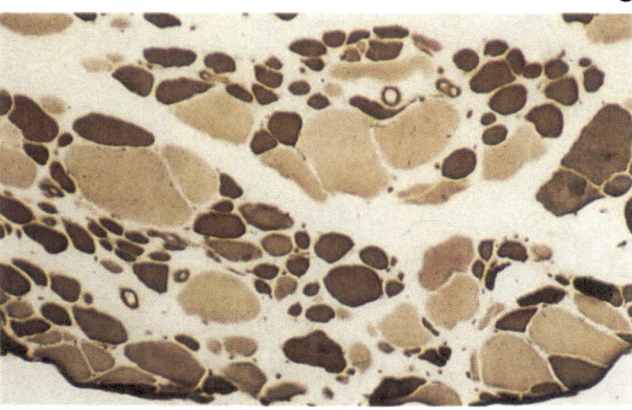

Figure 10.8 Limb girdle syndrome. Serial section to Figure 10.7. In this field the hypertrophied fibres are type 2A. ATP-ase pH 4.6 × 75

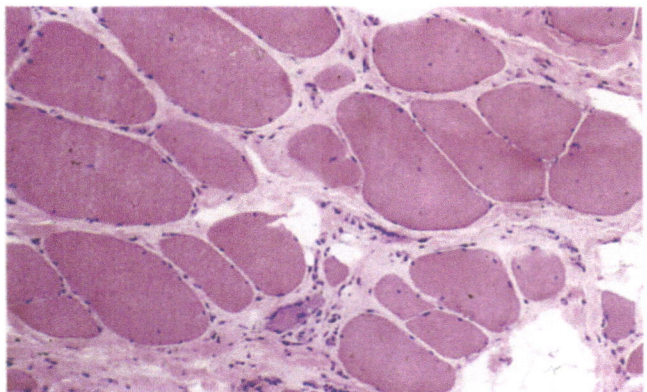

Figure 10.9 Limb girdle syndrome. Greatly hypertrophied fibres with surrounding, endomysial fibrosis. H & E × 180

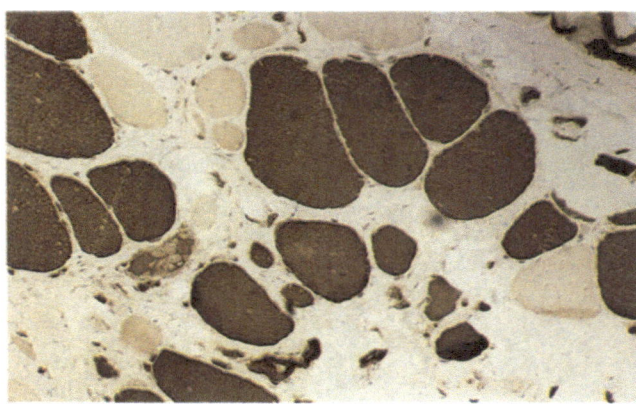

Figure 10.10 Limb girdle syndrome. Serial section to Figure 10.9. Hypertrophied type 1 fibres. Some of the small fibres with a rounded outline are probably derived from fibre splitting. ATP-ase pH 4.6 × 180

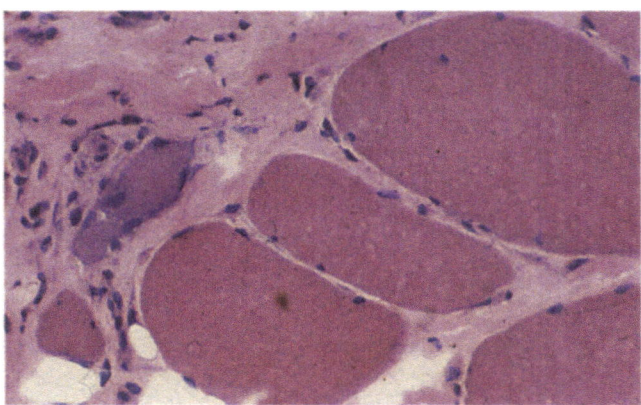

Figure 10.11 Limb girdle syndrome. A small basophilic regenerative fibre amongst the hypertrophied fibres. Necrosis and subsequent regeneration may well result from the functional stresses imposed upon surviving fibres. H & E × 450

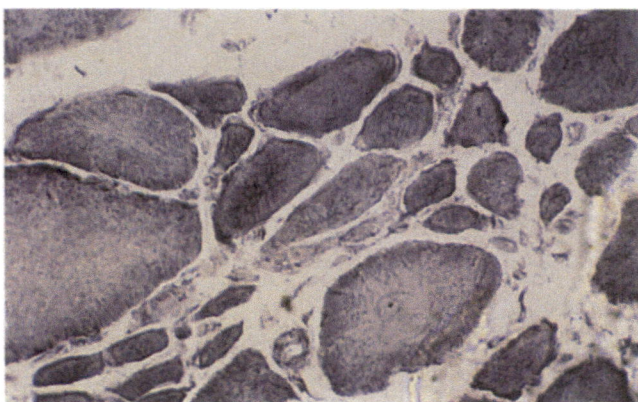

Figure 10.12 Limb girdle syndrome. A ring fibre and others with irregular myofibrillar architecture and a tiny group of angular atrophic fibres. Changes such as these led to the original designation of limb girdle dystrophy, but the clinical asymmetry and histological contrast between groups of grossly hypertrophied fibres and minute atrophic fibres suggest this is a chronic denervating disease. It is probably one of the mild variants of spinal muscular atrophy. NADH-TR × 300

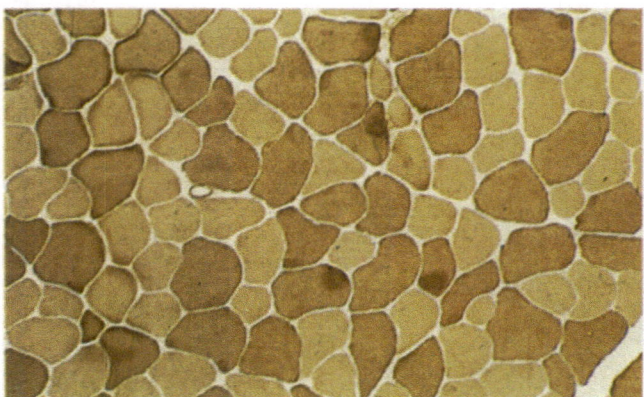

Figure 10.13 Deltoid biopsy from a 47-year-old man with mild proximal weakness, chiefly in a scapulohumeral distribution. EMG revealed convincing changes of denervation. An elder brother, with onset of weakness in his thirties had been diagnosed as facioscapulohumeral dystrophy and became wheelchair-bound in his sixth decade. There was no history of weakness in the parents or other close relatives. This biopsy shows none of the typical changes of denervation atrophy, but an almost selective type 1 atrophy. (Same case shown in Figures 10.14 and 10.15.) ATP-ase pH 9.4 × 180

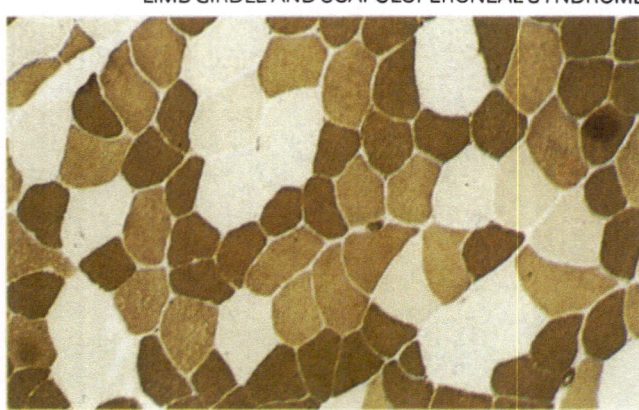

Figure 10.14 Selective type 1 atrophy and mild type 2A hypertrophy. ATP-ase pH 4.5 × 180

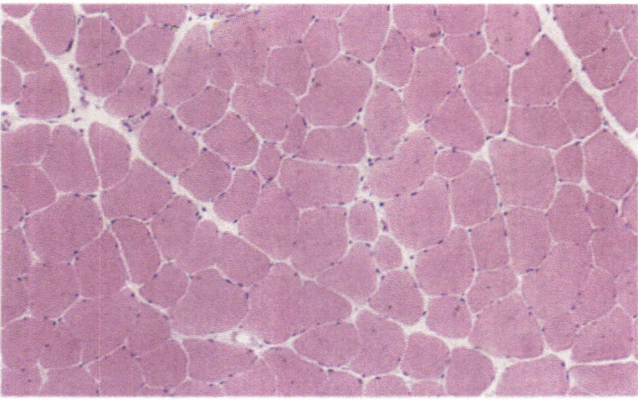

Figure 10.15 In addition to a dual fibre population there are a few central nuclei but no other changes. Despite the uncharacteristic histology the firm EMG evidence of denervation in a late onset slowly progressive disorder suggests this is adult onset spinal muscular atrophy, with autosomal recessive inheritance. H & E × 180

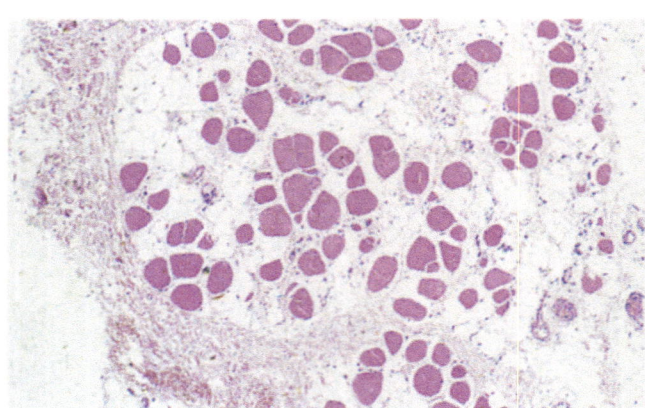

Figure 10.16 Deltoid biopsy of the brother of patient with scapulohumeral weakness, shown in Figures 10.13–10.15. He was diagnosed clinically as facioscapulohumeral dystrophy and is more severely affected than his younger brother. The biopsy shows great loss of muscle fibres with fatty replacement. The residual fibres are most greatly hypertrophied. There are a few tiny fibres which fit closely against the large fibres, suggesting they have been formed by splitting.   H & E × 30

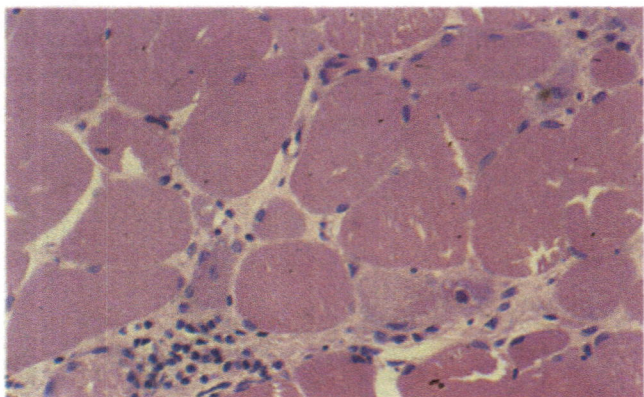

Figure 10.17 Limb girdle syndrome in a man of 27 years, with 3-year history of weakness. Deltoid biopsy shows increased variability in fibre size, but no grouped atrophy. The larger fibres are mildly hypertrophied. Several of the small fibres are basophilic regenerating fibres. On the basis of this biopsy polymyositis was diagnosed. Despite steroid therapy his weakness has progressed slowly and intermittently. His condition was reassessed 15 years later and the revised diagnosis was adult onset spinal muscular atrophy. (Later biopsies of this case shown in Figures 10.18–10.20.)   H & E × 300

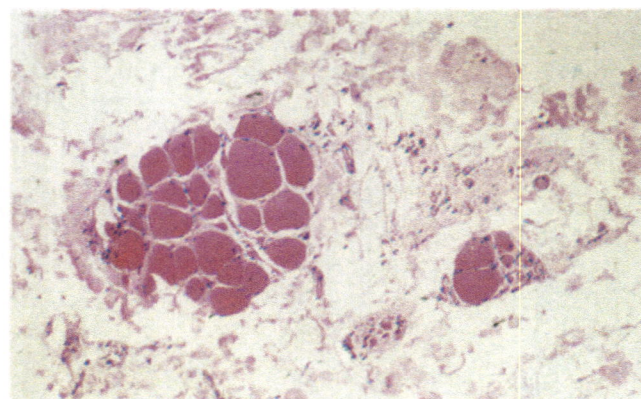

Figure 10.18 Second deltoid biopsy in man with 18-year history of limb girdle weakness whose original biopsy is shown in the previous figure. There is extensive loss of muscle fibres, with fibro-fatty replacement. Two islands of surviving residual fibres show hypertrophy, together with a few tiny fibres. In addition there are a few severely atrophic fibres, just visible within the fibrous connective tissue. (Same case shown in Figures 10.19 and 10.20) H & E × 30

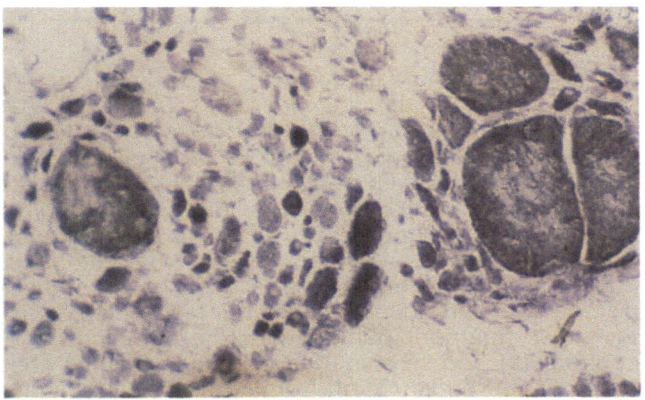

Figure 10.19 The hypertrophied fibres show patchy staining with the oxidative enzyme reaction, indicating an abnormal myofibrillar arrangement, probably a myopathic change in overloaded fibres. NADH-TR × 180

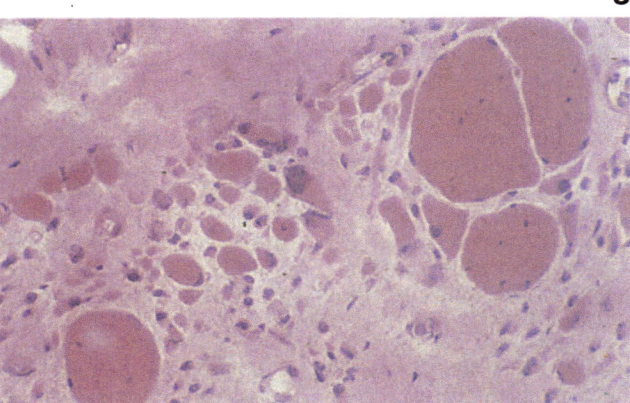

Figure 10.20 A few residual grossly hypertrophied normal fibres surrounded by groups of severely atrophic fibres and increased endomysial connective tissue. There is no evidence of inflammation, necrosis or regeneration. The histology in conjunction with clinical deterioration, despite steroid therapy suggests this is a variant of spinal muscular atrophy, rather than inflammatory myopathy. H & E × 180

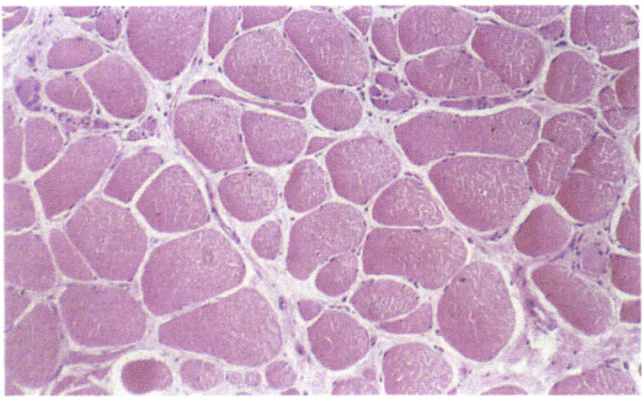

Figure 10.21 Quadriceps biopsy from an 11-year-old boy, originally diagnosed as having limb girdle dystrophy. He was observed to run oddly at age 9 and complained of stiff legs after exercise. He showed proximal muscle weakness and mild asymmetrical calf muscle hypertrophy. CPK only moderately elevated. No family history. 2 years later there has been no progression of his disease. The biopsy shows great variation in fibre size, with many hypertrophied fibres and several rounded atrophic fibres, which may be due to splitting. (Same case shown in Figures 10.22–10.24.) H & E × 180

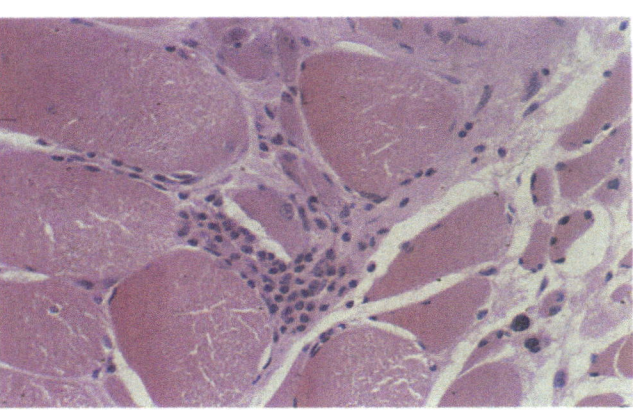

Figure 10.22 Focus of lymphocytes surrounding an atrophic fibre and a group of small angular fibres. In addition this biopsy contained isolated necrotic and regenerating fibres. H & E × 300

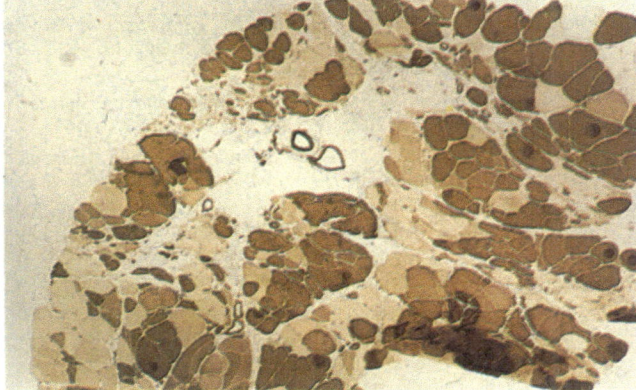

Figure 10.23 The myosin ATP-ase reaction shows that hypertrophic and atrophic fibres are both type 1 and type 2. There is no definite fibre type predominance or type grouping. Myosin ATP-ase pH 4.6 × 30

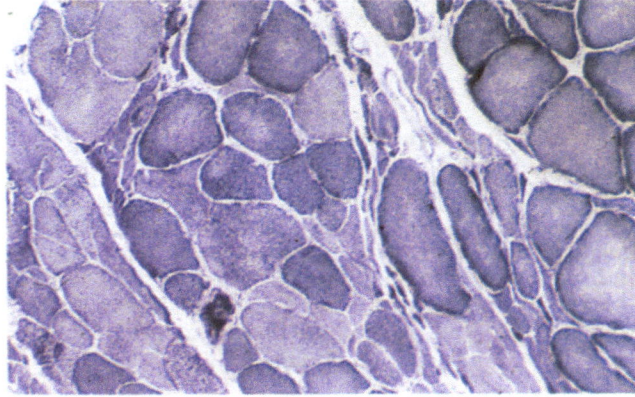

Figure 10.24 In some fascicles in the biopsy of this child with a limb girdle syndrome there is very definite grouped atrophy. This pattern supports a diagnosis of mild chronic spinal muscular atrophy with secondary myopathic changes. NADH-TR × 180

10.17). Inflammatory infiltrates are rarely conspicuous, but small aggregates are quite common[3] (Figure 10.22). The progressive fibre atrophy is accompanied by an increase in fibro-fatty interstitial connective tissue (Figures 10.15, 10.16, and 10.18–10.20).

Electron microscopy also reveals a wide variety of non-specific abnormalities, particularly disorganization of myofibrils. Mitochondrial aggregates may be found, but they have a normal appearance.

Motor end point biopsy: This investigation may provide the only firm morphological evidence of denervation. Subterminal collateral sprouting and an increase in the terminal innervation ratio are diagnostic of denervation[7]. However, even here the changes are not always clear-cut and ramifying, unemployed nerve endings in dystrophic muscle could be misinterpreted as collateral sprouting.

Differential Diagnosis

Disorders such as acid maltase deficiency or mitochondrial myopathy may have some clinical overlap but do not present problems on biopsy. Histologically it may be difficult to distinguish manifesting carriers of Duchenne dystrophy, males with Becker dystrophy and patients with chronic polymyositis. Only 10% of carriers of Duchenne dystrophy have overt clinical weakness and this tendency also runs in families[8]. Sadly wrong genetic advice will be given to a carrier if she is mistakenly assumed to have an autosomal recessive limb girdle syndrome. Hyaline fibres may occur in both conditions, but if they are conspicuous and evidence of denervation is lacking the carrier state must be considered and, in a man, Becker dystrophy (see Chapter 8). Polymyositis is described in Chapter 13. Untreated, chronic polymyositis may have histological similarities. Inflammatory aggregates can occur in both, but the grossly hypertrophied fibres, often very conspicuous in a limb girdle syndrome, are rarely seen in polymyositis. The scapuloperoneal syndromes have clinical overlap with facioscapulohumeral dystrophy. All the changes that have been ascribed to facioscapulohumeral dystrophy can be found in chronic denervating disease. I suspect that many patients with this localized distribution of muscle weakness have a form of chronic spinal muscular atrophy, rather than a truly dystrophic disorder.

Emery–Dreifuss Dystrophy

This is yet another rare condition within the group of 'is it dystrophic or neurogenic?' disorders. The eponym is given to a slowly progressive X-linked muscle disease associated with childhood contractures and cardiac conduction abnormalities[9]. The muscle weakness affects proximal arm muscles and distal leg muscles. Muscle biopsy has revealed chronic myopathic type changes without specific features, but EMG has suggested denervation[9]. The unusual constellation of clinical features has been cited as proof of a distinct entity, but a very similar disorder has been reported with autosomal dominant inheritance[10] and there is clinico-pathologic overlap with the scapuloperoneal syndromes[3,5]. Thus, until the fundamental pathologic defects are uncovered the relationships between these disorders remain uncertain. For the individual patient, the most important point is that the combination of contractures and chronic myopathy indicates the need for an ECG. Sudden death from an associated cardiac conduction defect can hopefully be prevented with a pacemaker[10].

Quadriceps Myopathy

There have been several reports of a hereditary myopathy restricted to the quadriceps. The pathological basis of this disorder is not well documented and it has been suggested that the condition is a variant of chronic SMA. Swash describes a man with weakness and wasting confined to quadriceps for nearly 30 years before progression to affect limb girdle muscles[11]. Histology of the deltoid muscle showed mild myopathic abnormalities in keeping with that of a limb girdle syndrome.

References

1. Walton, J. (1983). Changing concepts of neuromuscular disease. *Hospital Update*, **9**, 949–58

2. Gardener-Medwin, D. (1980). Clinical features and classification of the muscular dystrophies. *Br. Med. Bull.*, **36**, 109–15

3. Jennekens, F. G. I. *et al.* (1975). Inflammatory myopathy in scapulo-ilio-peroneal atrophy with cardiopathy. *Brain*, **98**, 709–22

4. Thomas, P. K., Schott, G. D. and Morgan-Hughes, J. A. (1975). Adult onset scapulo-peroneal myopathy. *J. Neurol. Neurosurg. Psychiatry*, **38**, 1008–15

5. Takahashi, K. *et al.* (1974). Scapulo-peroneal dystrophy associated with neurogenic changes. *J. Neurol. Sci.*, **23**, 575–83

6. Thomas, P. K., Calne, D. B. and Elliott, C. F. (1972). X-linked scapulo-peroneal syndrome. *J. Neurol. Neurosurg. Psychiatry*, **35**, 208–15

7. Mastaglia, F. L. and Walton, J. (1982). *Intramuscular Nerves and Nerve Terminals in Skeletal Muscle Pathology.* pp. 497–8. (Edinburgh: Churchill Livingstone)

8. Moser, H. and Emery, A. E. H. (1974). The manifesting carrier in Duchenne muscular dystrophy. *Clin. Genet.*, **5**, 271–84

9. Rowland, L. P. *et al.* (1979). Emery–Dreifuss muscular dystrophy. *Ann. Neurol.*, **5**, 111–17

10. Fenichel, G. M. *et al.* (1982). An autosomal-dominant dystrophy with humeropelvic distribution and cardiomyopathy. *Neurology*, **32**, 1399–401

11. Swash, M. and Heathfield, K. W. G. (1983). Quadriceps myopathy: a variant of the limb girdle syndrome. *J. Neurol. Neurosurg. Psychiatry*, **46**. 355–7

Myotonia is the inability to relax after voluntary contraction, most often manifest as inability to relax the fingers after a tight handshake. Myotonia can also be elicited by percussion of the muscle. The phenomenon diminishes with both repetitive percussion or voluntary activity. EMG findings are characteristic. Insertion of the needle and voluntary contraction provoke bursts of repetitive activity, initially of high amplitude, but gradually diminishing and slowing. A sound recording produces an extraordinary effect, likened to a dive bomber. Myotonia is found in several completely separate disorders, but myotonic dystrophy is by far the commonest and also the most serious, progressive condition.

Myotonic Dystrophy

Myotonic dystrophy is an inherited, progressive muscle disease, that is clinically and pathologically quite distinct from the other dystrophies. Myotonia and progressive weakness of the facial muscles are the hallmarks of the disorder, which may be associated with a variety of systemic abnormalities, including cataracts, premature balding, cardiac arrhythmias and endocrine disturbances[1]. It is postulated that a cell membrane defect affects skeletal muscle and other tissue, but the nature of this abnormality and how it predisposes to both myotonia and muscle wasting is still unknown. One hypothesis suggests there is reduced density or impaired function of aminergic and peptidergic (hormonal) receptors throughout the body[2]. Clearly, the membrane abnormality is quite different from the postulated defect of Duchenne dystrophy.

The onset of clinical symptoms is most often between 20 and 30 years, although myotonia may cause little inconvenience and is often disregarded by patients, who therefore do not seek medical aid until muscular weakness becomes disabling in middle age or even later. The combination of muscular weakness and myotonia is distinctive and diagnostic, but one or other may be difficult to discern in the early clinical stages. EMG studies are very helpful. Repetitive electrical discharge is pathognomonic of myotonia, but this alone does not distinguish myotonic dystrophy from the other rarer causes of myotonia. Muscle biopsy can confirm the diagnosis; however, it is important to take the biopsy from a clinically affected muscle, otherwise misleading normal histology may be obtained.

Whilst unsuitable for biopsy, weak facial muscles are responsible for the characteristic appearance of these patients, who develop hollow cheeks and drooping eyelids. Harper illustrates how the family album may portray these changes[1]. Sternomastoid weakness may appear at an early stage. In the limbs early involvement

of distal muscles is usual and thus differs from other dystrophies. It is not, however, as severe as in peroneal muscular atrophy and pes cavus is not a feature.

Systemic abnormalities are numerous and diverse, but less often the cause of presenting symptoms. Occasionally, cataracts may cause visual impairment at a time when muscle symptoms are minimal. In addition, when myotonia is detected, the identification of symptomless lens opacities by slit lamp examination provides valuable diagnostic confirmation of myotonic dystrophy. Retinal degenerative changes may also develop. Frontal balding in men is a well recognized association, but is much too common in the normal population to be a diagnostic guide. It has rarely been described in females. Testicular atrophy is quite common. There is a raised plasma FSH and testicular histology resembles that of Klinefelter's syndrome. A minority develop clinical diabetes mellitus. More often only biochemical abnormalities are demonstrated, particularly an abnormal insulin response to a glucose load. Symptomatic cardiac disease is also a minority finding, but a much larger proportion show some ECG abnormality, usually a conduction defect. Sudden death is a recognized complication. ECG changes are quite non-specific and Harper suggests that ECG abnormalities alone in an otherwise normal member of a dystrophic family should not be taken as positive evidence of the disease. Cardiomyopathy and mitral valve prolapse are unusual complications of myotonic dystrophy[3], as is the strange association with multiple pilomatricomas.

The clinical expression of myotonic dystrophy within a family can be very variable. In a large kinship some members may have only minor signs and even myotonia may be absent[4]. Nevertheless, children of parents with a mild disease can still develop typical myotonic dystrophy.

Congenital Myotonic Dystrophy

In classical myotonic dystrophy early development is normal. Only occasionally are the first signs detected in late childhood; the onset is usually later[1]. However, the disorder can present at birth, but with very different clinical features. Although myotonic dystrophy is an autosomal dominant disorder the congenital form is always maternally transmitted, suggesting there is some intrauterine disturbance in addition to the genetic factor. In the affected neonate there is generalized hypotonia, with difficulties in sucking and swallowing and often severe respiratory problems. Talipes is common and arthrogryposis is found in a small proportion. There is a considerable neonatal mortality, but those who survive show delayed motor development

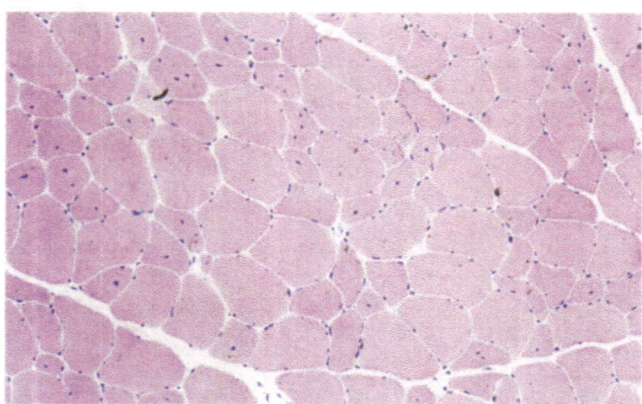

Figure 11.1 Myotonic dystrophy in a 27-year-old man, with a 3-year history of inability to relax grip. He has a family history of myotonia and cataracts. Deltoid muscle biopsy shows a dual population of small rounded fibres and larger fibres. Many of the small fibres have central nuclei. (Same case is shown in Figures 11.2–11.8.)   H & E × 180

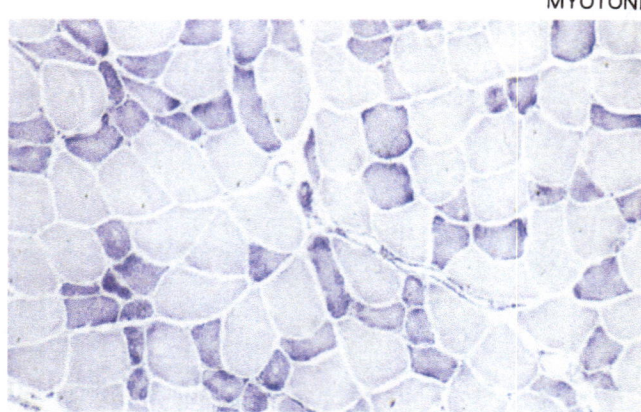

Figure 11.2 Myotonic dystrophy. The small fibres are uniformly type 1 fibres, whereas the large fibres are type 2.   NADH-TR × 180

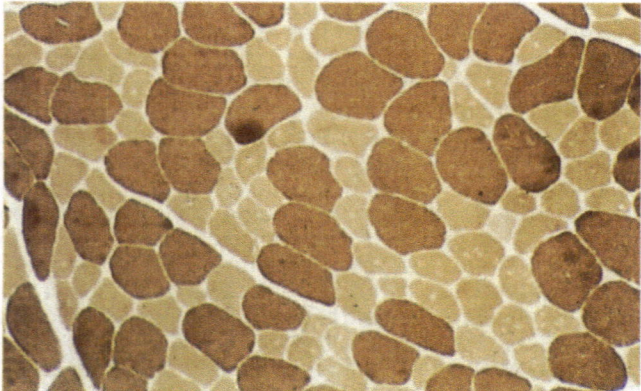

Figure 11.3 Myotonic dystrophy. Small fibres are uniformly type 1 (light) with the routine myosin ATP-ase reaction.   ATP-ase pH 9.4 × 180

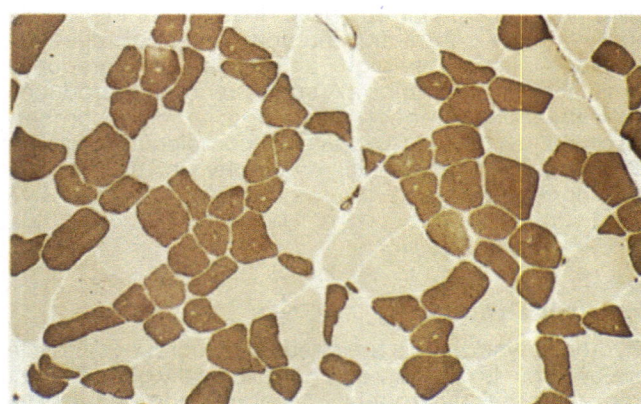

Figure 11.4 Myotonic dystrophy. Small type 1 fibres (dark). The larger fibres are type 2A. There are no type 2B fibres in this field.   ATP-ase pH 4.6 × 180

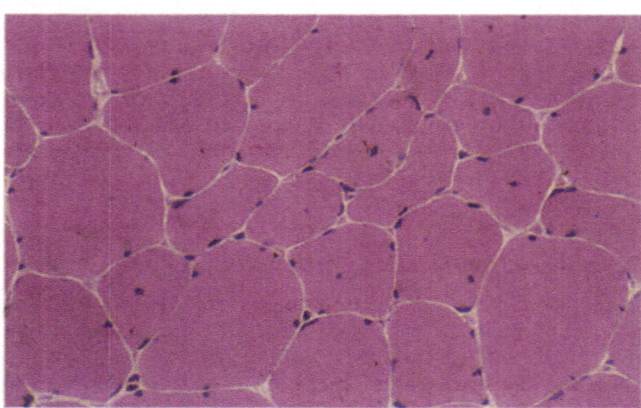

Figure 11.5 Myotonic dystrophy. Many of the smaller fibres contain a central nucleus.   H & E × 300

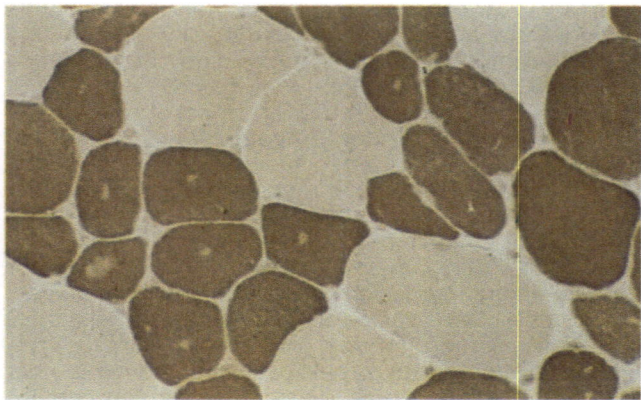

Figure 11.6 Myotonic dystrophy. The small type 1 fibres have a tiny central unstained area, which corresponds with the central nucleus. Although the majority of type 1 fibres are atrophic, a few normal size fibres remain. The type 2A fibres are mildly hypertrophied.   ATP-ase pH × 300

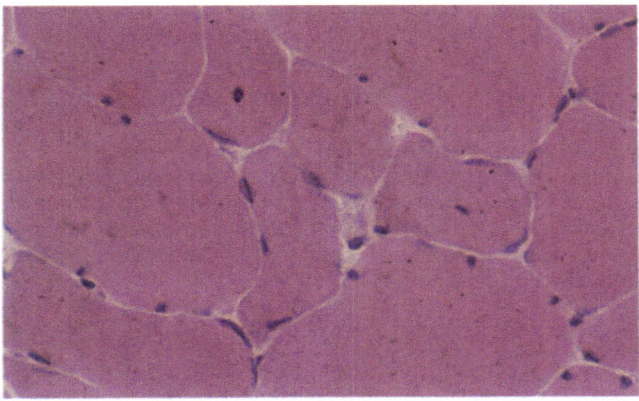

Figure 11.7 Myotonic dystrophy. An eosinophilic bleb at the periphery of an atrophic fibre in the centre of the field corresponds with a sarcoplasmic mass. H & E × 450

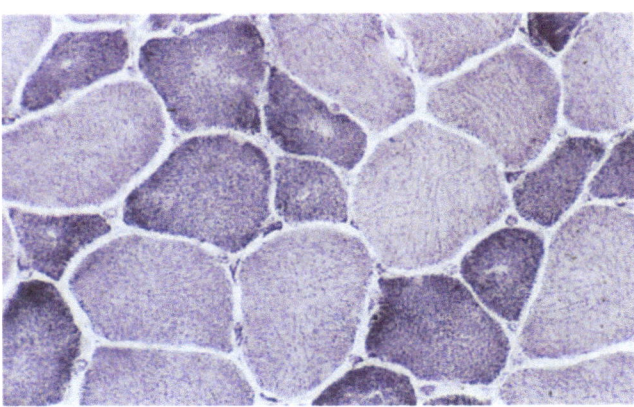

Figure 11.8 Myotonic dystrophy. In this biopsy, taken early in the course of the disease, apart from slight condensation of the stain at the periphery of small fibres, there is virtually normal cell architecture. NADH-TR × 300

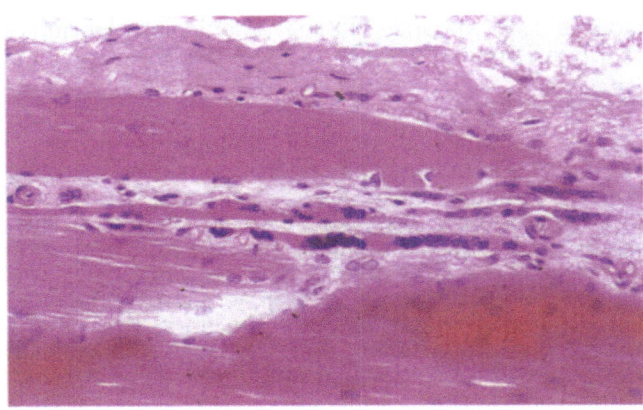

Figure 11.9 Longstanding myotonic dystrophy. Several atrophic thin fibres contain columns of central nuclei H & E × 300

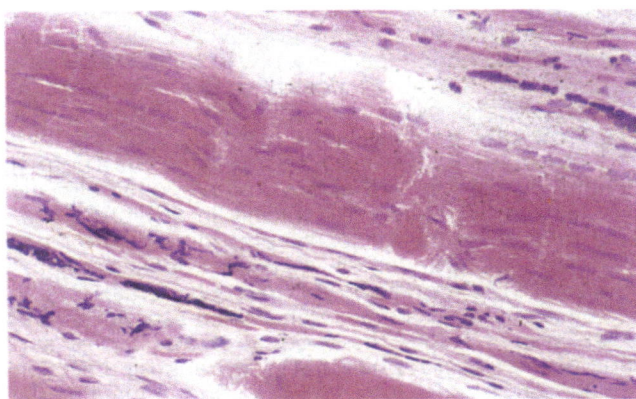

Figure 11.10 Longstanding myotonic dystrophy. Numerous severely atrophic fibres with columns of central nuclei, alongside a single hypertrophic fibre. H & E × 300

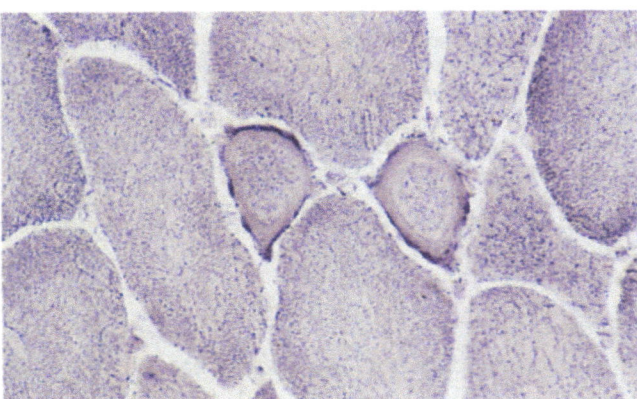

Figure 11.11 Ring fibres in myotonic dystrophy. A few small fibres show abnormal, myofibrillar architecture. These fibres show a peripheral concentric arrangement of myofibrils, around normal internal architecture. NADH-TR × 300

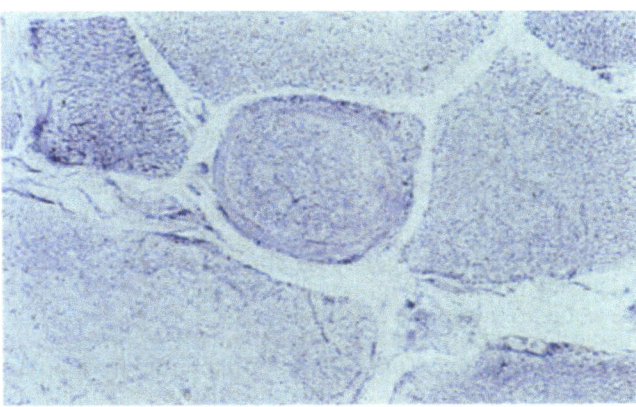

Figure 11.12 Ring fibre in myotonic dystrophy. A narrow, peripheral rim of myofibrils with a concentric arrangement. Abnormalities of fibre architecture are best demonstrated with the NADH-TR reaction. NADH-TR × 750

and are often mentally retarded. There is a characteristic facial appearance with an open droopy mouth, but clinical myotonia is absent. EMG evidence is sometimes obtained but paradoxically clinical myotonia in a young infant virtually excludes dystrophy and favours one of the other rarer myotonic disorders such as myotonia congenita. The affected children eventually learn to walk and motor skills seem to improve; however, inevitably they develop all the signs of the progressive disorder, with onset of overt myotonia between 5 and 10 years. Muscle biopsy in the neonate is abnormal, but very different from the later picture.

Biopsy – Myotonic Dystrophy

The need to biopsy an affected muscle must be emphasized. In the adult onset disorder, the earliest detectable change is a selective atrophy of type 1 fibres, combined with hypertrophy of type 2 fibres (Figures 11.1–11.4). The changes are usually obvious from simple inspection but when mild can be confirmed by measurement of fibre diameters. Type 2 fibre hypertrophy may precede type 1 atrophy and there may be a paucity of type 2B fibres, possibly because conversion of 2A to 2B accompanies hypertrophy (Figure 11.4). Type 2 atrophy is definitely not a feature[5]. Type 1 fibre predominance may be found, but often there is a normal distribution. Central nuclei are another characteristic early feature (Figure 11.5). Initially in any one transverse section central nuclei are present in only a small proportion of the small type 1 fibres (Figures 11.5–11.8). Progression of muscular weakness is associated with a considerable increase in central nuclei. In later stages the majority of small fibres and many of the hypertrophied fibres in transverse section contain one or more internal nuclei and in longitudinal section long chains of nuclei are seen in thin atrophic fibres (Figures 11.9 and 11.10). These nuclear chains are virtually pathognomic of myotonic dystrophy, but they are not found until the disease is well advanced and the clinical diagnosis is obvious. Thus the pathologist should not expect to find them in a biopsy which seeks to confirm myotonic dystrophy in its early clinical stage.

Fibre architectural abnormalities: These become more obvious with progression of the disease. However, even in early clinical stages a careful search will reveal some changes. Levels through a biopsy are often helpful. The NADH-TR reaction may reveal occasional moth-eaten or targetoid fibres, generally in type 1 fibres. The oxidative enzyme reaction may also demonstrate small angular darkly stained fibres, but these are scattered and not in the groups that characterize denervation atrophy. Ring fibres are particularly common in myotonic dystrophy[1]. The circumferential arrangement of peripheral myofibrils is probably best seen with the NADH-TR reaction (Figures 11.11 11.12), but they are visible in a good H & E stained section. Unlike most muscle fibre abnormalities ring fibres are often easy to see in formalin fixed tissue because there is frequently artifactual separation of the malaligned peripheral myofibrils from the central column. It has been suggested that ring fibres themselves are artifactual, produced by handling the muscle during biopsy; nevertheless, they probably reflect the great irritability of muscle fibres in myotonic dystrophy and when numerous they are a valuable histological clue. Sarcoplasmic masses represent yet another cellular disturbance that is particularly characteristic of

myotonic dystrophy. In transverse section with H & E staining, these are subsarcolemmal blebs of homogeneous eosinophilic cytoplasm (Figure 11.13), which are also PAS positive. With the NADH-TR reaction they usually appear as pale staining crescents or even complete haloes, although conversely, there is sometimes increased peripheral oxidative enzyme activity (Figure 11.14).

Electron microscopy

Electron microscopy of the peripheral zone reveals a great paucity of myofilaments but accumulation of lysosomes, honeycomb-like proliferation of the sarcoplasmic reticulum (SR) and glycogen granules[5] (Figures 11.25 and 11.26). Focal subsarcolemmal mitochondrial aggregates explain the patchy increased oxidative enzyme activity. By light microscopy tiny peripheral foci of acid phosphatase reactivity are described and apparently correlate with lysosomes and membrane profiles of the SR system. In the interior of the fibre, an early change detected by electron microscopy is disappearance of thin filaments and swelling of the SR system in the region of the 1 band[5].

Fibre necrosis

This is a relatively unusual feature of myotonic dystrophy. However, both necrotic and regenerating fibres are occasionally found, particularly in more advanced disease. As with other slowly progressive, wasting diseases the physical stresses imposed upon surviving fibres may themselves be responsible for necrosis and subsequent regeneration. Advanced disease shows great variation in fibre size, many severely atrophic fibres and, as with all wasting diseases, a considerable increase in fibro-fatty connective tissue.

Muscle spindles

In myotonic dystrophy the intrafusal fibres also show characteristic changes but spindles are encountered relatively infrequently in a small biopsy and again the changes are more conspicuous in established muscle disease. The intrafusal fibres show longitudinal splitting and fragmentation, particularly in the polar regions of the spindle and particularly in spindles of the distal limb muscles[6] (Figure 11.15). Whilst a normal spindle contains around seven (range 3–14) intrafusal fibres, transverse section through the polar region in myotonic dystrophy may reveal 20–30 minute fragments. Even so, the change is patchy and even within the same muscle all spindles are not affected. The spindle abnormality has been interpreted as a consequence of the mechanical stress of sustained myotonic contractions. However, this is not the whole answer because Swash has recently shown that spindles are normal in myotonia congenita[7].

Intramuscular nerves

Large, elongated motor end plates may be found in myotonic dystrophy (Figure 11.16). These are probably a modification induced by myotonic contractions, rather than a primary abnormality.

The plethora of histological changes in myotonic dystrophy cannot be fully explained in pathogenetic terms, but it may be that sarcoplasmic masses are a direct indication of defective muscle fibres, whilst hypertrophy, ring fibres and fibre splitting are all superimposed changes due to the sustained contractions. Myotonia itself is believed to result from a cell membrane abnormality, but this has no consistent morphological counterpart. Other myotonic disorders do not show the same histological changes and are probably due to completely different biochemical defects. It is only myotonic dystrophy that affects both membrane function and cellular organization. Astrom and Adams postulate that there is a primary failure of myofilament synthesis and organization and that central nuclei reflect the inability of the muscle cell to overcome this defect[8].

Biopsy – Congenital Myotonic Dystrophy

Congenital myotonic dystrophy presents somewhat different histology, in which the essential abnormality seems to be immaturity. There may be variation in fibre size with large central nuclei in a small proportion (Figures 11.17 and 11.18). The ATP-ase reaction shows clear-cut fibre type differentiation (Figures 11.19 and 11.20), sometimes with type 1 predominance. Fibres with central nuclei resemble myotubes, with a central zone devoid of myosin ATP-ase activity (Figures 11.19 and 11.27). In the neonate there is no constant relationship between abnormality of fibre size and fibre type. Type 1 fibres may be slightly smaller than type 2 (Figures 11.19 and 11.20), but the reverse is also described[9]. The definite selective type 1 atrophy of adult disease is most unusual, but it has been reported and of course resembles congenital fibre type disproportion[10]. A most distinctive appearance is seen with the NADH-TR reaction, in which the majority of fibres have a thin, unstained peripheral halo. This halo is not demonstrated by H & E or the ATP-ase reaction. Electron microscopy shows that the peripheral sarcoplasm is almost totally devoid of myofibrils and mitochondria and contains only glycogen granules and a few vesicles[9] (Figure 11.28). Satellite cells are numerous, a point of distinction from myotubular myopathy, which has very similar histology. The concept of immaturity is supported by studies of affected premature infants, which show late differentiation of fibre type, retention of central nuclei in extrafusal fibres[11] and late completion of the spindle[12]. Co-existent congenital anomalies, such as patent ductus arteriosus, cryptorchidism, nesidioblastosis and persistent fetal glomeruli, suggest the maturational defect may be more widespread[13]. There is a high neonatal mortality[1] but infants who survive eventually develop the typical progressive changes of adult onset disease (Figures 11.21–11.24). The similarity between the peripheral haloes of infant muscle cells and the sarcoplasmic masses of adult fibres is worthy of comment. Whilst the former seems to be arrested development and the latter acquired disorganization they may well reflect the same fundamental defect.

Myotonia Congenita

This is a rare disorder. In comparison with myotonic dystrophy, the myotonia is usually more severe, tends to interfere with daily life and is frequently exacerbated by cold[1]. The condition has a variable pattern of inheritance; dominant, recessive and sporadic cases are described. The history is usually one of muscle stiffness, an inability to get going, which dates from childhood and is occasionally noted from birth. Progressive muscle weakness does not occur and there are no associated systemic problems. The clinical demonstration of myotonia in early childhood virtually excludes myotonic dystrophy, but at a late stage the distinction can be difficult. Patients with myotonia congenita sometimes show striking, generalized muscle hypertrophy, EMG readily confirms myotonia and muscle enzymes are normal.

Muscle biopsy can be completely normal or show only minimal abnormalities with H & E. However, muscle hypertrophy is frequently present. With the ATP-ase reaction a complete absence of 2B fibres seems to be a consistent finding. It is suggested that 2A fibres are converted to 2B fibres by repetitive electrical activity, a theory borne out by an increase in the proportion of 2A fibres. If this is true one might also anticipate that biopsy of myotonia congenita early in childhood will sometimes reveal 2B fibres. In longstanding disease, there may be other abnormalities, especially atrophic fibres and some internal nuclei. However, these changes are not as marked as in established myotonic dystrophy and there are no architectural abnormalities. Sarcoplasmic masses are not seen and there is a normal pattern with the oxidative enzyme reaction. Swash has recently reported normal muscle spindles in myotonia congenita[7]; however, this was a small sample and an extensive survey has not been carried out.

Rare Myotonic Disorders Including Periodic Paralysis

The other myotonic disorders are also inherited but exceptionally rare and with a clinical history that usually distinguishes them from myotonic dystrophy[1].

Paramyotonia congenita gives a prolonged myotonic reaction triggered by cold and, in contrast to myotonic dystrophy, it is aggravated by repetitive movements. Muscle hypertrophy may develop, but there is no progressive weakness and no systemic symptoms. Biopsy has been recorded as normal or with variation in fibre size, with both hypertrophic and atrophic fibres. The disorder may be related to the equally rare, periodic paralyses. Myotonia is but a minor clinical component of these disorders in which episodes of flaccid weakness, lasting from an hour or two to a few days are the major problem. Cell membrane dysfunction is usually associated with changes in the serum potassium level. The picture is very similar with hyperkalaemic, hypokalaemic or occasionally normokalaemic periodic paralysis, but the episodes of weakness are often more severe when associated with a hypokalaemic state. There are rare instances of death from respiratory muscle involvement or cardiac arrhythmia with hypokalaemic paralysis. However, in all of these disorders the majority of patients recover completely and only a few show any progressive weakness. A persistently raised CPK has been described in one family.

In all forms of periodic paralysis histology is characterized by vacuolar myopathy. This is most striking in a biopsy taken during an attack, when vacuoles may be found in almost all fibres. The number and size of vacuoles diminish between attacks and they may in fact be absent. Electron microscopy reveals vacuoles which appear to arise from the sarcoplasmic reticulum and T tubules. An initial cluster of small vesicles evolves into a vacuole up to $100\,\mu m$ diameter, which is membrane band and contains granular material. Continuity between the extracellular space and T system has been demonstrated with electron-dense tracers. In addition collections of long, straight

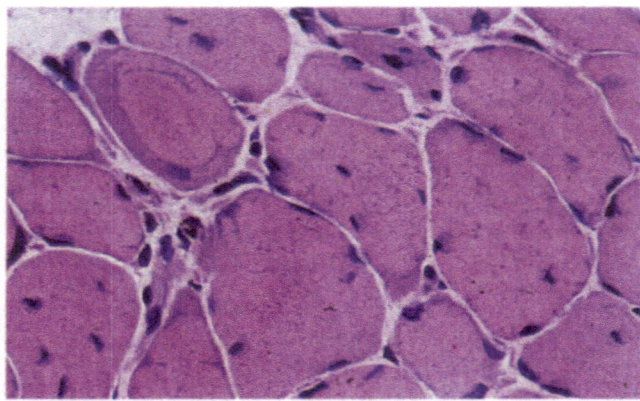

Figure 11.13 Sarcoplasmic masses in myotonic dystrophy. Biopsy from tibialis anterior of a 25-year-old-woman. Several fibres show basophilic blebs of cytoplasm and in one fibre a complete halo.   H & E × 300 (serial section shown in Figure 11.14)

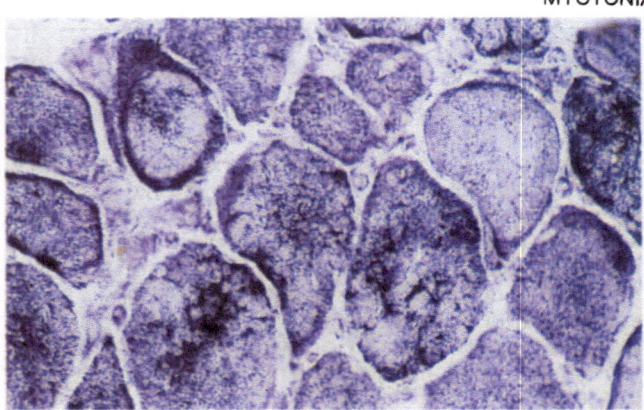

Figure 11.14 Sarcoplasmic masses showing a strongly positive oxidative enzyme reaction. In addition this stain reveals internal derangement of myofibrillar pattern in several fibres.   NADH-TR × 300

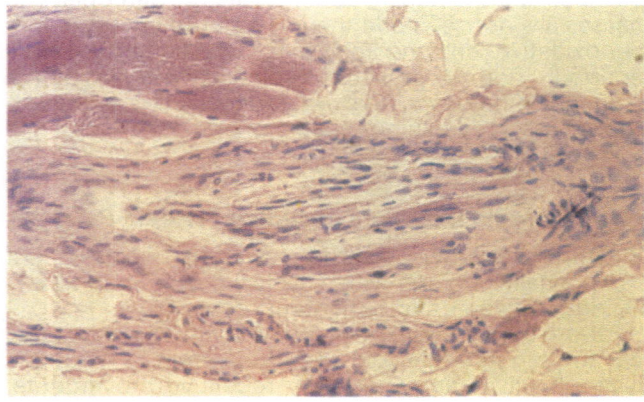

Figure 11.15 Muscle spindle in advanced myotonic dystrophy. Longitudinal section of the spindle from a distal leg muscle in advanced disease shows splitting with numerous abnormally thin intrafusal fibres.   H & E × 180

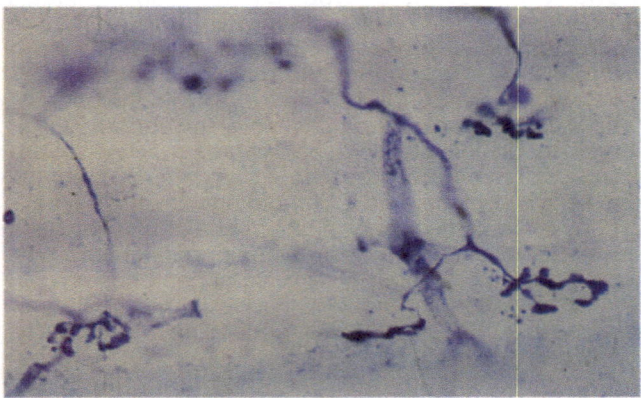

Figure 11.16 Motor end plate in longstanding myotonic dystrophy. The end plate appears elongated. This change is probably secondary to myotonic contractions. Methylene blue vital staining × 300

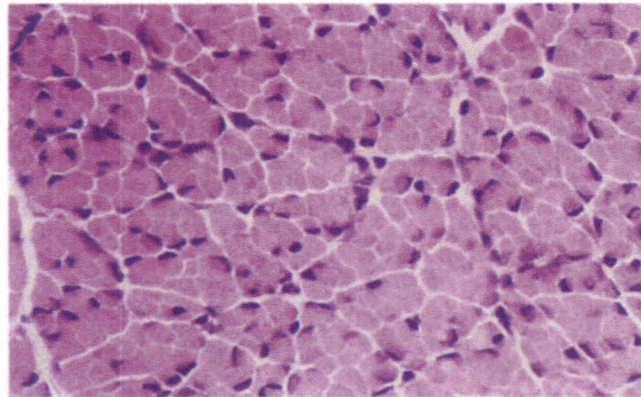

Figure 11.17 Congenital myotonic dystrophy. Quadriceps biopsy from a severely hypotonic neonate, dying in the second week of life of respiratory difficulty. The biopsy shows variation in fibre size with some large central nuclei. Myotonic dystrophy in the mother was not recognized until after the birth of the baby.   H & E × 300

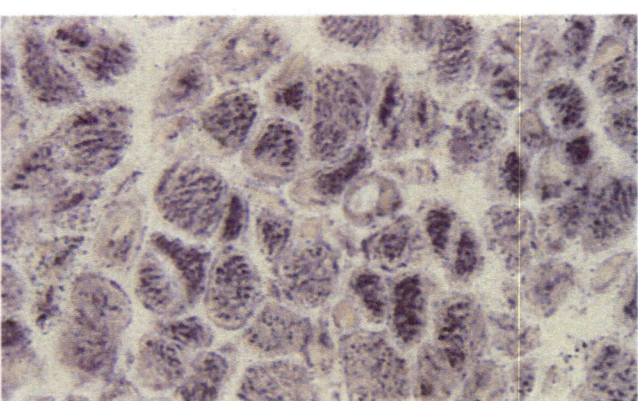

Figure 11.18 Congenital myotonic dystrophy. Variation in fibre size and peripheral unstained haloes, devoid of enzyme activity.   NADH-TR × 750

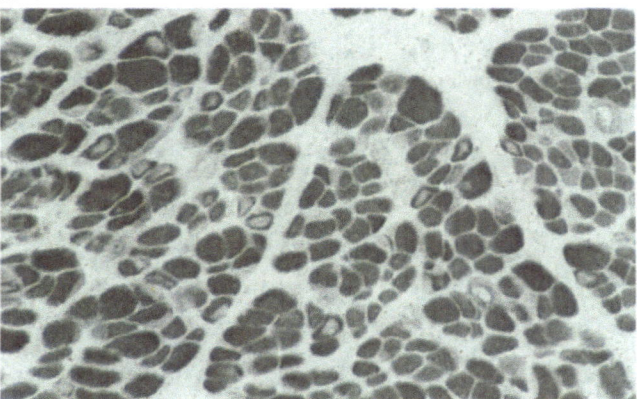

Figure 11.19 Congenital myotonic dystrophy. Variation in fibre size. Type 1 and 2 differentiation is poor, but this is postmortem muscle. Differentiation is usually normal in muscle obtained by biopsy. In addition, several fibres resemble myotubes, with unstained central zones.   ATP-ase pH 9.4 × 300

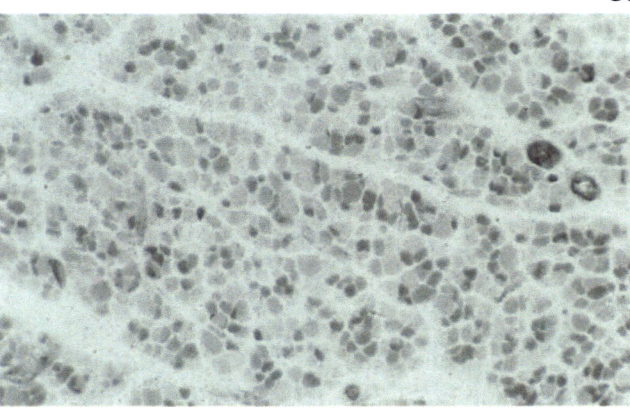

Figure 11.20 Congenital myotonic dystrophy. There is variation in fibre size with no selective fibre atrophy.   ATP-ase pH 4.1 × 300

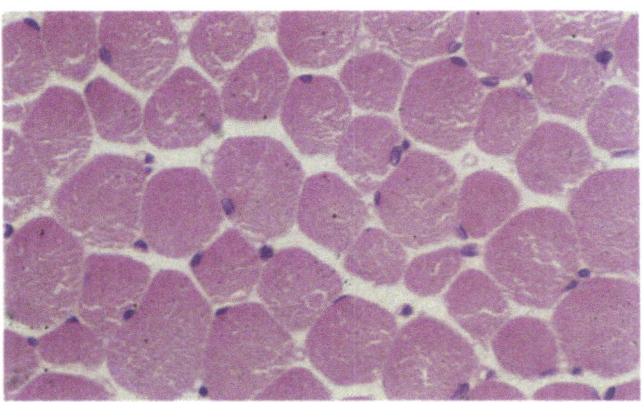

Figure 11.21 Congenital myotonic dystrophy in a 3-year-old boy. He had the characteristic myopathic facies with droopy mouth. On examination his mother proved to have myotonia and distal wasting. Her disorder was not recognized until her children were examined. Deltoid biopsy in the 3-year-old son shows only mild variation in fibre size.   H & E × 180

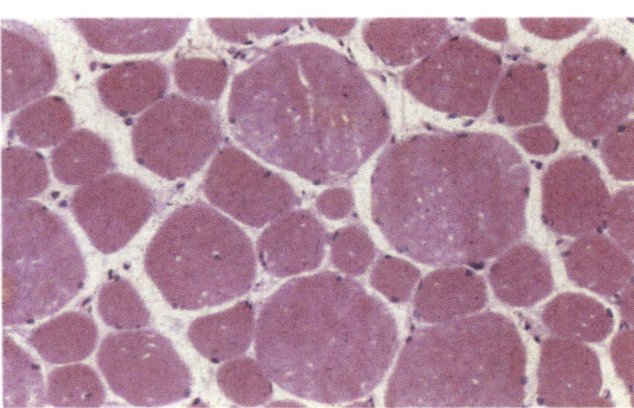

Figure 11.22 Congenital myotonic dystrophy. Deltoid biopsy of 6-year-old brother of case shown in Figure 11.21. There is marked variation in fibre size, with small rounded atrophic fibres, amidst hypertrophied fibres. (Same case shown in Figures 11.23 and 11.24.)   H & E × 300

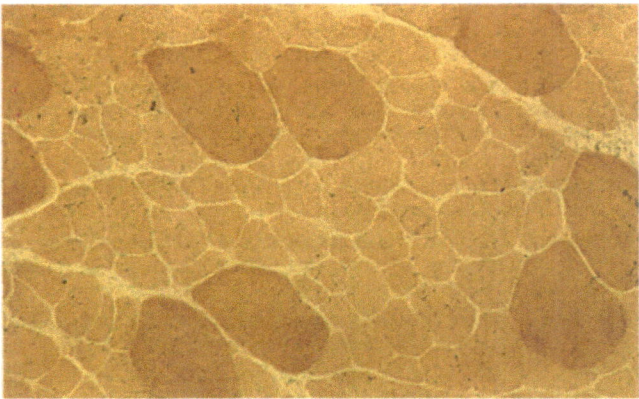

Figure 11.23 Congenital myotonic dystrophy. Small fibres are exclusively type 1. The type 2A fibres are moderately hypertrophied.   ATP-ase pH 9.4 × 300

Figure 11.24 Congenital myotonic dystrophy. Small fibres are type 1 and hypertrophied fibres are type 2A. These changes are already quite characteristic of myotonic dystrophy.   ATP-ase pH 4.6 × 300

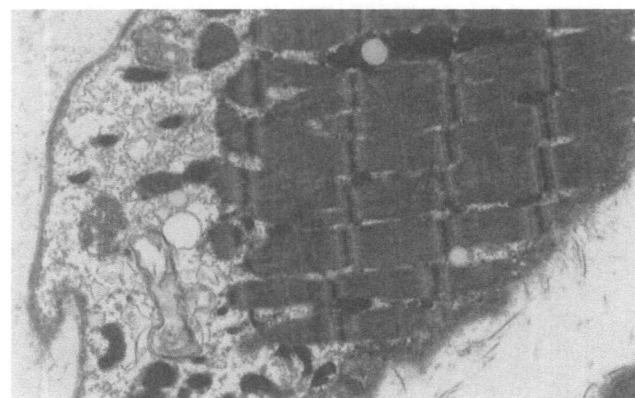

Figure 11.25 Sarcoplasmic mass in adult myotonic dystrophy. The peripheral cytoplasm is devoid of myofibrils and contains glycogen granules and several membranous whorls.   EM × 7100

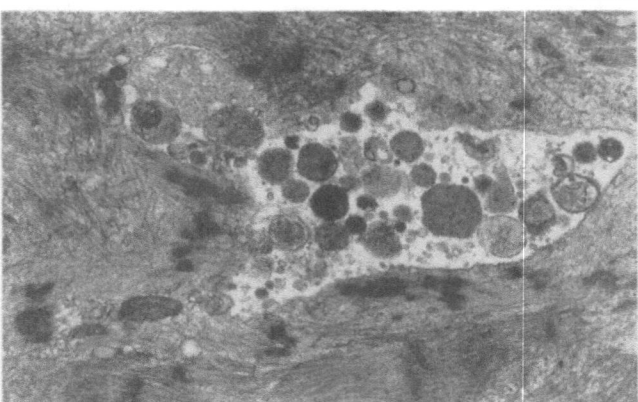

Figure 11.26 Disorganization of normal cell architecture in adult myotonic dystrophy. There is myofibrillar disarray and a collection of lysosomes in the peripheral cytoplasm.   EM × 11 000

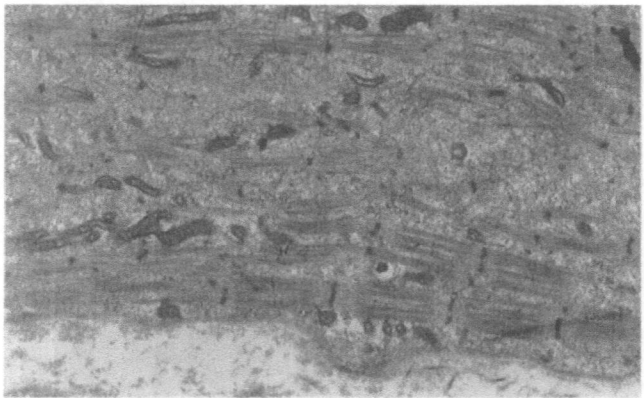

Figure 11.27 Myotube-like fibre in congenital myotonic dystrophy. The central zone contains only scanty myofibrils.   EM × 7100

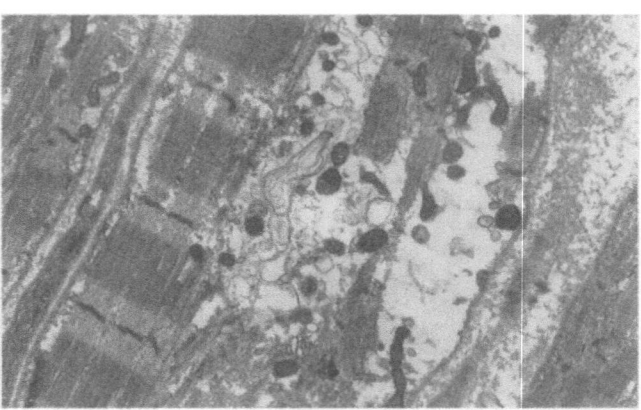

Figure 11.28 Peripheral cytoplasmic haloes in congenital myotonic dystrophy are due to absence of myofibrils in this zone. Part of the peripheral cytoplasm is practically devoid of organelles. The central part contains a few membranous whorls.   EM × 5100

tubules, referred to as tubular aggregates, are a frequent finding in the periodic paralyses. These tubular aggregates lie around the edge of fibres and also appear to originate from the sarcoplasmic reticulum. Morphological changes in the membranous structures involved in conduction are common to the myotonic disorders, but nevertheless it seems almost certain that each represents a different, genetically programmed, biochemical defect and the visible changes are secondary effects.

References

1. Harper, P. S. (1979). Myotonic dystrophy. In *Major Problems in Neurology 9* (Philadelphia: W. B. Saunders)

2. Brumback, R. A. *et al.* (1981). Myotonic dystrophy: a disease of abnormal membrane receptors: an hypothesis of pathophysiology and a new approach to treatment. *Med. Hypotheses*, **7**, 1059–66

3. Morris, L. K., Cuetter, A. C. and Gunderson, C. H. (1982). Myotonic dystrophy, mitral valve prolapse and cerebral embolism. *Stroke*, **13**, 93–4

4. Phillips, W. P., Johnson, G. J. and Larsen, B. (1982). Incomplete manifestations of myotonic dystrophy in large kinship in Labrador. *Ann. Neurol.*, **11**, 582–91

5. Casanova, G. and Jerusalem, F. (1979). Myopathology of myotonic dystrophy. A morphometric study. *Acta Neuropathol. (Berl.)*, **45**, 231–40

6. Swash, M. (1972). The morphology and innervation of the muscle spindle in dystrophia myotonica. *Brain*, **95**, 357–68

7. Swash, M. *et al.* (1983). Normal muscle spindle morphology in myotonia congenita. The spindle abnormality in myotonic dystrophy is not due to myotonia alone. *Clin. Neuropathol.*, **2**, 75–8

8. Astrom and Adams (1982). Myotonic disorders. In Mastaglia and Walton (eds.) *Skeletal Muscle Pathology*. pp. 266–83

9. Farkas, E. *et al.* (1974). Histochemical and ultrastructural study of muscle biopsies in 3 cases of dystrophia myotonica in the newborn child. *J. Neurol. Sci.*, **21**, 273–88

10. Argov, Z. *et al.* (1980). Congenital myotonic dystrophy. Fiber type abnormalities in two cases. *Arch. Neurol.*, **37**, 693–6

11. Sahgal, V. *et al.* (1983). Skeletal muscle in preterm infants with congenital myotonic dystrophy. Morphologic and histochemical study. *J. Neurol. Sci.*, **59**, 47–55

12. Sahgal, V. *et al.* (1983). Ultrastructure of muscle spindle in congenital myotonic dystrophy. A study of preterm infant muscle spindles. *Acta Neuropathol.* (Berl.), **61**, 207–13.

13. Young, R. S. K. *et al.* (1981). Dysmaturation in infants of mothers with myotonic dystrophy. *Arch. Neurol.*, **38**, 716–19

Congenital Myopathies

Introduction

The congenital myopathies are a group of neuromuscular disorders presenting early in childhood, but frequently showing static or only slowly progressive muscle weakness. They are often familial but quite distinct from both the progressive muscular dystrophies and the severely disabling spinal muscular atrophies. Congenital myopathies are characterized by histochemical type 1 fibre predominance and by a variety of peculiar structural changes within the fibre, upon which nomenclature and classification are based. The pathological changes have suggested a common pathogenesis of maturation arrest. Amongst these early onset myopathies there are several, if not many, different nosological entities, but they show considerable clinical and pathological overlap. Although usually of childhood onset, identical histology is occasionally found in an adult onset myopathy. Thus a problem of terminology and which disorders to include can perhaps be solved by borrowing Brooke's title of 'Congenital (more or less) muscle diseases'[1]. The myopathies described in this chapter all have distinctive morphological features, but whilst they may be suspected clinically they can only be identified with certainty by biopsy.

Pathogenesis

The original description of myotubular myopathy by Spiro drew a parallel with fetal myotubes[2]. Although later studies have sometimes rejected this comparison, recent authors have returned to the theme of maturation arrest. In developing human muscle primitive myotubes have large central nuclei, which later migrate to a peripheral position. Fetal muscle fibres initially show uniform type 2C histochemical properties. Type 1 fibres are the first mature fibres to appear, followed later in gestation by 2A and 2B. Fardeau has suggested that each congenital myopathy may be considered as arrested or aberrant development at a particular step in the normal sequence[3]. Thus myotubular myopathy may reflect interference with an early stage of myogenesis, whereas impaired maturation at a later stage could give rise to myopathies with type 1 predominance. This is a useful, unifying concept, which as its author emphasizes will probably be modified and expanded as our knowledge increases. Normal development could be impaired by intrinsic defects of developing muscle cells or by defective innervation. Although minor changes have occasionally been reported, there are no consistent morphological abnormalities in motor nerves and the precise pathogenetic mechanisms that operate in congenital myopathies have yet to be determined.

Centronuclear Myopathy – Myotubular Myopathy

Multiple central nuclei are the main pathological feature of a centronuclear myopathy. Fibres with central nuclei in neonatal disease resemble fetal myotubes, hence the name myotubular myopathy. However, genuine fetal nature is unproven and the less specific term – centronuclear myopathy – is often preferred. It is apparent from clinical and genetic diversity that this histological picture does not denote a single entity, but includes several different disorders. Two well-defined groups with consistent clinical and biopsy findings have emerged, but there remain a large number of both sporadic and familial cases which are difficult to classify. The two distinct subgroups are a severe, sex-linked recessive disorder, presenting with profound neonatal hypotonia[4,5] (Figures 12.1–12.6) and a somewhat milder childhood form with variable inheritance[6,7]. Ophthalmoplegia, ptosis and facial weakness are characteristic clinical features of both groups. In the severe neonatal form respiratory problems are frequently responsible for early death of the affected males[5]. A few infants who have survived have been able to walk[4]. Female carriers may have mild facial weakness and minor abnormalities on muscle biopsy. In the milder form males and females are affected and again floppiness may be noted at birth[6] or they present with weakness in childhood[7]. Despite this motor development is normal or only slightly delayed. However, there is often slow progression and some patients are quite severely disabled in the second or third decade[8]. A dominant mode of inheritance has been found in some families. Others appear to be autosomal recessive[8] and there are many sporadic cases.

Patients with multiple central nuclei on biopsy who do not fit into either of these groups include cases of neonatal and childhood onset myopathy without ophthalmoplegia or facial weakness[9,10] and cases of adult onset disease[11]. Although this is a heterogeneous group most patients exhibit generalized weakness and slow clinical progression. Many show the additional biopsy feature of type 1 fibre hypotrophy[9,10,12]. A few cases of early onset have been associated with a cardiomyopathy[13] (Figures 12.13–12.22). Centronuclear myopathy has also been described with onset in late adult life, when the patient may become quite severely weak and unable to walk (Figures 12.23–12.28). Some adult cases have shown pseudohypertrophy of the calves[11,14].

Muscle Biopsy

By definition the key feature of the muscle biopsy of all cases of centronuclear myopathy is a high percentage

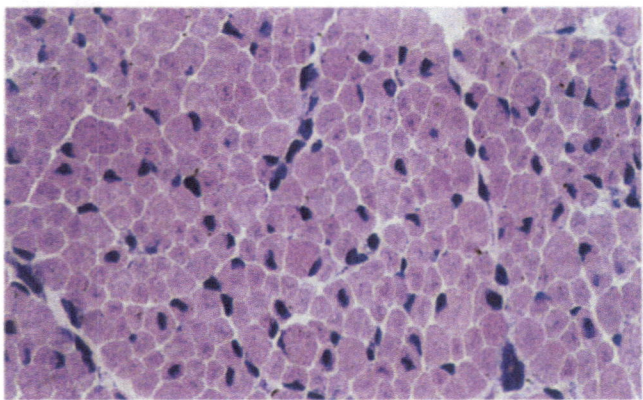

Figure 12.1 Myotubular myopathy. 3-day-old male infant with profound hypotonia. No clinical abnormalities detected in the mother. Biopsy of quadriceps muscles shows many tiny fibres, some with large central nuclei. This child had repeated respiratory infections and died in the first year of life. (Same case shown in Figures 12.2–12.6.)   H & E × 300

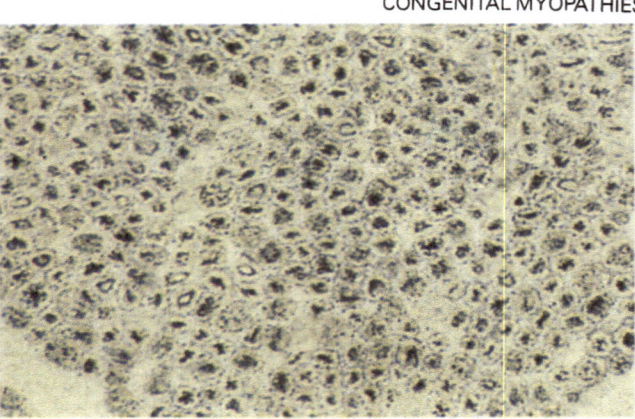

Figure 12.2 Myotubular myopathy. With the oxidative enzyme reaction most fibres appear to have an unstained peripheral halo.   NADH-TR × 300

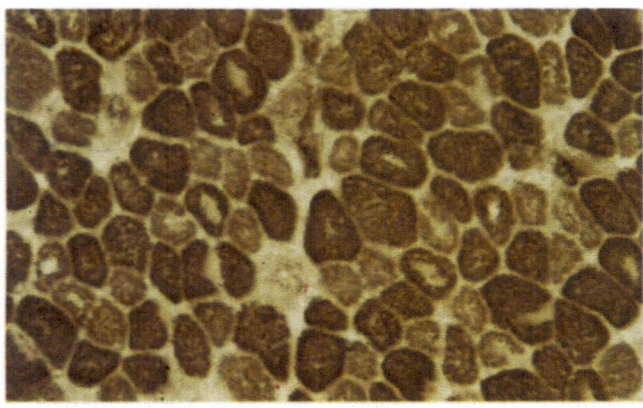

Figure 12.3 Myotubular myopathy. Unstained central zone with myosin-ATP-ase present in many fibres, both type 1 and type 2. Type 1 fibres are slightly smaller than type 2.   Myosin ATP-ase pH 9.4 × 750

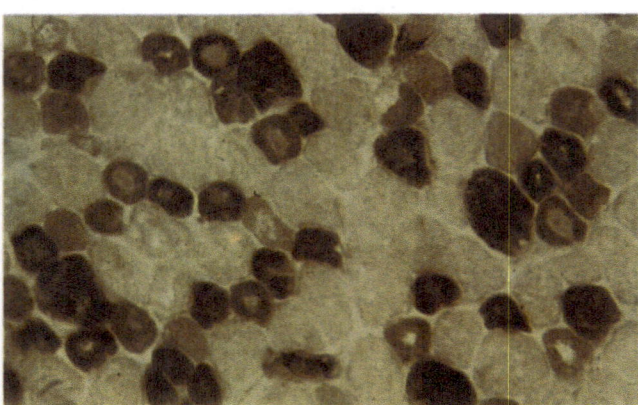

Figure 12.4 Myotubular myopathy. Unstained central zones show up in small type 1 fibres. Fibres with intermediate staining reaction are probably 2C fibres.   Myosin ATP-ase pH 4.1 × 750

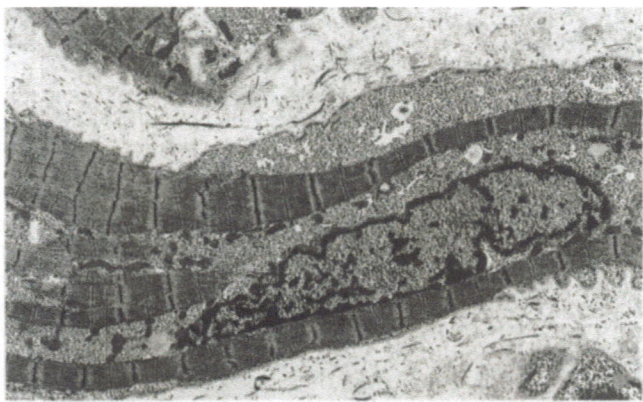

Figure 12.5 Myotubular myopathy. Electron micrograph of myotube-like fibre in longitudinal section showing a centrally placed nucleus, with a perinuclear halo and peripheral zone devoid of myofibrils and filled with glycogen granules.   EM × 3400

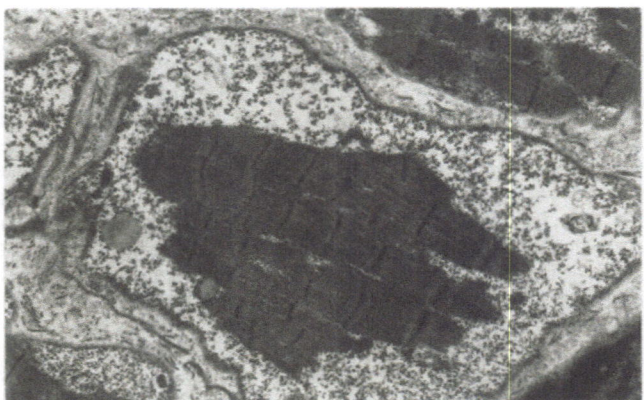

Figure 12.6 Myotubular myopathy. Electron micrography of myotube-like fibre in transverse section showing central myofibrils and wide peripheral zone devoid of organelles and filled with glycogen granules.   EM × 4500

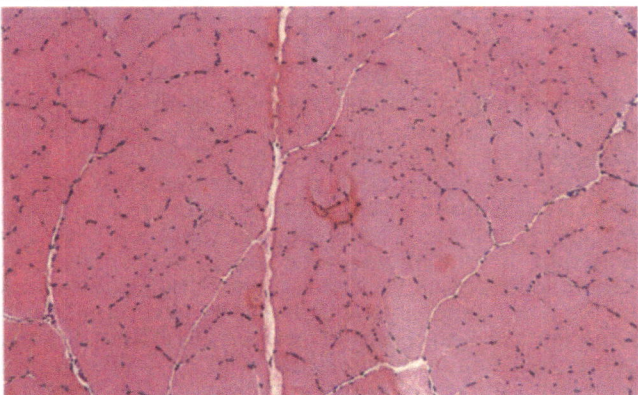

Figure 12.7 Congenital fibre type disproportion. Quadriceps biopsy for reassessment of a·10-year-old girl, who was quite severely hypotonic at birth and diagnosed as acute, infantile spinal muscular atrophy. Sat alone at 9 months, walked at 18 months, but remained hypotonic and weak, clumsy and unable to run during childhood. Long narrow face, slight ptosis, poor muscle bulk generally and absent tendon reflexes. EMG – no denervation. CPK – normal. Now aged 14 years, her strength has improved considerably and she is able to ride a bicycle. (Same case shown in Figures 12.8–12.12.) H & E × 180

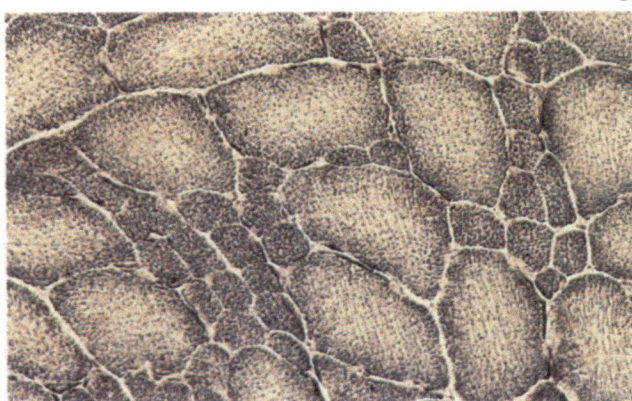

Figure 12.8 Congenital fibre type disproportion. Disparity in fibre size, which can be difficult to see with H & E (as in Figure 12.7) is well demonstrated by the histochemical reactions. There are no abnormalities of cell architecture. NADH-TR × 300

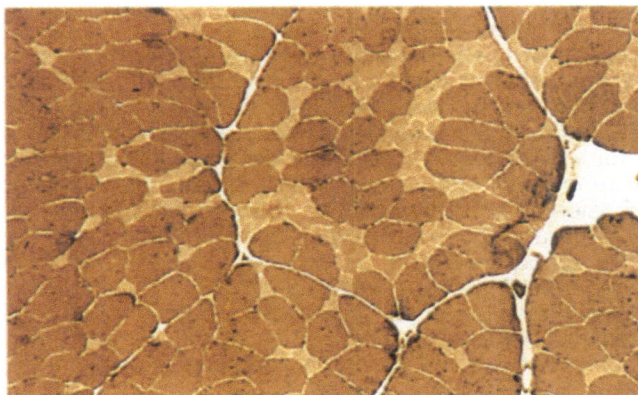

Figure 12.9 Congenital fibre type disproportion. The myosin ATP-ase reaction shows that type 1 fibres (pale) are universally small, whereas type 2 fibres (dark) are mildly hypertrophied. Myosin ATP-ase pH 9.4 × 180

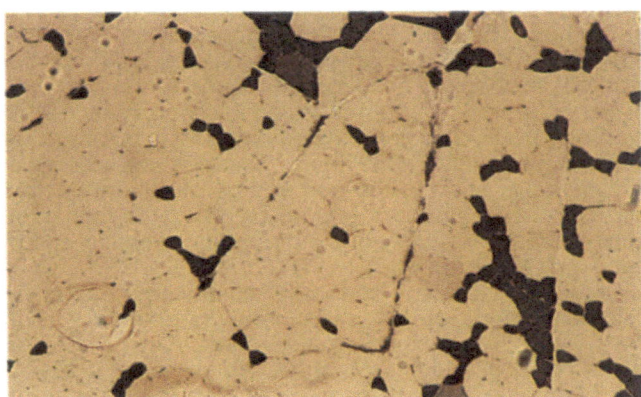

Figure 12.10 Congenital fibre type disproportion. Uniformly small (dark) type 1 fibres. There is a suggestion of mild type 2A predominance. Type 2B fibres are scarce. Myosin ATP-ase pH 4.6 × 180

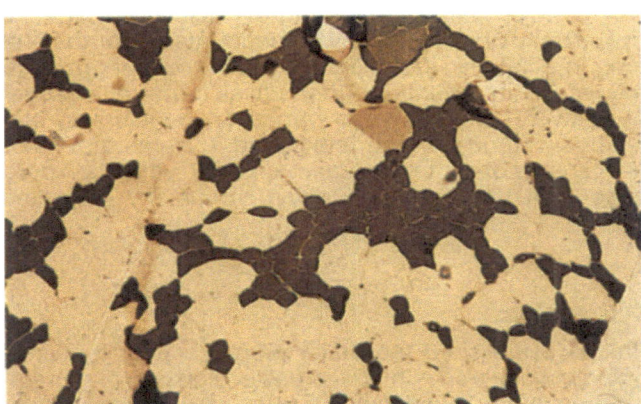

Figure 12.11 Congenital fibre type disproportion. In places groups of small type 1 fibres are present amongst the larger type 2A fibres. Myosin ATP-ase pH 4.6 × 180

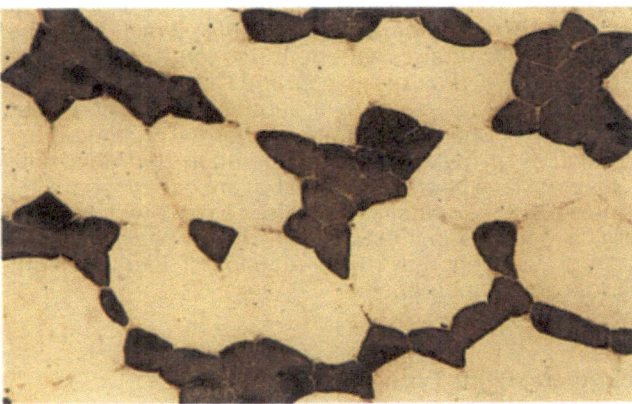

Figure 12.12 Congenital fibre type disproportion. Considerable difference in size of type 1 and 2 fibres. The relative hypertrophy of type 2 fibres probably accounts for clinical improvement, that was already apparent at 10 years in this patient. Myosin ATP-ase pH 4.6 × 300

of central nuclei. Central nuclei appear in small numbers in many myopathic disorders, but in centronuclear myopathy usually at least 25% and sometimes up to 90% of fibres in any one transverse section have a central nucleus. Signs of degeneration or regeneration are noticeably absent. The central nuclei may be found in type 1 and type 2 fibres, but frequently predominate in or are exclusive to type 1 fibres. Peripheral sarcolemmal nuclei may co-exist with central nuclei. In longitudinal sections central nuclei appear as long chains. Fibres with central nuclei may also show a perinuclear zone, devoid of myofibrils, but containing glycogen and mitochondria. This central zone extends for a variable distance along the fibre and creates a resemblance to the fetal myotube. The centre of the fibre stains deeply with the NADH-TR reaction and with PAS, but is unstained with myosin ATP-ase. In transverse section the NADH-TR reaction may reveal a radial striate pattern because the inner myofibrils are smaller than those at the periphery[15]. Differentiation with myosin ATP-ase may be poor but there is usually type 1 predominance[7] and sometimes type 1 uniformity. The type 1 fibres are generally smaller than type 2 and in some instances this discrepancy may be marked producing a bimodal distribution. Type 1 hypotrophy has been emphasized in reports of patients with hypotonia and generalized weakness, but without oculofacial involvement[9,10,12]. There is considerable individual variation in the percentage of central nuclei, degree of type 1 hypotrophy and type 1 predominance and there are no clear-cut differences between childhood and adult forms.

Only the severe, neonatal sex-linked, recessive disorder is sufficiently distinctive to be identified from the biopsy[4,5,18]. In these male infants the majority of fibres have a striking myotube appearance (Figures 12.1 and 12.2). In transverse section there are both peripheral and central nuclei, but with the myosin ATP-ase reaction almost every fibre contains either a large central or perinuclear clear zone (Figures 12.3 and 12.4). The oxidative enzyme reaction shows a reversed pattern, with a thin pale staining peripheral rim and a dark centre (Figure 12.2). There may be normal differentiation of type 1 and type 2 fibres or type 1 predominance and type 1 fibres are usually smaller than type 2 (Figures 12.3 and 12.4).

Electron microscopy confirms the absence of myofibrils from the centre of the fibre, which contains glycogen, normal mitochondria and sometimes lysosomes[12,16] (Figures 12.5 and 12.6). Myofibrillar disruption may be seen in the centre of the fibre, but peripheral myofibrils usually show normal architecture[7]. Larger foci of myofibrillar degeneration and abnormal inclusions have been described but are exceptional[10,17]. In the severe, neonatal form there is a paucity of satellite cells, a point of distinction from congenital myotonic dystrophy which may have an almost identical light microscopic appearance.

Congenital Fibre Type Disproportion

Brooke introduced the term 'congenital fibre type disproportion' for a relatively benign, hypotonic neuromuscular disorder of childhood, in which the sole pathological change was reduction in size of type 1 fibres[19]. Initially this appeared to be a consistent clinicopathological entity, but later reports reveal wide clinical variation and cast doubts on the specificity of small or hypoplastic type 1 fibres[20,21,31]. In myopathies with

generalized architectural changes, such as nemaline and centronuclear myopathy, type 1 fibres are frequently slightly smaller than type 2. However, there are also cases described in which nemaline rods or central nuclei form a very minor component of a biopsy displaying marked fibre type disproportion[23,24]. It is apparent from patients who have had multiple or sequential biopsies that whilst type 1 hypotrophy may be the only change in one site, additional morphological changes can be present elsewhere. Similarly, a family study has shown only small type 1 fibres in one member, but central nuclei in another[13]. Nevertheless, it is probable that a group exists in which fibre type disproportion is the only abnormality.

The patients with congenital fibre type disproportion described originally by Brooke and those in several later reports were infants with congenital hypotonia, frequently noted after a breech or other complicated delivery[19,20]. Respiratory difficulties in the immediate neonatal period were a problem in one case only and, compared with centronuclear myopathy, this seems to be an unusual feature[20]. Congenital dislocation of the hip and other skeletal deformities, including talipes and high arched palate, were not uncommon. Contractures, which were not present at birth frequently developed in the first few months. Limb and truncal weakness and occasionally facial weakness were observed in infancy. Motor milestones were delayed, but there was no deterioration after 2 years and most cases showed considerable improvement. The condition may be familial and both autosomal dominant and recessive inheritance have been described. A very few cases of congenital hypotonia with an initial biopsy picture of congenital fibre type disproportion have followed a downhill, eventually fatal, course, but in all cases postmortem studies have shown additional morphological abnormalities in the muscle[20,22].

In summary, provided that congenital dystrophia myotonica is excluded, congenital hypotonia with type 1 fibre hypotrophy is highly suggestive of a congenital myopathy, but it is a heterogeneous group. Despite this, in most cases where type 1 hypotrophy is the only or the dominant pathological change a favourable outcome can be anticipated. However, because a small percentage have shown progressive disease, the initial prognosis must be guarded.

A similar biopsy picture of selective type 1 hypotrophy or atrophy may be encountered for the first time in adult life, in patients with a slowly progressive myopathy. In several reported cases numerous central nuclei were also present or were seen in the biopsy of a younger member of the family and it seems that most are variants of centronuclear myopathy rather than pure congenital fibre type disproportion[12,13] (Figures 12.13–12.28).

Muscle Biopsy

Brooke established the major biopsy criteria by histographic analysis[25]. In the muscle biopsies of normal children type 1 and type 2 fibres are approximately equal in size, but in congenital fibre type disproportion type 1 fibres are smaller than type 2 by more than 12% of the average diameter of the larger fibre (Figures 12.7–12.12). Type 2 fibres are often hypertrophied, but are of uniform size. The coefficient of variability of type 2 fibres is less than 0.25. Thus even with H & E a dual fibre population of large and small fibres is usually apparent and contrasts with the great variability in fibre size observed in muscular dystrophies (Figure 12.7). Although disparity in size of type 1 and type 2 fibres is usually quite obvious with the ATP-ase reaction (Figures 12.9 and 12.10), it is advisable to make accurate measurements of fibre diameters and construct a histogram to confirm the bimodal distribution. This is particularly valuable in neonatal biopsies where the difference in fibre size is less obvious than in older children. It seems likely that whilst type 1 fibres remain hypoplastic, type 2 fibres hypertrophy with age, perhaps accounting for clinical improvement and increasing the disparity in size observed in the biopsy[26].

In pure congenital fibre type disproportion, as originally described, there is no other obvious histologic abnormality. However, it is probably artificial to define such strict pathological limits because of the cases with sparse nemaline rods or central nuclei which fall between two categories[23,24]. Type 1 hypoplasia appears to be the basic defect which links these disorders and classification is determined by the proportion of fibres with the additional morphologic abnormalities. 'Moth-eaten' fibres have, on occasion, been described[20] but congenital fibre type disproportion is not associated with necrosis or regeneration or any increase in endomysial connective tissue. Such changes almost certainly negate the diagnosis and in a neonate suggest congenital muscular dystrophy. Mild type 1 fibre predominance is sometimes found[21] and a small percentage of 2C fibres may be present in the young infant.

Nemaline Myopathy

Shy first recognized abnormal rod or thread like structures as a peculiarity in the skeletal muscle fibres of a hypotonic infant and introduced the descriptive term 'nemaline myopathy' (Greek, nema = thread)[26]. Numerous reports have confirmed that congenital nemaline myopathy is a distinct clinicopathological entity, although rods are not unique to this disorder and have been identified in a variety of myopathic and neurogenic diseases[27]. There is a clinical spectrum, but most cases are characterized by neonatal hypotonia and delayed motor milestones. Diminished fetal movements have been reported[28]. Muscle weakness is generalized, but particularly affects the paraspinal and proximal limb musculature. Facial weakness is not uncommon. Diminished muscle bulk may be striking and appears out of proportion to the relatively mild muscle weakness. Deep tendon reflexes are usually absent or reduced. There are frequently associated skeletal abnormalities, particularly high arched palate and a long thin face and not uncommonly kyphoscoliosis and pes cavus[29]. Weakness of respiratory muscles is an important clinical feature, responsible in a few instances for death in the neonatal period[28,30]. Even in less severely affected patients repeated respiratory infections in childhood are a common and sometimes serious problem. Death due to pneumonia has been reported in late childhood and 'teens[29,31]. There is also unpredictable variation in progression of the limb and truncal weakness. Some cases appear to be static. Others show slow progression, which may not be apparent until middle age[32,33]. A congenital heart lesion such as ventricular septal defect or patent ductus has been present in a few cases, but there is no constant cardiac anomaly and the cardiac muscle fibres do not contain nemaline rods[29]. The inheritance pattern is also variable[30]. Autosomal

dominant and recessive pedigrees are reported, in addition to sporadic cases. It seems that affected siblings usually follow a similar course, but there may be wide disparity between different generations of the same family.

Muscle Biopsy

The histologic changes of nemaline myopathy are distinctive and unmistakable provided that appropriate special stains are employed, but they are easily missed in H & E sections (Figure 12.29). Nemaline rods are tiny, thread-like cytoplasmic bodies, which stain blue-purple against a green background with the modified Gomori's trichrome technique in cryostat sections (Figure 12.31). With H & E stained cryostat sections, the rods are inconspicuous, although large clusters may produce red patches in the peripheral cytoplasm (Figure 12.32). In H & E stained paraffin sections rods are practically invisible. The rods may show up with phase contrast[34], but this is not a consistent finding. Special stains are undoubtedly the most reliable method of detection. If only paraffin-embedded tissue is available rods can usually be demonstrated with the trichrome method and also with PTAH (rods are bluish-black), although results are not as good as in cryostat sections.

In a congenital nemaline myopathy rods are usually found in a large percentage of fibres and sometimes in every fibre (Figures 12.31 and 12.32). Postmortem reports of a few fatal cases have shown that rods are widespread in skeletal muscles, including diaphragm, oesophagus and pharyngeal muscles but there is considerable variation in the extent of rod formation in different muscles[28,32]. Also, there is no clear correlation between the number of rod-containing fibres and the degree of clinical weakness.

Rods are most numerous at the periphery of affected cells and may form large subsarcolemmal collections (Figures 12.31 and 12.32). Smaller clusters and single rods may be dispersed amongst the myofibrils. Nemaline rods often impart a speckled appearance at low magnification (Figure 12.33) and occasionally occupy up to three-quarters of the cross-sectional area of a single fibre.

Nemaline rods can be found in both type 1 and type 2 fibres, but there is frequently a type 1 uniformity (Figure 12.30). There may be considerable variation in fibre distribution between adjacent fascicles, from a normal mosaic to type 1 uniformity. The fibres may be of uniform size, but some cases have shown type 1 atrophy or hypoplasia and a bimodal distribution (Figure 12.34). There are often small numbers of central nuclei and the sarcolemmal nuclei may be large and vesicular with prominent nucleoli. Rods are also found in intra-fusal fibres.

Electron microscopy reveals that rods are electron-dense bodies of irregular size and shape, with variation in pattern according to the plane of section (Figure 12.35). In longitudinal section the rods are roughly rectangular and appear to be an array of parallel filaments with regular cross-striations, whereas in transverse section there is a polygonal outline and a basketweave or lattice pattern. Individual rods vary between 2 and 5 μm in length and 0.15 and 1.5 μm in width. Beneath the sarcolemma the rods have a haphazard arrangement, but in the centre of the fibre they are often orientated longitudinally. Clusters of rods may be associated with myofibrillar degeneration. Single rods can be found within myofibrils in continuity

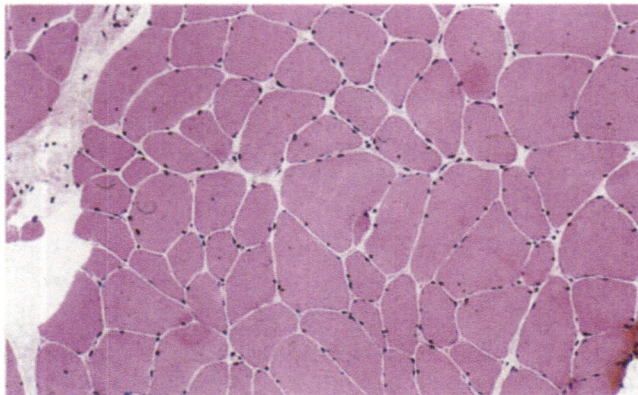

Figure 12.13 Familial type 1 atrophy, associated with cardiomyopathy. 30-year-old man with mild proximal muscle weakness. Family history disclosed that six other members of his family were similarly affected, suggesting autosomal dominant inheritance (see diagram of family tree, Figure 12.22). In addition to skeletal muscle disease he has a large heart and ECG evidence of a conduction defect. The proximal myopathy appears to be only slowly progressive, but two brothers have died at an early age from cardio-myopathy. Quadriceps biopsy shows a dual population of small and large fibres with a few central nuclei. (Same case is shown in Figures 12.14–12.18.)   H & E × 180

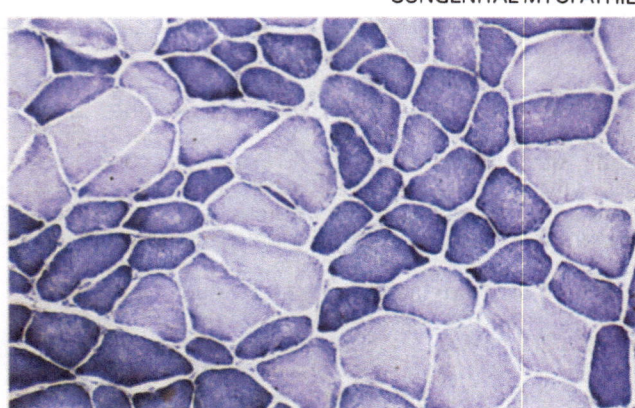

Figure 12.14 Familial type 1 atrophy. Almost all type 1 fibres are small, whereas many type 2 fibres are mildly hypertrophied.   NADH-TR × 180

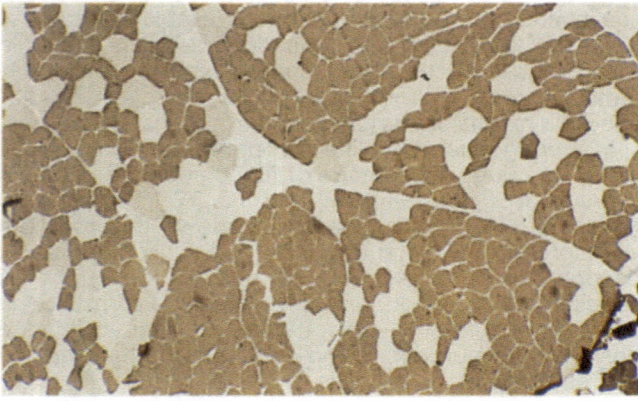

Figure 12.15 Familial type 1 atrophy showing type 1 predominance. (Type 1 – dark).   Myosin ATP-ase pH 4.6 × 30

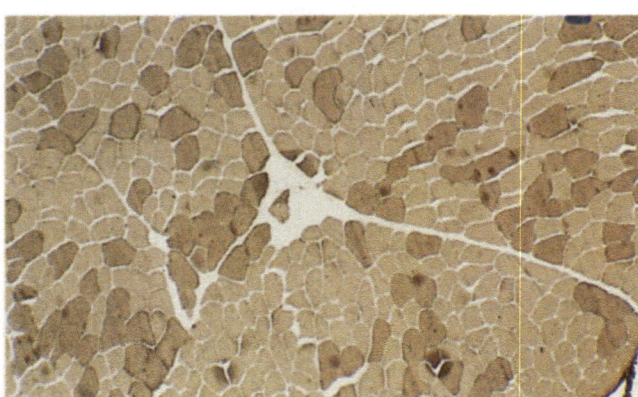

Figure 12.16 Familial type 1 atrophy. Serial section to Figure 12.15. There is moderate type 1 predominance. (Type 1 – light).   Myosin ATP-ase pH 9.4 × 30

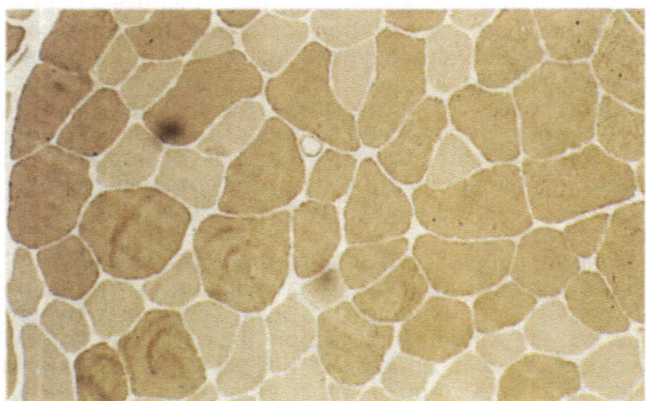

Figure 12.17 Familial type 1 atrophy. Myosin ATP-ase reveals the dual fibre population. Type 1 fibres are uniformly small, whereas type 2 fibres are mildly hypertrophied.   Myosin ATP-ase pH 9.4 × 180

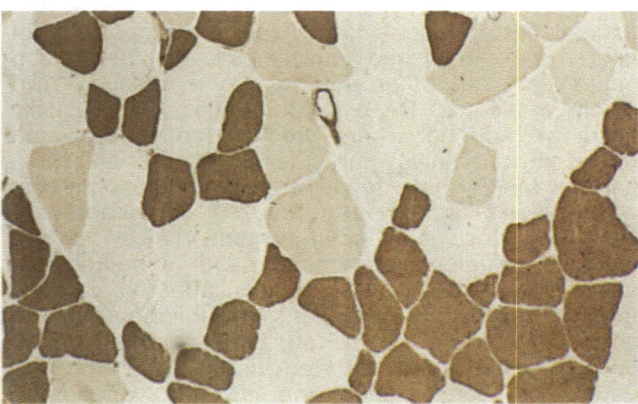

Figure 12.18 Familial type 1 atrophy. Serial section to Figure 12.17. Both type 2A and 2B fibres are present.   Myosin ATP-ase pH 4.6 × 180

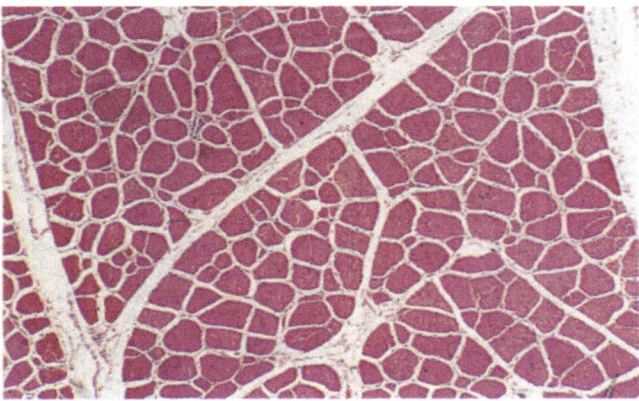

Figure 12.19 Familial type 1 atrophy associated with cardiomyopathy. Quadriceps muscle obtained at postmortem from 38-year-old brother of case shown in Figures 12.13–12.18. Death was due to cardiac failure. He was only mildly incapacitated by proximal muscle weakness. The biopsy shows a similar dual fibre population to that of the younger brother, but with greater disparity in fibre size.   H & E × 75

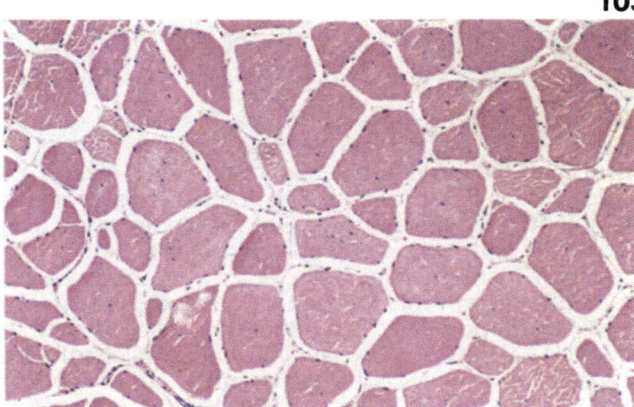

Figure 12.20 Same case as in Figure 12.19 shows an increase in central nuclei. There are occasional split fibres, presumably due to functional overloading of the larger fibres, but widespread degenerative changes are notably absent.   H & E × 180

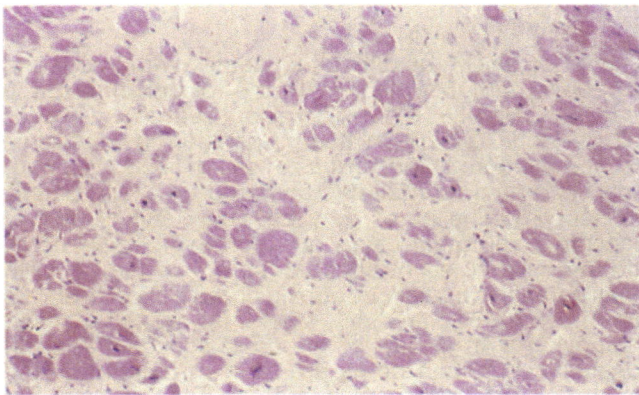

Figure 12.21 Heart muscle from case shown in Figures 12.19 and 12.20. At postmortem there was a greatly enlarged heart with dilatation of all chambers. The myocardium shows diffuse interstitial fibrosis. The coronary arteries were not significantly atheromatous. This family illustrates the occasional association between cardiomyopathy and congenital myopathy in the fibre type disproportion/centronuclear myopathy category. The pathogenesis of myocardial disease is unknown, but it is the more sinister lesion.   H & E × 75

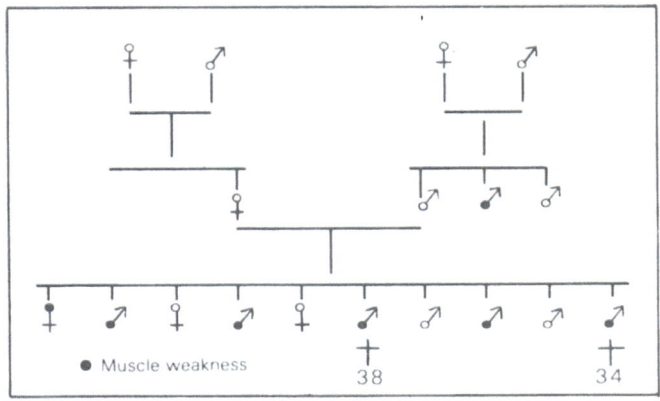

Figure 12.22 Family tree of the two brothers with type 1 atrophy and cardiomyopathy shown in Figures 12.13–12.21. Affected members are indicated by solid symbols

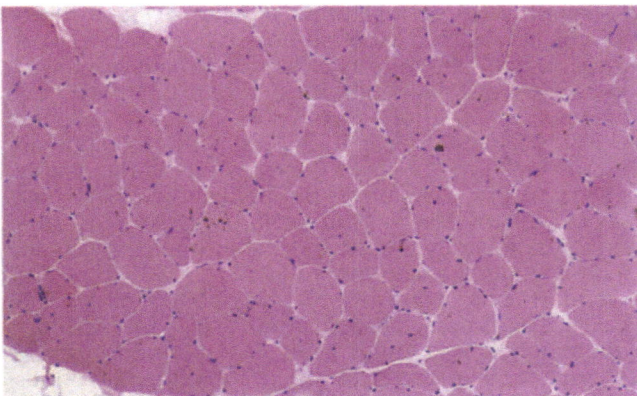

Figure 12.23 Type 1 fibre atrophy with central nuclei. Deltoid biopsy from a 40-year-old woman aware of mild weakness for several years. She had never been able to run properly. She showed mild generalized weakness, including facial weakness. Deep tendon reflexes were absent in the lower limbs. In addition she had ECG evidence of a cardiac conduction defect. No known family history. The biopsy shows small and normal size fibres with no evidence of degenerative changes. (Same case shown in Figures 12.24–12.28.)   H & E × 180

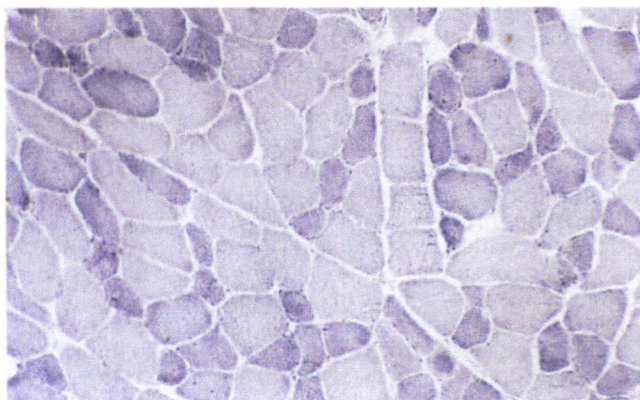

Figure 12.24 Type 1 fibre atrophy with central nuclei. The small fibres are all type 1 fibres.   NADH-TR × 180

with the Z band (Figure 12.36) and sometimes there appears to be a gradation between slightly thickened Z bands and the larger well-defined rods. This location, a structural similarity and similar response to protease treatment, support the view that rod bodies are Z line anomalies, probably lateral polymers of the Z line unit[35]. The long filaments are actin and small cross-linking filaments, responsible for the basketweave pattern, are α-actinin. Tropomyosin is probably also a component. It seems likely that all rods have the same basic structure and that conflicting reports of measurements of filament width and periodicity can be explained by differences in the angle of sectioning. Although the cause of rod formation is still unknown, a defect in regulation of actin filament length in diseased muscle has been suggested[35].

Although nemaline rods in profusion are characteristic of congenital nemaline myopathy, they occasionally appear in other disorders, such as polymyositis, drug-induced myopathy and chronic peripheral neuropathy and even in the normal myotendinous junction[27]. Thus the presence of nemaline rods must not distract the observer from evidence of another type of neuromuscular disease, especially in patients presenting after early childhood. Inflammation and fibrosis are not features of the congenital myopathy and do not appear in adult life.

Nemaline rods have not been described in smooth muscle. They have been identified in cardiac muscle, often in hypertrophied fibres in cases quite unrelated to skeletal muscle nemaline myopathy. Generally there is no relationship between the nemaline myopathy of skeletal muscle and the appearance of rods in cardiac muscle. However, there is one recent report of rods in myocardial conducting tissue of a patient who died of cardiac failure and also had rods in skeletal muscle[36].

Central Core Disease

A central core aptly describes a well demarcated central zone, devoid of normal histochemical reactivity that extends longitudinally throughout most of the fibre. In contrast to other forms of congenital myopathy the majority of reported cases are familial, with a consistent autosomal dominant pattern of inheritance, suggesting a single nosological entity[37]. However, there are a few exceptions: cases with a different genetic background and cases showing morphological overlap with other disorders.

Central core disease is not a cause of severe neonatal hypotonia or birth asphyxia. In some patients motor development is retarded and in others motor milestones are normal and weakness is not apparent until after the child has begun walking[37-38]. There is frequently an association with congenital dislocation of the hips, which may of itself delay walking. Pes cavus and kyphoscoliosis are also quite common[39]. The weakness is mild and symmetrical and chiefly affects proximal muscles. Facial weakness is often present. Patients may be thin, but do not usually show any significant muscle wasting. An exceptional and probably autosomal recessive sibship showing focal, asymmetrical muscle wasting has been described[40]. Deep tendon reflexes are absent in some patients and preserved in others. In almost all cases weakness is static or at the most slowly progressive[41]. Survival into the eighties is recorded[37]. Genuine onset, as opposed to recognition in adult life seems to be most unusual, but has been reported in one family[42].

Undoubtedly the most important association is with malignant hyperpyrexia. Many patients who show susceptibility to malignant hyperpyrexia do not have a distinctive neuromuscular disease and biopsy changes are non-specific. Central core disease is the only well defined myopathy known to carry a risk. The malignant hyperthermia trait has been identified in patients with typical childhood onset central core disease[43]. A raised CPK has been present in some but not all of these susceptible patients. Orthopaedic problems requiring surgical correction are common amongst the congenital myopathies. The association of central core disease and malignant hyperpyrexia emphasizes the need for preliminary muscle biopsy under local or, if necessary, carefully monitored general anaesthesia (see Chapter 16). Biopsy is the only sure way of distinguishing between these myopathies and identifying patients with central core disease who are at risk from a fatal complication of an otherwise benign disorder.

Muscle Biopsy

Central cores can be difficult to identify with H & E and are best demonstrated with the oxidative enzyme reaction (NADH-TR) in cryostat sections (Figures 12.37 and 12.38). In this preparation in transverse section the core stands out as a well-defined, rounded, unstained area, sometimes bordered by a thin deeply stained rim. The cores may be single and central or eccentric[37]. In other cases between two and six cores are present in each affected fibre[41]. There is also considerable variation in core diameter. Some are as small as 4 μm diameter, others up to 30 μm and occupying a large part of the cross-sectional area. In longitudinal section cores are seen to extend for the length of the biopsy and are thus thought to run continuously throughout the whole muscle fibre. With H & E the core region has a homogeneous appearance and stains more deeply than the rest of the fibre. Cores are pale staining with PAS and phosphorylase. With myosin ATP-ase cores again may be pale, but are sometimes barely detectable. Biopsy studies have shown that the proportion of muscle fibres containing cores has varied widely from case to case and there is no correlation between the number of cores and the degree of weakness. In most instances at least 40% of fibres have been affected and sometimes almost 100%. However, there are reports of families where biopsy of a parent has revealed numerous cores, but they have been sparse or non-existent in clinically affected children[38]. This suggests that the core is not the primary abnormality, but an associated architectural change that develops with age. Sequential biopsies have revealed this evolution in at least one case. Nevertheless, in the majority extensive core formation is already apparent in early childhood[39].

Cores are only found in type 1 fibres and in all cases of typical central core disease there is a marked type 1 predominance and often type 1 uniformity. Type 1 predominance appears to be a fundamental abnormality. It is present early in childhood even in those cases with sparse cores. The only exceptions, to have shown normal fibre type differentiation, are cases with unusual clinical features and these are probably separate entities.

In central core disease there is usually abnormal variation in fibre size (Figure 12.37). A small proportion of type 1 fibres may be quite severely atrophic or hypoplastic, but they are not grouped and retain a rounded outline. There are often small numbers of central sarcolemmal nuclei. Nemaline rods have occasionally been seen in isolated fibres. There is no regeneration, necrosis or inflammation. Mild interstitial fibrosis is sometimes present in the adult biopsy.

Electron microscopy reveals variable structural disorganization within the core. Mitochondria, glycogen and sarcotubular profiles are absent, although T-tubules persist. The filamentous organization of the sarcomeres may be well preserved and striations retained, but the sarcomeres are abnormally short and the Z lines often have a zig-zag appearance. In other cores there is severe disruption of the myofibrils and Z lines are completely absent. These two patterns have been referred to as 'structured' and 'unstructured' cores, but this distinction has no diagnostic significance[44]. All degrees of filamentous disruption may co-exist in the same biopsy and even in different parts of the same fibre. The transition from the core to normal fibre is usually abrupt. There may be a slight accumulation of mitochondria around the core, responsible for the dark rim seen with the NADH-TR reaction. The structural similarity between the core and the target fibre of denervation (see Chapter 3) raises the possibility of a neural defect in central core disease.

Multicore Disease

Multicore disease is a less well-defined clinico-pathological entity than central core disease. The name was first introduced by Engel[45] to describe a benign congenital myopathy associated with multiple tiny foci of myofibrillar disruption. Multicores are quite distinct from central cores, which are larger and extend the full length of a fibre. The name 'minicore' seems far more appropriate and less confusing than 'multicore', but it has not been widely adopted. There is no clear pattern of inheritance of multicore disease. Sporadic and familial cases are reported, but no large family trees[46]. Clinically there is usually mild neonatal hypotonia. Early motor development is a little slow and the young child appears clumsy[46]. Muscle weakness is mild and generalized and in most cases non-progressive. Facial muscles are occasionally involved. Exceptions to this benign pattern are severe and fatal weakness reported in a Chinese infant[47] and a progressive case of adult onset[48].

Biopsy

Multicores (or minicores) refer to multiple small foci of loss of cross-striation with loss of activity of oxidative enzymes and myofibrillar ATP-ase. These defects are of course difficult to recognize in an H & E section, except with polarized light, when they appear as oval dark defects (Figure 12.39). With the oxidative enzyme reaction in transverse section there are tiny unstained discoid foci (usually around $2-8\,\mu$m diameter and almost always less than $15\,\mu$m diameter). These are irregularly distributed throughout the sarcoplasm creating a rather smudgy appearance (Figure 12.40). Some lesions may have a targetoid appearance with a peripheral dark rim in the oxidative enzyme reaction. The cores are found in both type 1 and type 2 fibres in any one transverse section[49]. Pale areas are also seen with PAS staining and with myosin ATP-ase, but these do not always correspond with the areas that are negative for oxidative enzymes. In longitudinal section

the lesions are short and discontinuous, with variation in size and shape. Some are disc-shaped with transverse orientation, others are fusiform and parallel to the long axis of the fibre.

In addition, the biopsy shows features common to most congenital myopathies, a clear type 1 predominance, type 1 hypotrophy or atrophy and a small proportion of central nuclei[46]. There may be fairly marked variability in fibre size, with small type 1 fibres and hypertrophic type 2 fibres. A slight increase in endomysial connective tissue has been described, but the usual negatives apply, no necrosis, regeneration or inflammation.

Electron microscopy confirms the minicores are foci of myofilament disruption and Z band streaming. Mitochondria are usually absent. The structural disorganization only involves a few sarcomeres ($2-10$) in a very small group of adjacent myofibrils and is sharply demarcated from surrounding normal myofibrils.

Differential Diagnosis of Congenital Myopathies

The clinical differential diagnosis of congenital myopathy includes all causes of the floppy infant, cerebral and metabolic disorders, in addition to other neuromuscular diseases. These disorders can be very difficult to distinguish in the early months and muscle biopsy is often an essential investigation. Complicated delivery and birth asphyxia can occur with a congenital myopathy and should not be taken as proof of a cerebral cause. Facial weakness, ptosis and ophthalmoplegia are clinical features of particular diagnostic significance since they virtually exclude spinal muscular atrophy and are commonest in myotubular myopathy, congenital dystrophia myotonica and the mitochondrial myopathies. Investigation of a floppy infant must include a detailed family history and at least visual examination of both parents and any siblings. In some cases further investigation and even muscle biopsy of a parent may be appropriate.

In most cases, when the full range of histochemical stains is applied, congenital myopathies are easily recognized. Electron microscopy is particularly valuable in the neonate, as structural changes in tiny fibres are sometimes difficult to appreciate. Even if structural abnormalities are not detected, type 1 fibre predominance or small type 1 fibres strongly suggest a congenital myopathy. In contrast, CNS disorders often produce type 2 fibre atrophy (Figures 12.41–12.44). Fibrosis and inflammation positively exclude congenital myopathy and strongly suggest congenital muscular dystrophy.

Diagnostic problems may be encountered particularly in three areas.

(1) Distinction between congenital dystrophia myotonica and myotubular myopathy. In the neonate, congenital dystrophia myotonica and myotubular myopathy may have very similar histology. Electron microscopy reveals a paucity of satellite cells in myotubular myopathy. However, it would be absurd to rely upon this method when the disorders can be simply and reliably separated by examination of the mother. Congenital dystrophia myotonica is always due to maternal transmission.

(2) Distinction between congenital fibre type disproportion and spinal muscular atrophy. The problem should not be emphasized unduly, but

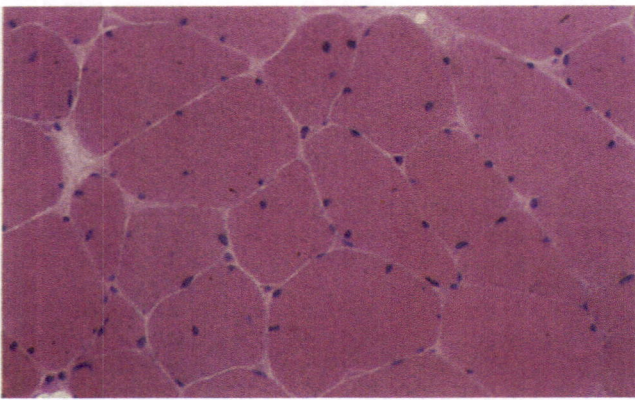

Figure 12.25 Type 1 fibre atrophy with central nuclei. Many of the smaller fibres have central nuclei. There is no evidence of fibrosis, inflammation, necrosis or regeneration.   H & E × 300

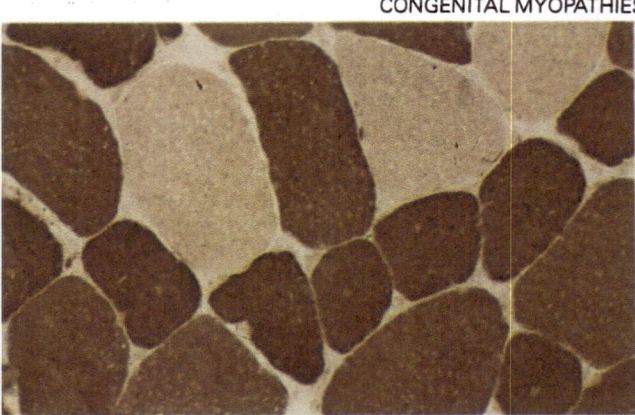

Figure 12.26 Type 1 atrophy with central nuclei. The myosin ATP-ase reaction shows that all the small, centrally nucleated fibres are type 1 fibres, although not every type 1 fibre is small. Type 2 fibres are of normal size.   ATP-ase pH 4.5 × 300

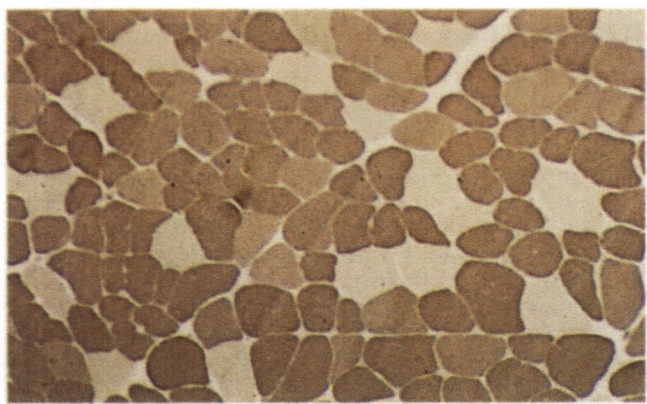

Figure 12.27 Type 1 fibre atrophy with central nuclei. There is mild type 1 fibre predominance.   ATP-ase pH 4.5 × 180

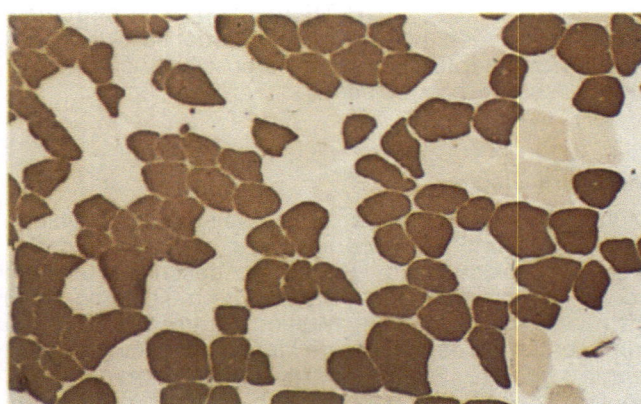

Figure 12.28 Type 1 fibre atrophy with central nuclei. Serial section to Figure 12.27. These abnormalities in conjunction with the clinical picture suggest this is a congenital myopathy in the centronuclear/congenital fibre type disproportion category. The story suggests there was mild weakness in childhood, but it did not become a problem until adult life.   ATP-ase pH 4.2 × 180

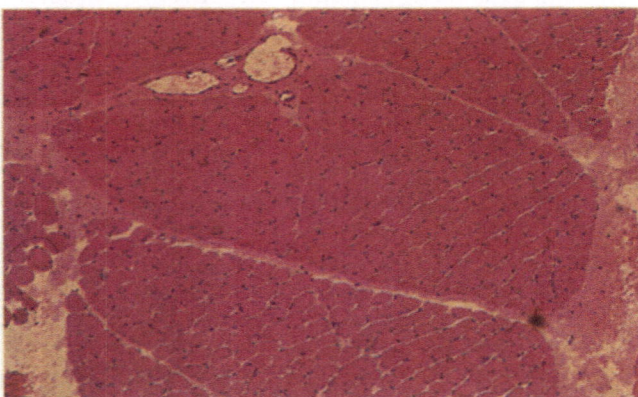

Figure 12.29 Nemaline myopathy. 9-year-old boy who attained normal early milestones, but was noted at school to be clumsy and poor at sport. He tired easily and complained of aching legs after exercise. He showed mild global weakness and hypotonia. There was slight facial weakness. Reflexes were difficult to elicit. CPK normal. His parents and one sister are clinically normal. 5 years later his condition is unchanged. Deltoid biopsy at low magnification shows no abnormality, apart from the fact that the fibres are smaller than expected for his age. (Same case shown in Figures 12.25–12.27, 12.30 and 12.31.)   H & E × 75

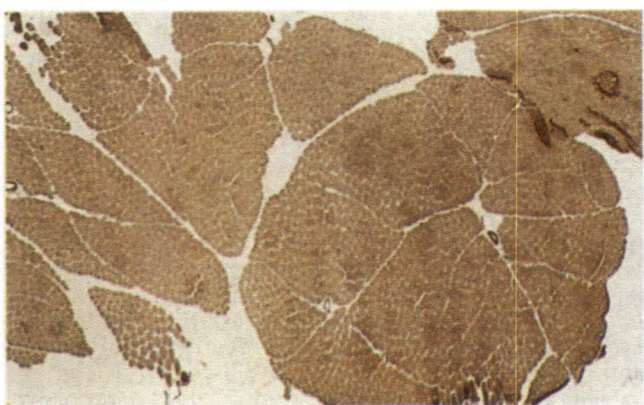

Figure 12.30 Nemaline myopathy. Uniform fibre typing with histochemical reaction of type 1 fibres. No type 2 fibres are present.   ATP-ase pH 9.4 × 30

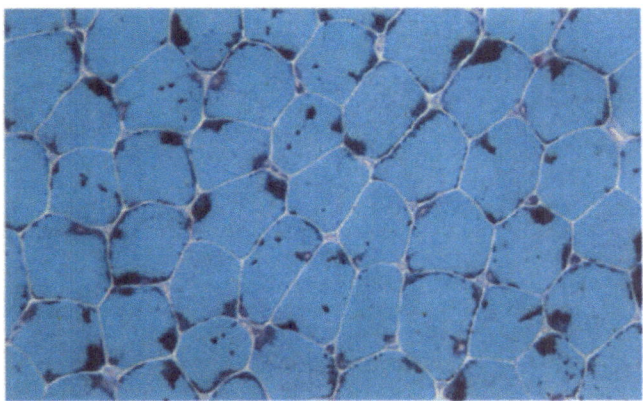

Figure 12.31 Nemaline myopathy. The small dark blue rod bodies stand out clearly against the green cytoplasm with the trichrome reaction. There are large peripheral clusters and a few smaller internal specks. Every fibre contains some rods.   Gomori's trichrome × 180

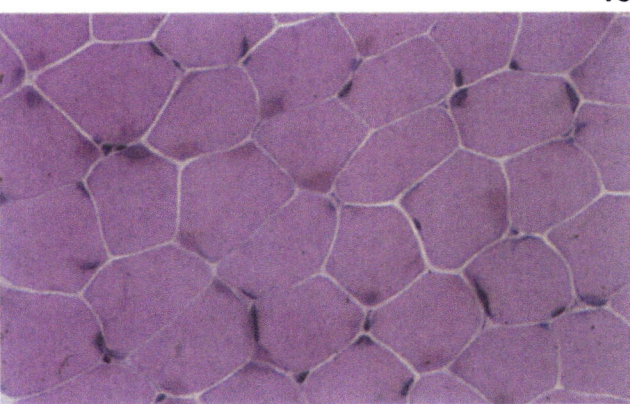

Figure 12.32 Nemaline myopathy. The rod bodies are much harder to detect with an H & E stain, but when numerous, as in this case, small peripheral eosinophilic smudges may be seen.   H & E × 300

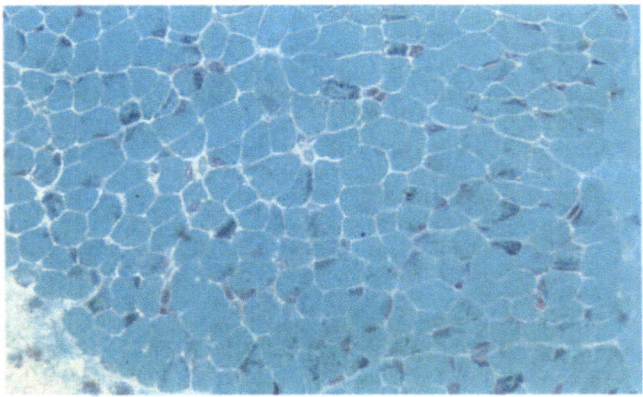

Figure 12.33 Nemaline myopathy. Quadriceps biopsy from a severely hypotonic, areflexic, 3-month-old baby girl. The trichrome preparation has a slightly speckled appearance. In this age group, when fibres are so tiny, rod bodies are easily overlooked. Electron microscopy provides useful confirmation. In this case the rods were numerous. (Same case shown in Figure 12.34.)   Gomori's trichrome × 180

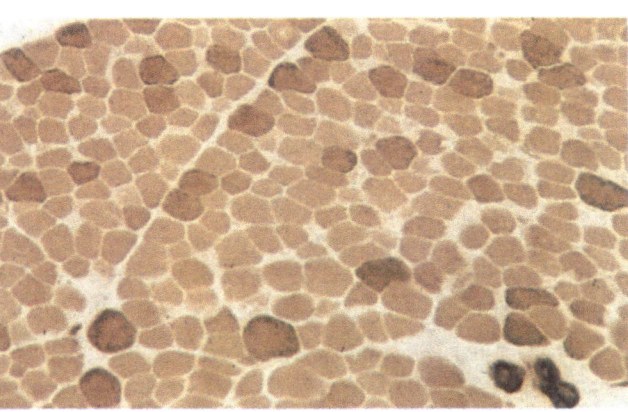

Figure 12.34 Nemaline myopathy in a 3-month-old girl. There is type 1 predominance with small type 1 fibres, similar to congenital fibre type disproportion. Nemaline myopathy may show this disparity in fibre size. The prognosis for rod body myopathy in the neonate is usually worse than for uncomplicated congenital fibre type disproportion, because the respiratory muscles are involved. This child suffered repeated respiratory infections and died at 2 years of age.   ATP-ase pH 9.4 × 180

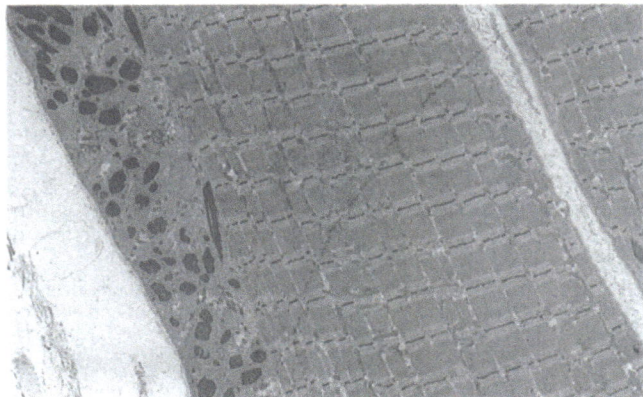

Figure 12.35 Nemaline rods. Electron-dense bodies, irregular in size and shape, clustered beneath the sarcolemma. Inner myofibrils have a normal arrangement.   EM × 5700

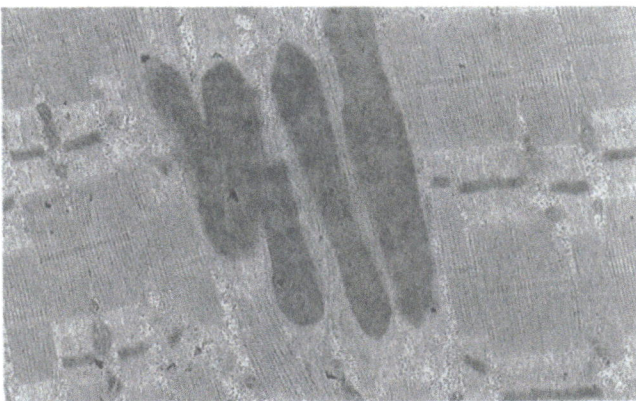

Figure 12.36 Nemaline rods. Electron-dense, rectangular arrays of parallel filaments, apparently replacing the Z band. This characteristic location supports the view that rods are polymers of the Z line unit.   EM × 19 000

the disorders might be confused in a neonatal biopsy before type grouping has developed in SMA. Even at this early stage some larger type 1 fibres can usually be found in SMA, but not in congenital fibre type disproportion, where the type 1 fibres are uniformly small.

(3) The category of benign congenital hypotonia. In a young infant the problem is sometimes to decide if minor biopsy changes are of any real significance. The term 'benign congenital hypotonia' was originally introduced by Walton to distinguish spinal muscular atrophy from non-progressive weakness. The advent of muscle histochemistry and recognition of the congenital myopathies greatly reduced the number of cases assigned to the non-specific category. However, undoubtedly there are some infants, usually with mild hypotonia and no other signs, who do not have distinctive histology although biopsy is not entirely normal (Figures 12.45–12.48). The biopsy may show residual large type 1 (Wolfhart B) fibres and sometimes mild type 2 atrophy. Progressive muscle disease is most unlikely and if there is no evidence of a CNS disorder guarded reassurance may be given. Perhaps these cases represent the mildest form of maturational delay and can justifiably be labelled 'benign congenital hypotonia'.

References

1. Brooke, M. H. (1977). Congenital (more or less) muscle diseases. In *A Clinician's View of Neuromuscular Diseases.* pp. 200–218. (Baltimore: Williams and Wilkins)

2. Spiro, A. J., Shy, G. M. and Gonatas, N. K. (1966). Myotubular myopathy. *Arch. Neurol. (Chic.),* **14**, 1–13

3. Fardeau, M. (1982). Congenital myopathies. In Mastaglia, F. L. and Walton, J. (eds.) *Skeletal Muscle Pathology.* pp. 161–203. (Edinburgh: Churchill Livingstone)

4. van Wijngaarden, G. K., Fleury, P., Bethlem, J. and Meijer, A. E. F. H. (1969). Familial myotubular myopathy. *Neurology,* **19**, 901–8.

5. Barth, P. G., van Wijngaarden, G. K. and Bethlem, J. (1975). X-linked myotubular myopathy with fatal neonatal asphyxia. *Neurology,* **25**, 531–6

6. Kinoshita, M. and Cadman, T. E. (1968). Myotubular myopathy. *Arch. Neurol. (Chic.),* **18**, 265–71

7. Bill, P. L. A., Cole, G. and Proctor, N. S. F. (1979). Centronuclear myopathy. *J. Neurol., Neurosurg. Psychiatry,* **42**, 548–56.

8. Bradley, W. G., Price, D. L. and Watanabe, C. K. (1970). Familial centronuclear myopathy. *J. Neurol., Neurosurg. Psychiatry,* **33**, 687–93

9. Engel, W. K., Gold, G. N. and Karpati, G. (1968). Type 1 fibre hypotrophy and central nuclei. *Arch. Neurol. (Chic.),* **18**, 435–44

10. Lee, Y.-S. and Yip, W. C. L. (1981). A fatal congenital myopathy with severe type 1 fibre atrophy, central nuclei and multicores. *J. Neurol. Sci.,* **50**, 277–90

11. Harriman, D. G. F. and Haleem, M. A. (1972). Centronuclear myopathy in old age. *J. Pathol.,* **108**, 237–48

12. Karpati, G., Carpenter, S. and Nelson, R. F. (1970). Type 1 muscle fibre atrophy and central nuclei. A rare familial neuromuscular disease. *J. Neurol. Sci.,* **10**, 489–500

13. Kinoshita, M., Satoyoshi, E. and Matsuo, N. (1975). Myotubular myopathy and type 1 fibre atrophy in a family. *J. Neurol. Sci.,* **26**, 575–82

14. Bethlem, J., Wijngaarden, G. K., Meijer, A. E. F. H. and Hulsmann, W. C. (1969). Neuromuscular disease with type 1 fibre atrophy, central nuclei and myotube-like structures. *Neurology,* **19**, 705–10

15. Bill, P., Cole, G., Proctor, N. S. F., Saffer, D. and Botes, A. (1979). Crural hypertrophy associated with centronuclear myopathy. *J. Neurol., Neurosurg. Psychiatry,* **42**, 542–7

16. Headington, J. T., McNamara, J. O. and Brownell, A. K. (1975). Centronuclear myopathy: histochemistry and electron microscopy. *Arch. Pathol. (Chic.),* **99**, 16–24

17. Jadro-Santel, D., Grcevic, N., Dogan, S., Franjic, J. and Benc, H. (1980). Centronuclear myopathy with type 1 fibre hypotrophy and fingerprint inclusions associated with Marfan's syndrome. *J. Neurol. Sci.,* **45**, 43–56

18. Askanas, V., Engel, W. K., Reddy, N. B., Barth, P. G., Bethlem, J., Krauss, D. R., Hibberd, M. E., Lawrence, J. V. and Carter, L. S. (1979). X-linked recessive congenital muscle fibre hypotrophy with central nuclei. *Arch. Neurol. (Chic.),* **36**, 604–9

19. Brooke, M. H. (1971). A neuromuscular disease characterised by fibre type disproportion. In Kakulas, B. A. (ed.) *Clinical Studies in Myology.* (Amsterdam: Excerpta Medica)

20. Cavanagh, N. P. C., Lake, B. D. and McMeniman, P. (1979). Congenital fibre type disproportion myopathy. *Arch. Dis. Childh.,* **54**, 735–43

21. Clancy, R. R., Kelts, K. A. and Oehlert, J. W. (1980). Clinical variability in congenital fiber type disproportion. *J. Neurol. Sci.,* **46**, 257–66

22. Spiro, A. J., Horoupian, D. S. and Snyder, D. R. (1977). Biopsy and autopsy studies of congenital muscle fiber type disproportion: a broadening concept. *Neurology,* **27**, 405

23. Sugie, H., Hanson, R., Rasmussen, G. and Verity, M. A. (1982). Congenital neuromuscular disease with type 1 fibre hypotrophy, ophthalmoplegia and myofibril degeneration. *J. Neurol., Neurosurg. Psychiatry,* **45**, 507–12

24. Kinoshita, M., Satoyoshi, E. and Kumagai, M. (1975). Familial type 1 fiber atrophy. *J. Neurol. Sci.,* **25**, 11–17

25. Brooke, M. H. and Engel, W. K. (1969). The histographic analysis of human muscle biopsies with regard to fiber types. 4. Children's biopsies. *Neurology,* **19**, 591–605

26. Shy, G. M., Engel, W. K., Somers, J. E. and Wanko, T. (1963). Nemaline myopathy: a new congenital myopathy. *Brain,* **86**, 793–807

27. Neustein, H. B. (1973). Nemaline myopathy: a family study with three autopsied cases. *Arch. Pathol. (Chic.),* **96**, 192–5

28. Hudgson, P., Gardner-Medwin, D., Fulthorpe, J. J. and Walton, J. N. (1967). Nemaline myopathy. *Neurology,* **17**, 1125–42

29. McComb, R. D., Marksbery, W. R. and O'Connor, W. N. (1979). Fatal neonatal nemaline myopathy with multiple congenital anomalies. *J. Pediatr.,* **94**, 47–51

30. Kondo, K. and Yuasa, T. (1980). Genetics of congenital nemaline myopathy. *Muscle Nerve,* **3**, 308–15

31. Dahl, D. S. and Klutzow, F. W. (1974). Congenital rod disease: further evidence of innervational abnormalities as the basis for the clinicopathologic features. *J. Neurol. Sci.,* **23**, 371–85

32. Hopkins, I. J., Russell Lindsey, J. and Ford, F. R. (1966). Nemaline myopathy: a long-term clinicopathologic study of affected mother and daughter. *Brain,* **89**, 299–311

33. Engel, A. G. (1966). Recent studies on neuromuscular disease. Late-onset rod myopathy (a new syndrome?). Light and electron microscopic observations in two cases. *Mayo Clin. Proc.,* **41**, 713–41

34. Fulthorpe, J. J., Gardner-Medwin, D., Hudgson, P. and Walton, J. N. (1968). Nemaline myopathy: a histological and ultrastructural study of skeletal muscle from a case presenting with infantile hypotonia. *Neurology,* **19**, 735–48

35. Yamaguchi, M., Robson, R. M., Stromer, M. H., Dahl, D. S. and Oda, T. (1982). Nemaline myopathy rod bodies: structure and composition. *J. Neurol. Sci.,* **56**, 35–56

36. Meier, C., Voellmy, W., Gertsch, M., Zimmerman, A. and Geissbuhler, J. (1984). Nemaline myopathy appearing in adults as cardiomyopathy. *Arch. Neurol.*, **41**, 443–5

37. Byrne, E., Blumbergs, P. C. and Hallpike, J. F. (1982). Central core disease: study of a family with five affected generations. *J. Neurol. Sci.*, **53**, 77–83

38. Morgan-Hughes, J. A., Brett, E. M., Lake, B. D. and Tome, F. M. S. (1973). Central core disease or not? Observations on a family with a non-progressive myopathy. *Brain*, **96**, 527–36

39. Armstrong, R. M., Koenigsberger, R., Mellinger, J. and Lovelace, R. E. (1971). Central core disease with congenital hip dislocation: study of two families. *Neurology*, **21**, 369–76

40. Dubowitz, V. and Platts, M. (1965). Central core disease of muscle with focal wasting. *J. Neurol., Neurosurg. Psychiatry*, **28**, 432–7

41. Isaacs, H., Heffron, J. J. A and Badenhorst, M. (1975). Central core disease: a correlated genetic, histochemical ultramicroscopic, and biochemical study. *J. Neurol., Neurosurg. Psychiatry*, **38**, 1177–86

42. Patterson, V. H., Hill, T. R. G., Fletcher, P. J. H. and Heron, J. R. (1979). Central core disease. Clinical and pathological evidence of progression within a family. *Brain*, **102**, 581–94

43. Eng, G. D., Epstein, B. S., Engel, W. K., McKay, D. W. and McKay, R. (1978). Malignant hyperthermia and central core disease in a child with congenital dislocating hips. *Arch. Neurol.*, **35**, 189–97

44. Neville, H. E. (1973). Ultrastructural changes in muscle disease. In Walton, J. N. (ed.) *Muscle Biopsy. A Modern Approach*. pp. 389–393. (Philadelphia: W. B. Saunders)

45. Engel, A. G., Gomez, M. R. and Groover, R. V. (1971). Multicore disease. A recently recognised congenital myopathy associated with multifocal degeneration of muscle fibres. *Mayo Clin. Proc.*, **46**, 666–81

46. Ricoy, J. R., Cabello, A. and Goizueta, G. (1980). Myopathy with multiple minicore. Report of two siblings. *J. Neurol. Sci.*, **48**, 81–92

47. Lee, Y. S. and Yip, W. C. L. (1981). A fatal congenital myopathy with severe type 1 fibre atrophy, central nuclei and multicores. *J. Neurol. Sci.*, **50**, 277–90

48. Bonnette, H., Roelofs, R. and Olson, W. H. (1974). Multicore disease: report of a case with onset in middle age. *Neurology*, **24**, 1039–44

49. Heffner, R., Cohen, M., Duffner, P. and Daigler, G. (1976). Multicore disease in twins. *J. Neurol., Neurosurg. Psychiatry*, **39**, 602–6

Figures 12.37–12.48 may be found overleaf.

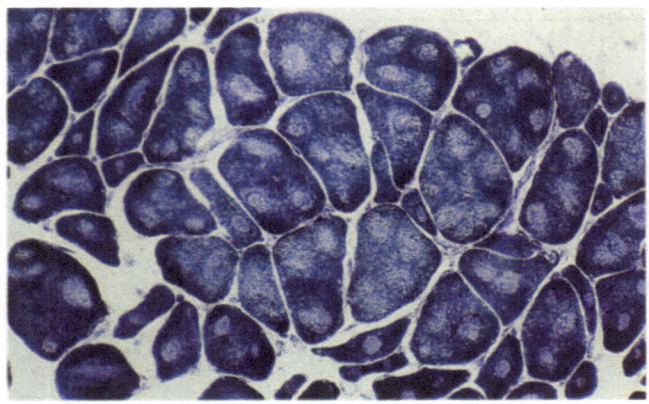

Figure 12.37   Central core disease. There is variation in fibre size and every fibre contains one or more cores.   NADH-TR × 180

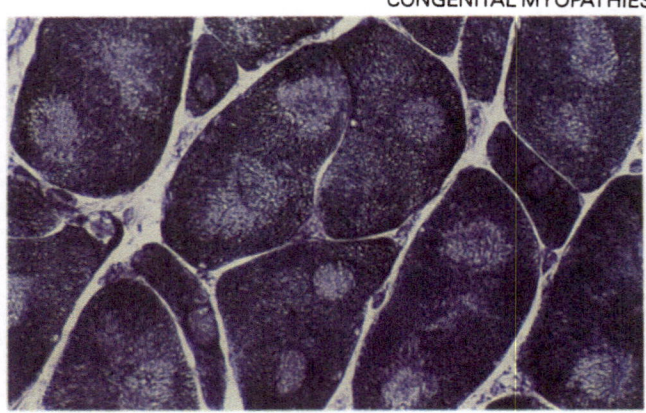

Figure 12.38   Central core disease. The cores are best demonstrated with the oxidative enzyme reaction, as well-circumscribed, rounded foci devoid of enzyme activity.   NADH-TR × 300

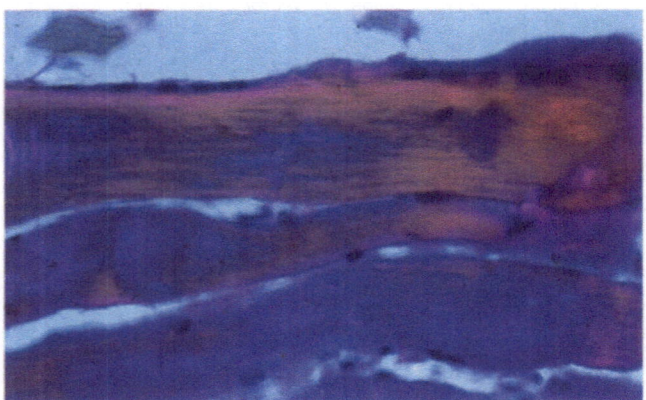

Figure 12.39   Minicore disease. Biopsy from a 5-year-old boy with delay in walking and then unsteady gait. His younger brother appears similarly affected. There is variation in fibre size and fibres contain minicores – oval areas devoid of normal myofibrils, which can be seen in longitudinal section under polarized light. (Same case shown in Figure 12.40.)   H & E × 300

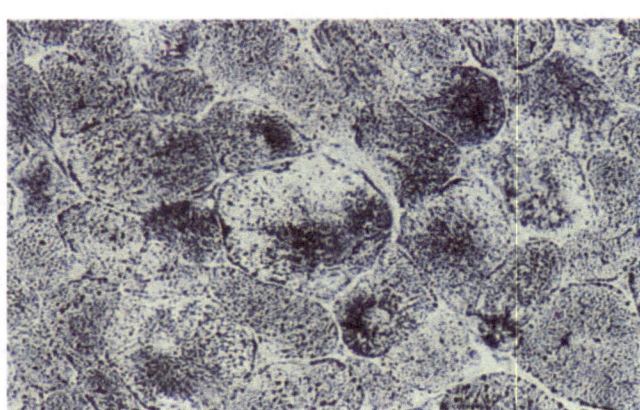

Figure 12.40   Minicore disease. There is variation in fibre size, but practically all the fibres are type 1. The oxidative enzyme reaction reveals patchy staining. There is no endomysial fibrosis.   NADH-TR × 300

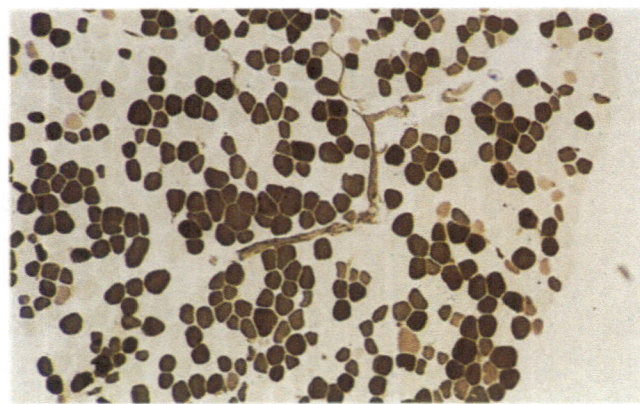

Figure 12.41   Congenital hypotonia associated with cerebral palsy. One-year-old boy who suffered birth injury. Hypotonia with delay in reaching motor milestones. Quadriceps biopsy shows moderate variation in fibre size, but no selective atrophy or hypertrophy. In this field the largest fibres are mostly type 1, but elsewhere, as shown in Figure 12.42, the type 2 fibres are larger. There is a mosaic distribution pattern and some 2C fibres are present. This varied pattern is not typical of any of the congenital myopathies, but is sometimes seen in association with central nervous system disease. (Same case shown in Figure 12.42.)   ATP-ase pH 4.1 × 180

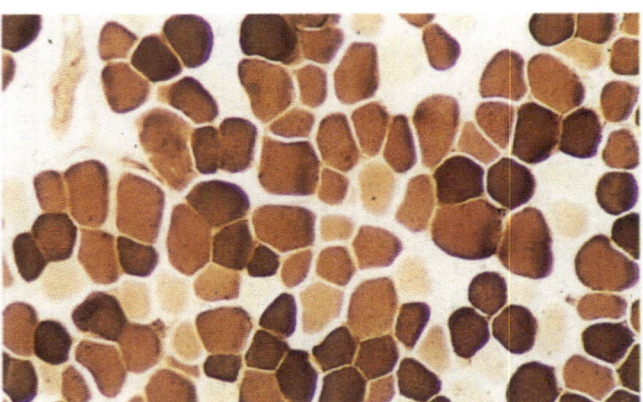

Figure 12.42   Congenital hypotonia of central origin. Variation in fibre size in which type 2 fibres are the largest. Some are 2C fibres.   ATP-ase pH 4.5 × 300

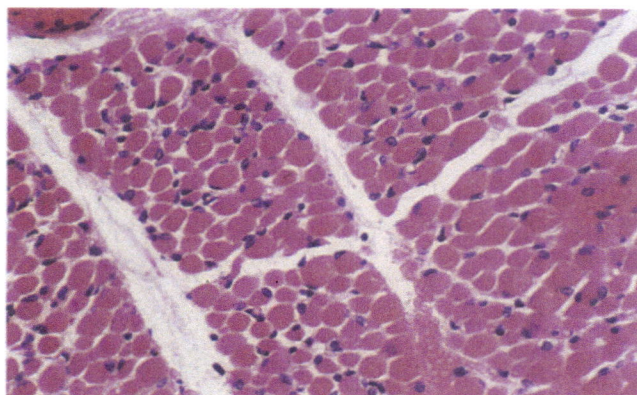

Figure 12.43 Quadriceps biopsy in a 15-month-old boy with mild hypotonia and delay in reaching motor milestones. He did not sit until 1 year and showed no sign of crawling at 15 months. The biopsy contains some small fibres, but no other abnormalities. The small fibres are all type 2 fibres. Subsequently, his motor skills improved. He eventually walked at 30 months, but he is mentally retarded. (Same case shown in Figure 12.44.) H & E × 180

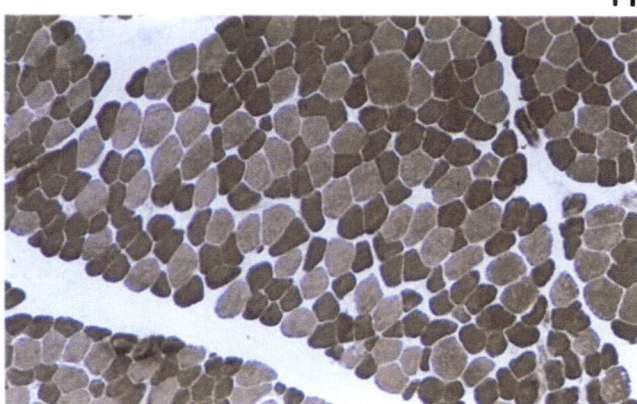

Figure 12.44 Mild congenital hypotonia. The small fibres are uniformly type 2 fibres. Type 1 fibres (light) are of normal size. ATP-ase pH 9.4 × 180

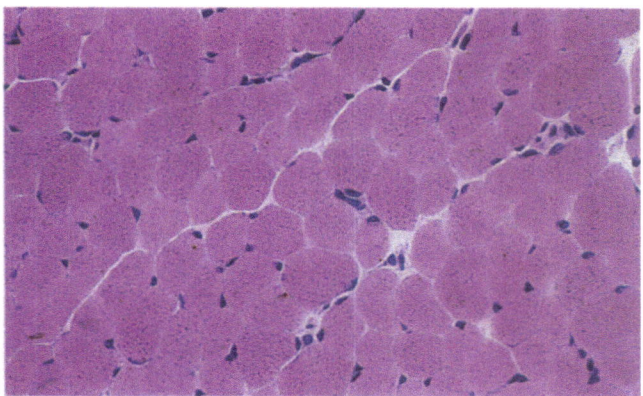

Figure 12.45 Benign congenital hypotonia. Quadriceps biopsy from an 18-month-old boy with mild hypotonia and delay in motor development. At the time of the biopsy he could sit unsupported, but was not crawling. There is slight variation in fibre size. His condition has since improved and he appears to be showing normal development. (Same case shown in Figures 12.46–12.48.) H & E × 300

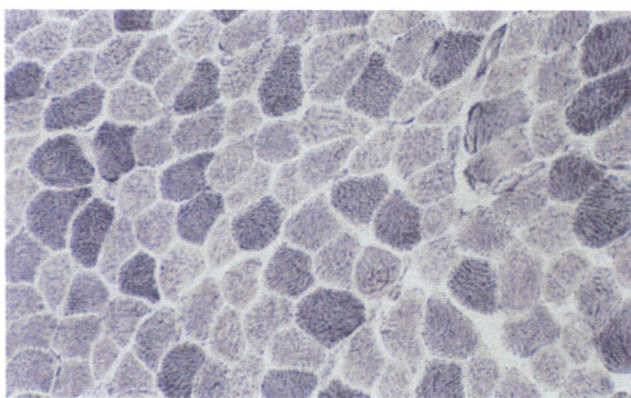

Figure 12.46 Benign congenital hypotonia. Slight variation in fibre size, without architectural abnormalities. The smaller fibres are mainly type 2 fibres. NADH-TR × 300

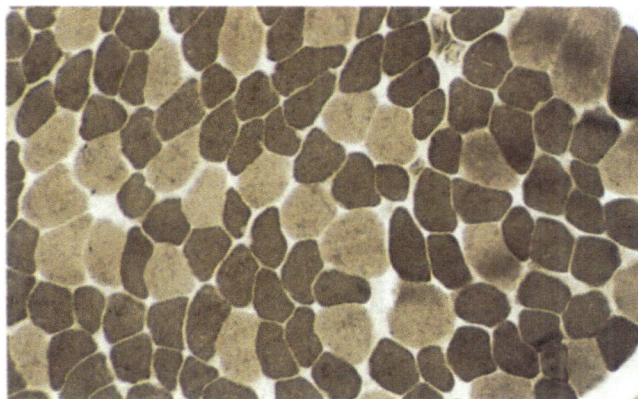

Figure 12.47 Benign congenital hypotonia. Small fibres are type 2 fibres. ATP-ase pH 9.4 × 300

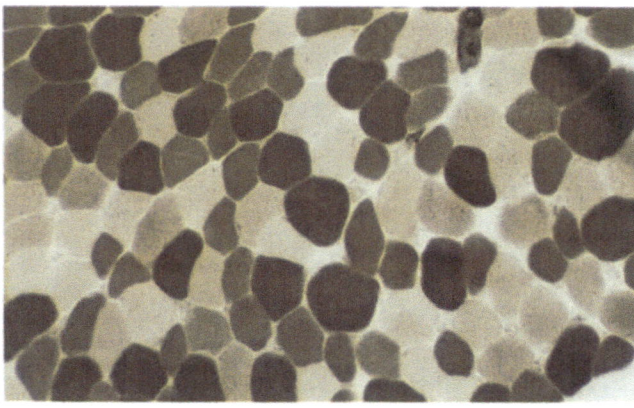

Figure 12.48 Differentiation of the type 2 fibres shows that the smallest are 2B fibres (intermediate staining). ATP-ase pH 4.6 × 300

Inflammatory myopathies are those in which muscle cell injury is largely attributable to an inflammatory reaction and inflammatory cells are invariably present in the muscle. The inflammatory response may be elicited by viral, bacterial or parasitic infestation of muscle. Bacterial and parasitic myositis prevail in the tropics, but are relatively infrequent causes in Western Europe. A systemic viral infection, such as influenza, is not uncommonly associated with or followed by an acute self-limiting myositis. However, the commonest clinically important inflammatory myopathies, responsible for debilitating and chronic disease, are the idiopathic disorders polymyositis and dermatomyositis.

Polymyositis and Dermatomyositis

Clinical Features and Presentation

These myopathies are generally believed to be immunological disorders. At present different prognostic groups can be recognized clinically, but there are no clear cut differences in muscle histology.

The classification of Bohan and Peters[1] is as follows:

Group 1 – primary, idiopathic polymyositis
Group 2 – primary, idiopathic dermatomyositis (adults)
Group 3 – dermatomyositis (or polymyositis) associated with neoplasia
Group 4 – childhood dermatomyositis associated with vasculitis
Group 5 – polymyositis or dermatomyositis associated with collagen vascular disease.

Recently Carpenter and Karpati attempted to correlate certain morphological features with different pathogenetic mechanisms[23]. This is an important fundamental approach, but does not consistently identify the different clinical groups. When biopsy confirms the presence of an inflammatory myopathy, further classification is dependent on the full clinical picture and the results of biochemical and immunological investigations.

Polymyositis and Adult Dermatomyositis

Clinical Picture and Investigations

Polymyositis is most often a progressive disorder of insidious onset, commonest in females and occurring at almost any age, but more often after 40 years. Clinically the most important sign is muscle weakness, usually symmetrical involvement of the pelvic and shoulder girdle muscles and frequently the anterior neck flexors. The deep tendon reflexes are preserved and atrophy is absent or slight at the onset. Muscle strength is notably diminished out of proportion to the degree of atrophy. Dysphagia and respiratory muscle weakness may occur but facial and ocular muscles are rarely involved. Muscle tenderness is often present but is not a major feature of the subacute or chronic disease. In the 'classic' case of polymyositis the serum CPK is moderately elevated, there are characteristic EMG abnormalities and the muscle biopsy shows evidence of inflammation, necrosis and regeneration.

Patients with dermatomyositis show all these changes and, in addition, typical skin lesions, consisting of lilac discolouration of the upper eyelids, periorbital oedema and an erythematous scaly rash on the dorsum of the hands, knees, elbows, medial malleoli, chest, neck and with butterfly distribution on the face. When all these criteria are fulfilled a firm diagnosis of polymyositis or dermatomyositis (if the rash is present) is easily made. However, in any one case and at any one time all the features may not be present and the diagnosis remains probable or only possible. Whilst dermatomyositis may be identified by the skin rash when there is only minor muscle involvement, it is rarely possible to substantiate a diagnosis of polymyositis in the absence of weakness. When there is a typical pattern of weakness a negative result from just one of the other investigations (i.e. serum enzymes, EMG or muscle biopsy) does not disprove the diagnosis, but if two of these tests are negative polymyositis becomes less probable[3].

Investigations

Elevation of sarcoplasmic enzymes in the serum, particularly creatine phosphokinase, is found in the great majority of cases of polymyositis and dermatomyositis, but in a small proportion a normal level remains. The serum aldolase, transaminase and lactic dehydrogenase are also frequently raised and their estimation may increase the diagnostic yield[3]. Although there is no close correlation between the actual CPK level and the severity of weakness, an elevated CPK does indicate active disease and decreased levels usually herald an improvement in muscle strength[2]. The ESR has little diagnostic value[3]. It is inconsistently raised and shows no correlation with disease activity. The majority of patients also show characteristic small amplitude, short duration polyphasic motor unit potentials on EMG, but, although it is difficult to explain, at least 10% of patients with otherwise classical disease have a completely normal EMG[3,4].

Biopsy site

Degenerative changes in the muscle may be focal and thus a normal biopsy obtained. Careful selection of the

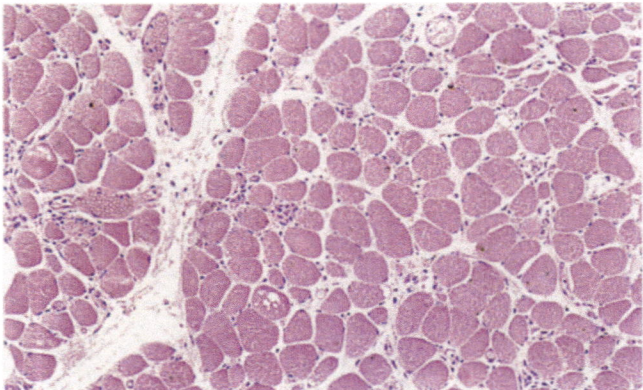

Figure 13.1   Irregularly scattered necrotic fibres in polymyositis. Deltoid biopsy from 64-year-old woman with proximal muscle weakness of recent onset and moderately raised CPK. Ovarian carcinoma resected 2 years previously.   H & E × 75

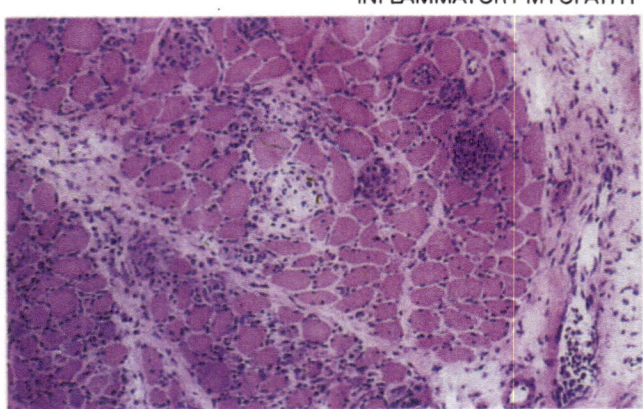

Figure 13.2   Necrosis and inflammation in quadriceps muscle of 57-year-old man with dermatomyositis. Recent, insidious onset of proximal muscle weakness and wasting together with a skin rash. (Same case as in Figures 13.8, 13.25 and 13.26.)   H & E × 75

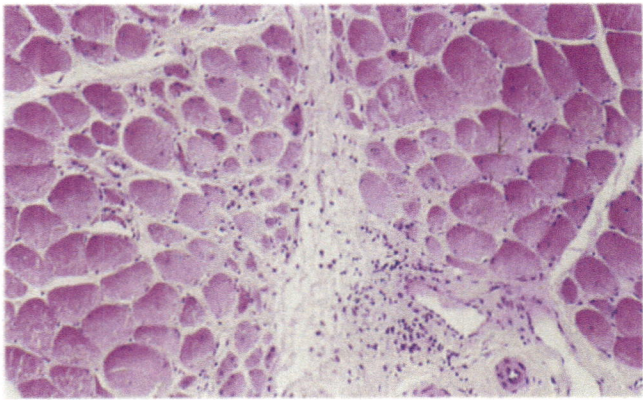

Figure 13.3   Mild perivascular chronic inflammatory cell infiltration within the fibrous septum and adjacent perifascicular muscle fibre atrophy. Deltoid muscle of 62-year-old man with proximal muscle weakness. No obvious skin rash. Carcinoma of the bronchus diagnosed 2 years previously. (Same case as in Figures 9.11, 9.27 and 9.28.)   H & E × 75

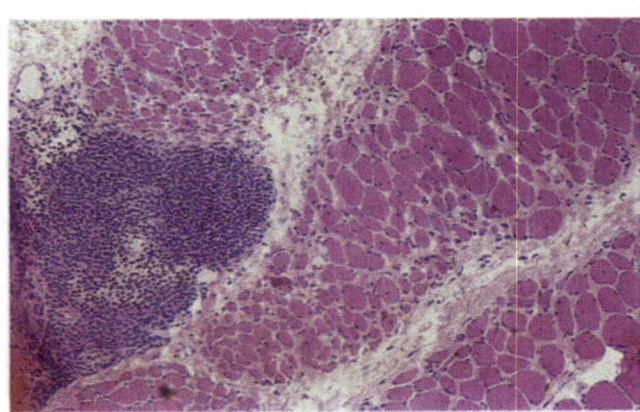

Figure 13.4   Interstitial lymphoid aggregate and perifascicular muscle fibre atrophy in young woman with polymyositis. Deltoid biopsy in 32-year-old woman with mild proximal muscle weakness. No skin rash observed. (Same case shown in Figures 13.5 and 13.6.)   H & E × 30

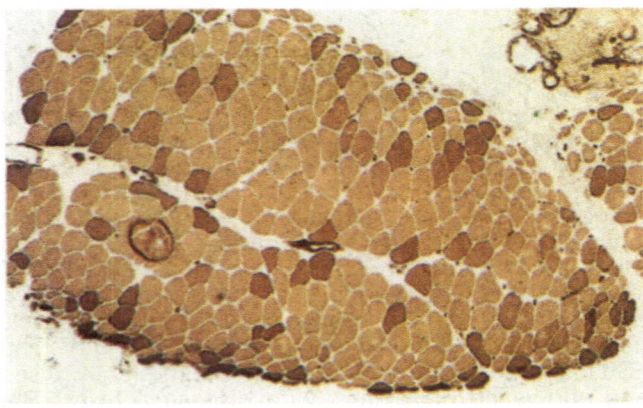

Figure 13.5   Perifascicular fibre atrophy involving both type 1 and type 2 fibres in polymyositis.   ATP-ase pH 9.4 × 30

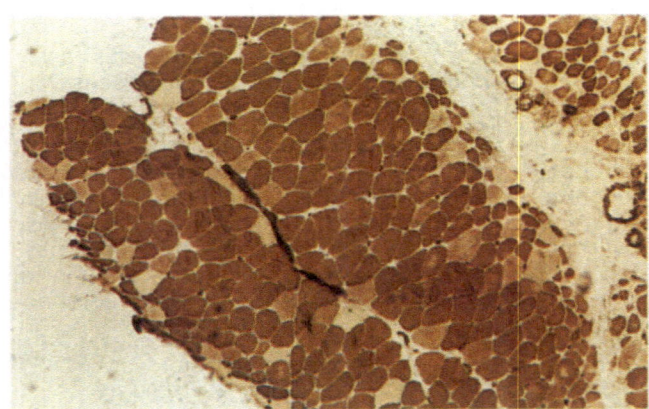

Figure 13.6   Serial section to Figure 13.5.   ATP-ase pH 4.5 × 30

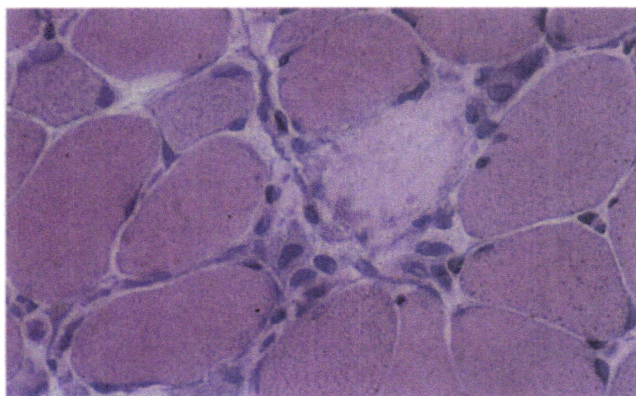

Figure 13.7 Fibre necrosis. Pale necrotic fibre in centre of the field. Surrounding mononuclear cells probably include mononuclear phagocytes and myoblasts. Deltoid biopsy in 64-year-old woman with polymyositis. (Same case as Figure 13.1.) H & E × 300

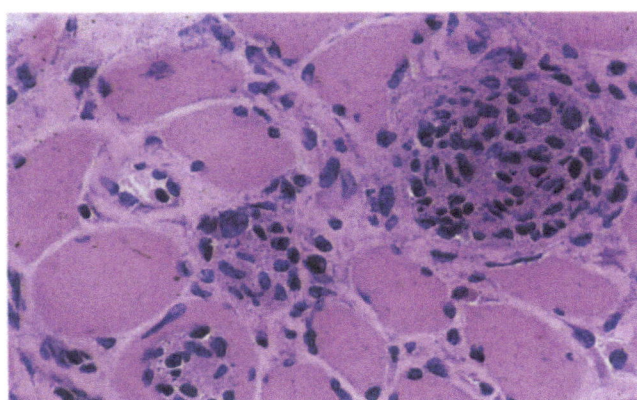

Figure 13.8 Phagocytosis of necrotic fibres. Cytoplasm of necrotic cells containing macrophages. Quadriceps muscle in 57-year-old man with dermatomyositis. (Same case as Figure 13.2.) H & E × 300

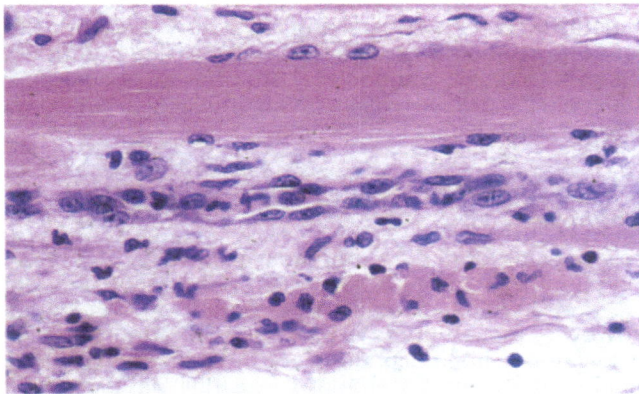

Figure 13.9 Regeneration. Mononuclear myoblasts lining up along the scaffold of a necrotic fibre. In the lower part of the field there is this phagocytic invasion of an eosinophilic necrotic fibre. Longitudinal section of deltoid muscle of elderly man with polymyositis. H & E × 300

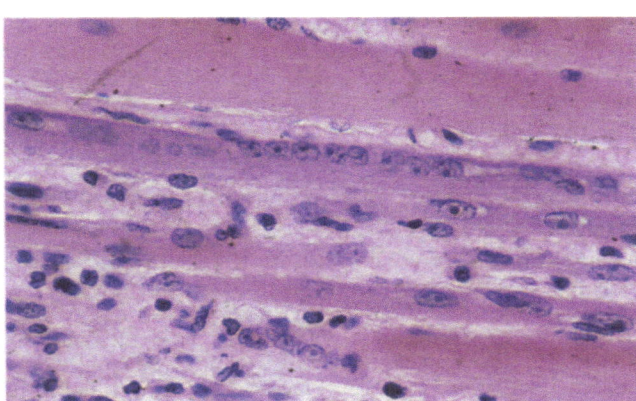

Figure 13.10 Regeneration. Fusion of myoblasts is complete. Myotubes are long thin fibres with faintly basophilic cytoplasm and fairly large nuclei. H & E × 300

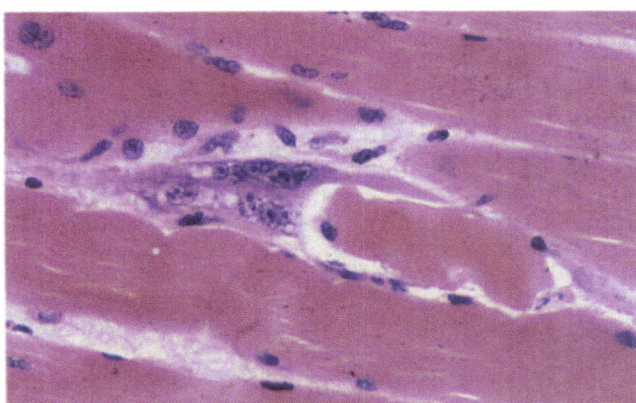

Figure 13.11 Necrosis and regeneration. Segment of eosinophilic necrotic cytoplasm, partly surrounded by basophilic regenerating myotubes. H & E × 300

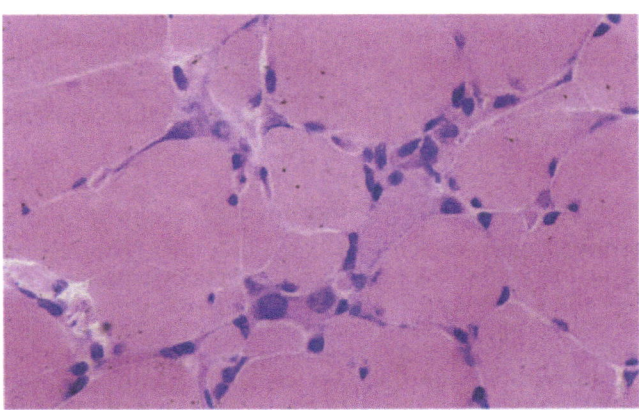

Figure 13.12 Regenerating myotubes. Small basophilic fibres amongst normal-sized fibres. Quadriceps muscle of 72-year-old woman with polymyositis. 10-week history of increasing proximal muscle weakness, with elevated CPK. No evidence of a skin rash. H & E × 300

biopsy site in relation to muscle weakness and EMG findings will increase the number with pathological abnormalities. In the two large series of inflammatory myopathies reported by Bohan *et al*. and by De Vere and Bradley, in which strict diagnostic criteria were applied, 17% and 12% of patients respectively had normal biopsies[3,4].

Unusual clinical presentation

Occasionally the onset of inflammatory myopathy is acute with diffuse and severe muscle weakness, pain, tenderness and subcutaneous oedema[5]. Myoglobinuria due to extensive muscle necrosis has also been attributed to polymyositis but this is very difficult to substantiate. Genuine cases may have occurred but the majority are probably examples of acute self-limiting viral myositis rather than a progressive disorder[6]. Other very unusual modes of presentation include a predominantly distal myopathy or a clinical picture that mimics facio-scapulohumeral dystrophy[7]. Rarely polymyositis begins as a localized tender swelling in a single muscle that clinically simulates a neoplasm, whilst histology shows degenerative and inflammatory changes[8]. This may remain a localized process or evolve into typical generalized polymyositis. Early elevation of the CPK may have predictive value[9].

Dermatomyositis (or Polymyositis) Associated With Malignancy

In adults dermatomyositis, and to a lesser extent polymyositis, has an association with internal malignancy such as carcinoma of the lung, colon and breast. There are no identifiable clinical or pathological differences between cases associated with malignancy and those without. In Bohan's series the patients with malignant disease were generally older (average age 62 years) than those with uncomplicated inflammatory myopathy (47 years). Malignant disease is not seen in childhood dermatomyositis and does not appear to be associated with overlap syndromes. The actual incidence of neoplasia is difficult to ascertain. De Vere and Bradley found a strong link between dermatomyositis and malignancy – 40% over 40 years[4]. In the larger series of Bohan *et al*. the incidence was much lower, approximately 15% of patients with classic dermatomyositis, but this may not be entirely accurate as some of their patients were lost to follow up[3]. The signs and symptoms of dermatomyositis frequently precede the manifestations of malignancy by a few months or up to a few years.

Childhood (Juvenile) Dermatomyositis

Childhood dermatomyositis, occurring mostly between 5 and 15 years, appears to be a distinct category of inflammatory myopathy which has a vascular basis[2]. The onset may be acute or insidious. The skin rash is similar, but contractures and subcutaneous calcinosis over the heels, elbows and knuckles, which appear late in the course of the disease, are more frequent than in adults. The major distinguishing feature is a necrotizing vasculitis that is responsible for muscle fibre damage and may cause systemic complications such as gastrointestinal perforation[11]. This group cannot be defined solely on the basis of age as similar pathology has been described in young adults. Juvenile type dermatomyositis is thus more appropriate. Chronic inflammatory myopathy other than dermatomyositis seems to

be very rare in childhood. A progressive myopathy of early onset that responds to steroids has on occasion been described[12]. Muscular dystrophy is the main differential diagnosis. The relationship of this disorder, which has been called infantile myositis, to congenital muscular dystrophy on the one hand and to polymyositis on the other is still uncertain.

Polymyositis or Dermatomyositis Associated With Collagen Vascular Disease

Muscle involvement occurs in many of the connective tissue diseases. This may be simply a mild degree of atrophy or patchy lymphocytic infiltration on biopsy, but some patients with well-documented multisystem disease such as rheumatoid arthritis, systemic lupus erythematosus, progressive systemic sclerosis or mixed connective tissue disease develop clinical and pathological changes indistinguishable from polymyositis[4]. Raynaud's phenomenon and ECG abnormalities may complicate simple polymyositis but are more usual in patients who have clinical and laboratory evidence of a separate connective tissue disorder. Similarly, although raised levels of antinuclear antibodies occasionally appear in pure polymyositis, the highest levels are found in the overlap group[3,10].

Prognosis

Polymyositis and dermatomyositis have a significant morbidity and mortality. An overall mortality between 14 and 40% has been reported in various series. However, these figures are heavily weighted by cases associated with malignancy as the majority of these patients die from dissemination of their neoplasm[3]. In the other groups the majority of patients show a favourable response to steroid therapy. This is particularly true in juveniles, who usually respond to a short course of low dose steroids[13] and death due to inflammatory myopathy is exceptional under 30 years. The majority of adults with uncomplicated polymyositis or dermatomyositis also show an improvement in muscle strength with prednisone, provided that treatment is begun early in the course of the disease. In many cases the disease appears to burn out and leaves no residual functional deficit[4]. In all cases the prognosis is far worse for patients treated late in the course of their illness, when extensive muscle breakdown and irreversible fibrosis may have already occurred and their disability persists. In the series of De Vere and Bradley, patients with rheumatoid arthritis and progressive systemic sclerosis were more disabled at presentation and throughout their illness than patients without an associated connective tissue disease[4]. Another series found a high mortality in patients with cardiac involvement[14]. Some adult patients prove refractory to steroid therapy but may still improve with immunosuppression[3,4,14].

Although increased mortality is reported in patients with inflammatory myopathy, relatively few deaths are directly attributable to muscle weakness. Apart from carcinoma, complications of other connective tissue diseases, side-effects of steroids and immunosuppressive agents and apparently unrelated causes such as coronary artery disease all contribute[4].

In summary idiopathic inflammatory myopathies can produce chronic, disabling and sometimes fatal disease. If suspected clinically every effort should be made to establish a firm early diagnosis, when necessary by repeating the essential investigations, in order to permit prompt therapy and provide the greatest chance of full recovery.

Aetiology

Polymyositis and dermatomyositis (PM and DM) are almost certainly syndromes with a variety of causes. At present the initiating factors are speculative but the histological evidence of mononuclear cell infiltration and the frequent association with autoimmune disorders suggests that immunologic reactions have a major pathogenetic role. Both humoral and cell mediated mechanisms may operate. The haplotype HLA-B8 which is associated with autoimmune diseases is also reported with increased frequency in PM and DM[15].

Vasculitis is sometimes a pathologic feature of inflammatory myopathies. It is particularly characteristic of juvenile dermatomyositis[16], where morphologic examination suggests that arterioles and capillaries are the main target of an inflammatory attack and muscle cell injury is the result of ischaemia[17]. The demonstration of immunoglobulin and complement in the walls of small intramuscular blood vessels supports an immune complex mediated vasculitis[18]. Glomerulonephritis, in which the role of immune complexes is well established, has occasionally been described in association with PM[19]. There are also rare examples of PM appearing in patients with hepatitis B antigenaemia[20] and in one case complexes containing HBsAg and complement were identified along the sarcolemma[21]. Thus it seems possible that in some patients immune complexes have a pathogenetic role, either by causing vasculitis or even by direct muscle cell injury.

In pure PM many investigations point towards cell-mediated immunity as the more important effector mechanism. Lymphocytes from affected patients have shown muscle cell cytotoxicity in tissue culture[22]. Microscopy reveals mononuclear inflammatory cells apparently invading intact muscle fibres and immunoperoxidase preparations reveal that T lymphocytes predominate in the cellular infiltrate[23,24]. An experimental animal model, similar to the human condition can be produced by inoculation of minced muscle in Freund's adjuvant[24]. The myositis can be transferred passively by lymphoid cells.

Although it is reasonably well established that muscle damage results from immunological injury, the antigens that trigger these diseases remain largely unknown. The association with malignancy, with autoimmune diseases and the examples of drug-induced myositis suggest that a wide variety of endogenous or exogenous antigens may be involved. Cutaneous hypersensitivity has occasionally been demonstrated in patients with dermatomyositis and malignancy[26]. In such cases a cross-reaction with tumour antigen or deposition of complexes containing tumour antigen can be postulated. Penicillamine occasionally induces an inflammatory myopathy which remits upon withdrawal of the drug[27]. Drugs may combine with self-antigens and act as haptens. However, in the large idiopathic group other factors must exist.

A viral aetiology seems a good suggestion but there is little proof. Peaks of onset of childhood dermatomyositis in the winter months raise the possibility of a precipitating viral (or bacterial) infection[28]. The onset of PM or DM may follow a childhood exanthem, but this is an exceptional occurrence[29]. The occasional association

with hepatitis B has already been mentioned. Several reports suggest there is actually direct viral invasion of muscle. Picorna and Coxsackie virus particles have been identified in muscle cells by electron microscopy[30,31] and in one instance the presence of virus antigen was confirmed by immunofluorescence[32]. Some support for a pathogenetic role for Coxsackie viruses is provided by the ability of this type of virus to produce myositis in animals[33]. However in man, despite the fine structural evidence, to date there has been only one successful virus isolation in chronic muscle disease. Tang et al. isolated Coxsackie virus type A9 from a young girl with chronic myopathy, but the clinical picture was not entirely typical of juvenile polymyositis[34]. There are other examples of virus isolation from muscle in patients with myositis, but all from cases with acute illness and mostly with evidence of a systemic viral infection[35,36].

Influenza viruses A and B not infrequently cause an acute myositis, which can be severe, but is short lived.[37] There is no real evidence to suggest that overt, acute viral myositis progresses to the more chronic form of PM or DM. If viruses are responsible for these progressive inflammatory myopathies it seems likely that the initial infection is subclinical and viral persistence is permitted by some immunological deficiency of the host. The most striking example of this sequence is seen in patients with hypogammaglobulinaemia in whom a dermatomyositis-like syndrome is sometimes a manifestation of chronic Echo virus infection[38]. The majority of patients with PM or DM do not have gross immunological deficiency, but subtle or transient deficiencies could be relevant. Dawkins has reported mild defects in humoral immunity in PM and DM patients[39].

Toxoplasma gondii is another infectious agent that has been incriminated in the aetiology of PM and DM. Acquired toxoplasmosis usually gives rise to lymphadenopathy and rarely it is a disseminated infection when organisms can be found in many organs, including skeletal muscle[40]. In contrast, patients in whom the only evidence of infection is a raised toxoplasma antibody titre sometimes have the typical clinical picture of PM or DM[41,42]. Muscle biopsy has shown inflammatory changes, but failed to reveal organisms and yet the myopathy responds to antitoxoplasma drug therapy[43]. Failure to demonstrate the parasite in areas of severe myositis suggests a hypersensitivity response to a small number of organisms.

In summary PM and DM probably represent the tissue response to immunological reactions which take place in muscle and can be initiated by a variety of aetiological agents.

Muscle Biopsy

Despite clinical differences and the evidence that different pathogenetic mechanisms operate in PM and DM, it is seldom possible to distinguish between these diseases by histology alone, particularly in a small biopsy. However, recent studies suggest that distinctive morphological features can sometimes be found in juvenile DM, less often in adult DM and PM[2]. These are discussed after the general description. No specific histological changes differentiate DM (or PM) associated with malignancy.

The main pathological changes of an inflammatory myopathy are muscle cell necrosis or degeneration and inflammatory cell infiltration (Figures 13.1–13.6).

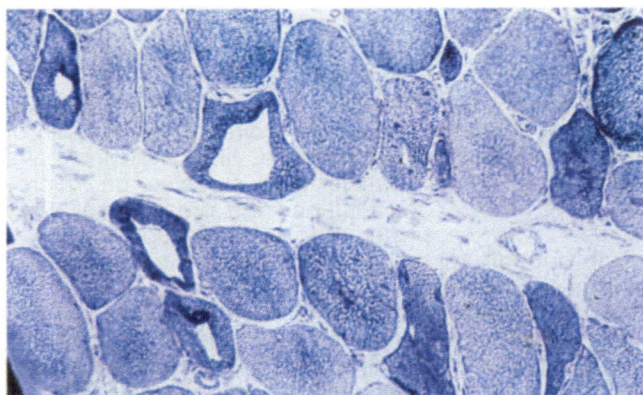

Figure 13.13 Vacuolar degeneration in polymyositis. Quadriceps biopsy from 54-year-old man with painful proximal muscles and increasing weakness. CPK moderately elevated. Initial improvement on steroids, but a carcinoma of bronchus, diagnosed 2 years later, rapidly caused death. (Same case shown in Figure 13.14.)   NADH-TR × 300

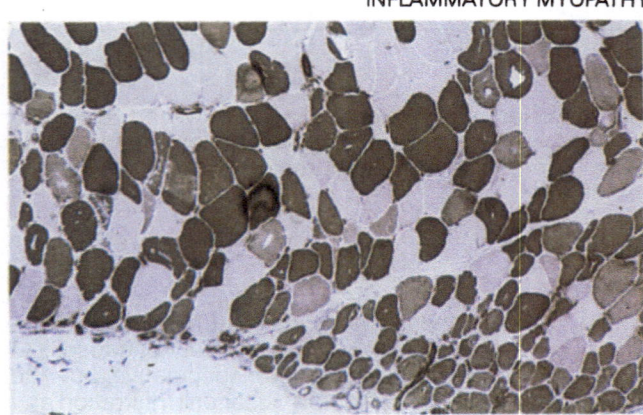

Figure 13.14 Vacuolar degeneration and patchy staining with myosin ATP-ase. Perifascicular pattern of fibre atrophy.   ATP-ase pH 4.5 × 75

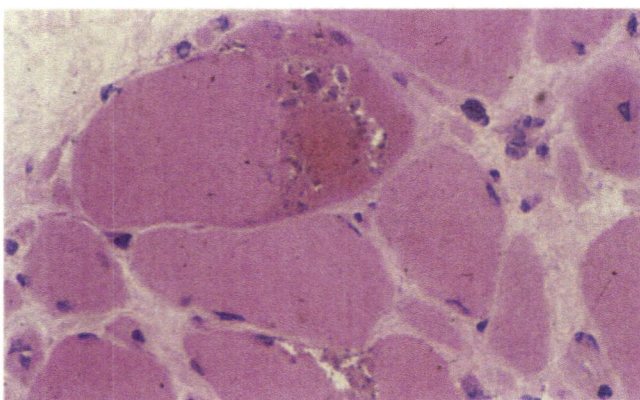

Figure 13.15 Eosinophilic cytoplasm inclusion and small vacuoles, probably lysosomes, containing dense granules. Quadriceps muscle of 73-year-old man with untreated chronic polymyositis. Five-year history of increasing proximal muscle weakness. (Same case shown in Figures 13.19–13.22, 13.31 and 13.32.)   H & E × 450

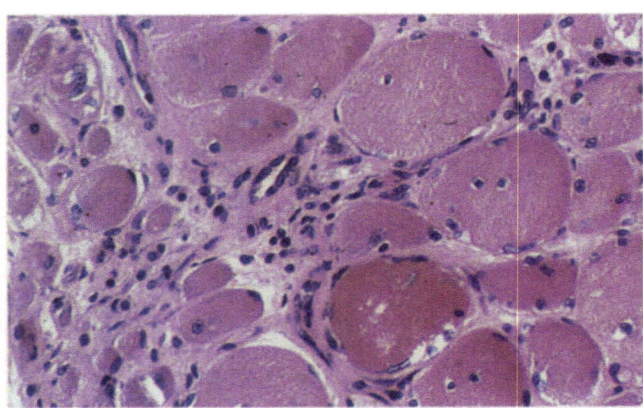

Figure 13.16 Multiple central nuclei in polymyositis. Elderly man with proximal muscle weakness, elevated CPK and carcinoma of the bronchus.   H & E × 300

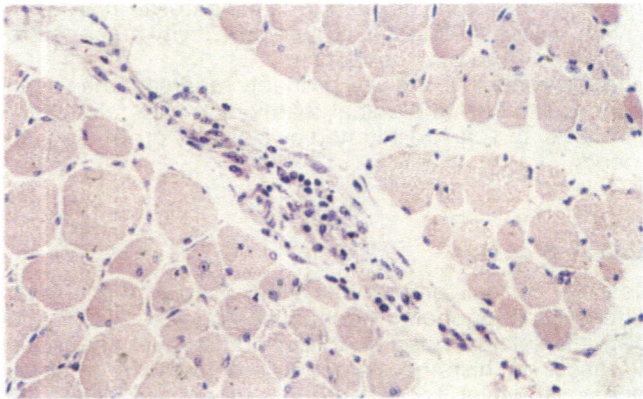

Figure 13.17 Mild perivascular septal chronic inflammation in deltoid biopsy of young woman with dermatomyositis. 32-year-old woman with 3-year history of muscle aches and pains, mild proximal weakness and typical erythematous skin rash on knuckles, elbows and knees. CPK normal at time of biopsy. (Same case shown in Figure 13.18.)   H & E × 75

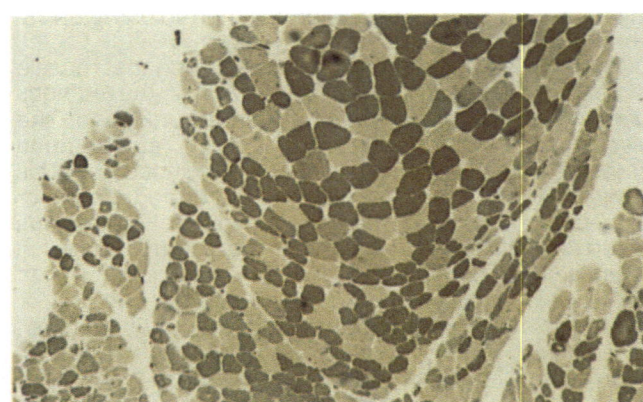

Figure 13.18 Perifascicular atrophy in dermatomyositis. ATP-ase pH 9.4 × 30

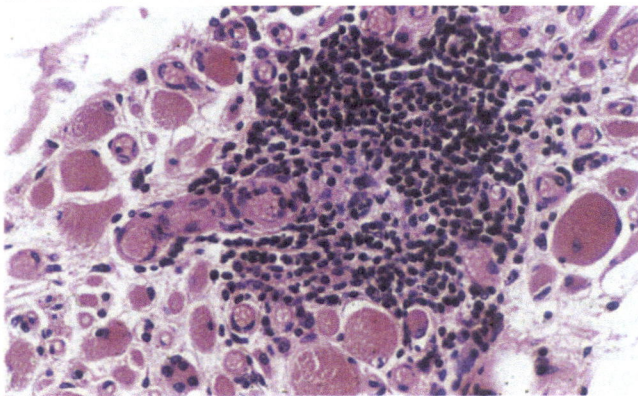

Figure 13.19 Lymphoid aggregate sheathing small blood vessel and spilling into fascicle amongst atrophic fibres. Chronic polymyositis in 73-year-old man. (Same case shown in Figures 13.20–13.22, 13.31 and 13.32.) H & E × 180

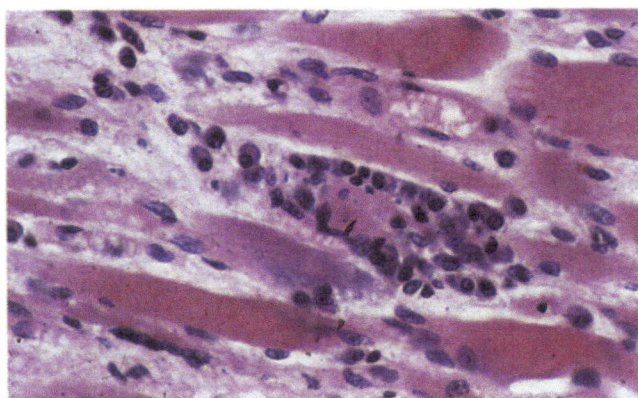

Figure 13.20 Lymphocytes and plasma cells clustered around a necrotic segment in chronic polymyositis. H & E × 300

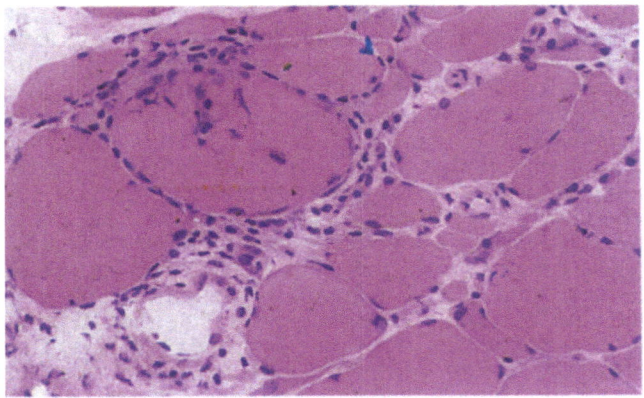

Figure 13.21 Mononuclear cells in the interstitium and within cytoplasm of one large fibre. H & E × 300

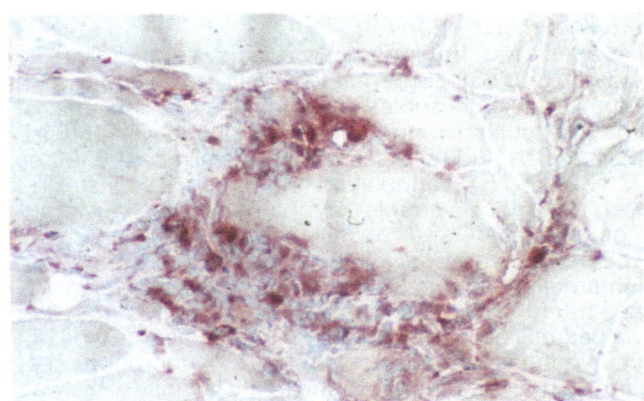

Figure 13.22 Adjacent section to Figure 13.21 showing acid-phosphatase activity (red) in infiltrating mononuclear phagocytes. Activity also present in periphery of degenerating fibres. Acid phosphatase is a lysosomal enzyme. Acid-phosphatase × 300

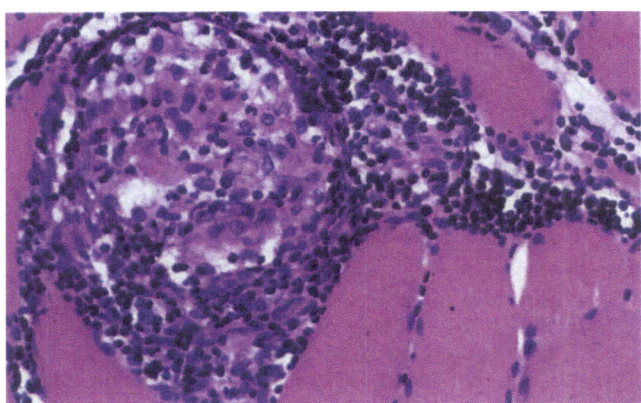

Figure 13.23 Epithelioid granuloma and infiltrating lymphocytes amongst intact muscle fibres. Patchy fibre atrophy is present elsewhere in this deltoid biopsy. 61-year-old man with diagnosis of polymyositis. Moderate weakness of all limbs. Moderately elevated CPK. Kveim test negative. Considerable improvement with steroids. (Same case shown in Figure 13.24.) H & E × 300

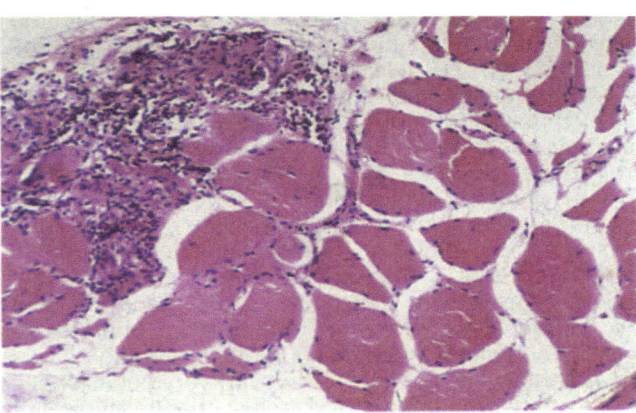

Figure 13.24 Polymyositis with granulomata. Granulomatous inflammation encroaching upon the fascicle, in which there are several atrophic fibres. H & E × 180

Regenerating fibres, atrophic fibres and fibres with architectural abnormalities are common (Figures 13.7–13.16). All of these abnormalities may not appear in a single positive biopsy. One or other change may predominate. In addition, the histopathology will vary according to the chronicity of the disease and will certainly be modified by treatment.

Necrosis and degeneration

Necrotic muscle fibres are identified by homogeneous, pale staining cytoplasm with H & E (Figure 13.7) and loss of enzyme activity in the histochemical preparations. Loss of striations is obvious in necrotic segments seen in longitudinal section. Phagocytic cells may be identified within degenerating cell cytoplasm (Figure 13.8). Where necrosis occurs, regeneration usually follows. Regenerating fibres are small and rounded, with basophilic cytoplasm, large vesicular nuclei and prominent nucleoli (Figures 13.9–13.12). A ring of regenerative myoblasts derived from satellite cells may be seen encircling a disintegrating necrotic fibre (Figure 13.11).

In addition to frank necrosis a variety of non-specific cytoarchitectural abnormalities may be found which probably indicate sublethal cell injury. By light microscopy vacuoles, abnormalities of myofibrillar pattern, central cores and cytoplasmic bodies all occur (Figures 13.13–13.15). Vacuolation is sometimes very striking and may mimic a vacuolar myopathy. Internal nuclei are often increased and occasionally numerous (Figure 13.16). Schwarz et al. have suggested that the number of internal nuclei may predict steroid responsiveness[44]. They found that improved muscle power was matched by a decrease in central nuclei and that patients who did not respond to steroids had a much higher proportion of centrally nucleated fibres in their initial biopsy. This was only a small series and the observations await confirmation.

Inflammation

Mononuclear inflammatory cell infiltration is an important diagnostic feature. The predominant cells are small lymphocytes, but large activated lymphocytes, histiocytes and plasma cells are also present. The infiltrate is usually patchy and either septal and perivascular (Figures 13.17 and 13.18) or within the fascicle surrounding individual muscle fibres (Figures 13.19 and 13.20). Histiocytes are well demonstrated by acid-phosphatase activity (Figures 13.21 and 13.22). Polymorphoneutrophil leukocytes are unusual, but may accompany florid, acute necrosis. Although lymphoid aggregates may be seen (Figures 13.4 and 13.19), germinal centres are excessively rare. A case is reported of polymyositis associated with gastric carcinoma in which the muscle contained lymphoid germinal centres[45]. Granulomata are also rare. Discrete epithelioid and giant cell granulomata, usually septal and without accompanying degenerative changes in muscle, suggest sarcoidosis or other granulomatous disease and not PM or DM. However, very occasionally sparse granulomata are found amidst changes typical of polymyositis (Figures 13.23 and 13.24). Even then the diagnosis should not be accepted before a search has been made for a granulomatous disorder.

Eosinophils are not usually a significant component of the cellular infiltrate in PM and DM. A few cases have been described with clinical features of polymyositis in which muscle cell necrosis was associated with a predominantly eosinophilic infiltrate[46]. These patients have had systemic illness, including myocarditis and usually a peripheral blood eosinophilia. It is suggested that this 'eosinophilic polymyositis' is part of the hypereosinophilic syndrome rather than classical PM or DM; however, it does respond to steroids.

Fibrosis

Fibrosis and fatty infiltration occur in chronic, untreated disease. This is not a feature of early PM or DM, but endomysial and perimysial fibrosis may follow extensive necrosis or longstanding atrophy (Figures 13.25 and 13.26).

Atrophy

Fibre atrophy is frequently present. The distribtuion of atrophic fibres can be perifascicular[47] (Figures 13.27 and 13.28) in clumps or irregularly scattered. In general, atrophic fibres have a rounded outline as opposed to the angular fibres characteristic of denervation. Occasionally, small group atrophy with angular fibres, suggesting denervation, is seen in an otherwise typical polymyositis and may be due to focal inflammatory lesions of intramuscular nerves. The term neuromyositis has been employed, but the change is not confined to any one category of PM or DM and does not have any particular clinical significance, except in rheumatoid arthritis, where a genuine peripheral neuropathy may co-exist. Selective atrophy of either type 1 or type 2 fibres is sometimes found (Figures 13.29 and 13.30). Neither is specific for inflammatory myopathy. Type 2 may be present ab initio, but can also occur as a consequence of steroid-induced myopathy. In patients showing a favourable response to steroids type 2 atrophy decreases, but in a poor responder it can be difficult to decide if selective type 2 atrophy indicates continuing disease activity or a corticosteroid-induced myopathy. The CPK is not usually raised in a steroid-induced myopathy. Comparison with a pretreatment biopsy is obviously of value. Inflammatory cell infiltration is not seen in steroid myopathy and type 2 atrophy combined with any residual inflammation points to continuing disease activity.

Hypertrophy: Fibre hypertrophy is generally absent in PM and DM. Hypertrophy is a useful distinguishing feature of Becker muscular dystrophy or chronic spinal muscular atrophy which show focal inflammation. However, exceptionally some hypertrophic fibres are present in chronic PM and DM in addition to the more characteristic changes.

Juvenile Dermatomyositis: In juvenile type DM, perifascicular atrophy involving both type 1 and type 2 fibres creates a very characteristic histological pattern (Figures 13.33 and 13.34). There may also be a few necrotic fibres at the periphery of the fascicle and others with cytoarchitectural abnormalities. Rarely a group of necrotic fibres resembling an infarct is found within a fascicle. Inflammatory cell infiltration is largely confined to the connective tissue septa and often quite sparse. Carpenter and Karpati demonstrated loss of capillaries in the peripheral zone of affected fascicles and suggested that fibre damage is due to ischaemia[2]. Banker first drew attention to vasculitic lesions in juvenile DM[48]. However, arteritis or even arteriolitis is a patchy process and very rarely detected in a small muscle biopsy, whereas capillary loss is an almost constant feature. Capillary vessels are difficult to identify in frozen sections and best assessed in semithin or plastic sections. Even so, reduction of capillaries is not pathognomonic of DM. It is possibly a primary event in juvenile DM, but can also be a consequence of any longstanding muscle atrophy.

Adult Polymyositis and Dermatomyositis

Most pathological accounts make no distinction between adult PM and DM. Carpenter and Karpati, in attempting this, found that capillary vascular damage and thus ischaemic changes were present in adult DM as in juvenile DM, but not in polymyositis[2]. However, the changes were patchy and the perifascicular distribution was less often present. In contrast, they found inflammatory cell infiltration within fascicles, rather than connective tissue septa, in polymyositis. They describe mononuclear inflammatory cells surrounding and apparently indenting the cytoplasm of a non-necrotic muscle cell as a characteristic feature. They report that zonal necrosis is unusual in PM and the pattern of fibre injury is generally one of spotty single fibre necrosis. Hughes and Esiri, in a fine structural study, also showed lymphocytes in intimate contact with the sarcolemmal sheath[49]. Other authors, with whom I concur, have not found consistent histological differences between PM and DM[44]. My own experience is that necrosis and regeneration are usually out of proportion to inflammation within the fascicle irrespective of the clinical picture (Figures 13.27 and 13.28). In most cases of adult inflammatory myopathy, muscle cell damage, whether spotty or zonal, is best explained by small vessel occlusion (Figures 13.35 and 13.36). Frequently mononuclear cells sheath capillaries as they approach the fascicle (Figure 13.35). Only a small proportion show intense inflammation within the fascicle and these also show perivascular inflammation (Figures 13.19, 13.20, 13.31 and 13.32).

Electron Microscopy

Electron microscopy has not revealed any specific features of necrotic or degenerating muscle cells in polymyositis or dermatomyositis. A plethora of fine structural abnormalities are described, ranging from minor focal changes to large segments of necrosis. In necrotic fibres the cytoplasm appears pale and structureless and macrophages engaged in phagocytic activity may be found beneath the sarcolemma (Figure 13.37). Other inflammatory cells, lymphocytes and plasma cells may be seen in close contact with the sarcolemmal sheath, but not within the interior of the cell.

Common degenerative changes are foci of Z band streaming and myofilament loss or disarray. Small rod bodies are occasionally found. The cytoplasm may contain quite numerous lysosomes, membranous whorls (Figures 13.38–13.41) and sometimes cytoplasmic bodies, consisting of a core of electron-dense material with a lighter periphery. Vacuoles, which are probably derived from the T system or sarcoplasmic reticulum are quite common (Figure 13.40). Chou, using a lanthanum tracer, demonstrated abnormal continuity between dilated T tubules and the sarcoplasmic reticulum and postulates this is a site of leakage of muscle enzymes[50]. The muscle cell basement membrane may show reduplication.

Regenerating myoblasts may also be found within the basement membrane derived from a necrotic fibre (Figure 13.39). Whereas macrophages contain many lysosomes and have complex cell processes, myoblasts are rounded cells with large nuclei, a few myofilaments and other scanty cytoplasmic organelles.

Filamentous inclusions have occasionally been identified in both nuclei and cytoplasm. Although bearing some relationship to virus particles their true nature remains uncertain. It seems most likely that these filaments are not virus proteins, but represent a cell response to injury.

Reduplication of capillary basement membrane is a common but non-specific abnormality in inflammatory myopathies. Collapsed rings of basement membrane material in the interstitium probably correspond to capillaries that have undergone complete necrosis (Figure 13.42). Carpenter and Karpati describe this as characteristic of dermatomyositis[2]. Tubular structures, referred to as tubular arrays or undulating tubules, have been frequently detected in the endoplasmic reticulum of endothelial cells in dermatomyositis (both juvenile and adult forms) but not in polymyositis[51] (Figures 13.43 and 13.44). Nevertheless, these structures are not pathognomic of dermatomyositis. They are well described in lupus erythematosus and have been found in other collagen vascular diseases. Their derivation is unknown, but it seems likely that they indicate some kind of cellular secretory activity.

Differential Diagnosis

Most of these conditions have already been discussed and are summarized here.

(1) Disorders with patchy inflammation
- other collagen disorders, e.g. rheumatoid arthritis
- chronic spinal muscular atrophy (the limb girdle syndrome)
- late onset muscular dystrophy (Becker dystrophy)
- inclusion body myositis.
(2) Disorders with type 2 fibre atrophy
- steroid myopathy
- cachexia
- osteomalacia
- polymyalgia rheumatica.
(3) Necrotizing myopathy due to drugs. Although necrosis is common in polymyositis it is rarely the florid diffuse involvement that occurs in certain toxic myopathies.
(4) Minor changes of doubtful significance. These are sometimes difficult to evaluate. In the absence of other firm diagnostic criteria, nonspecific changes, such as a few atrophic fibres or mild type 2 fibre atrophy, cannot be taken as evidence of polymyositis.

References

1. Bohan, A. and Peter, J. B. (1975). Polymyositis and dermatomyositis. *N. Engl. J. Med.*, **292**, 344–7 and 403–6

2. Carpenter, S. and Karpati, G. (1981). The major inflammatory myopathies of unknown cause. In Sommers, S. C. and Rosen, P. R. (eds.) *Pathology Annual*, **16** (New York: Appleton–Century–Crofts) pp. 205–37

3. Bohan, A., Peter, J. B., Bowman, R. L. and Pearson, C. M. (1977). A computer-assisted analysis of 153 patients with polymyositis and dermatomyositis. *Medicine*, **56**, 255–86

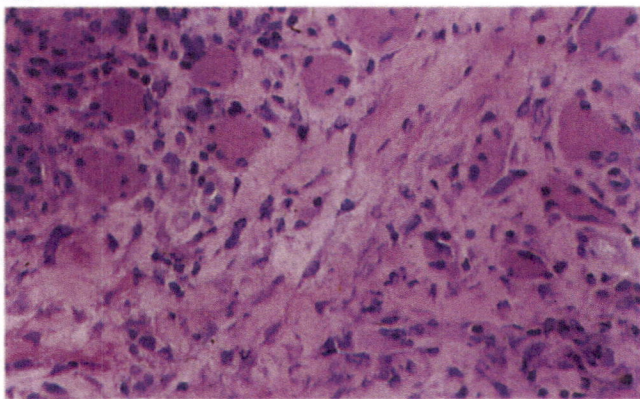

Figure 13.25 Fibrosis in chronic polymyositis. Atrophic fibres are widely separated by interstitial collagen. Fibrosis of this extent indicates chronic disease. Changes are largely irreversible and full clinical recovery cannot be expected. (Same case shown in Figure 13.26.) H & E × 180

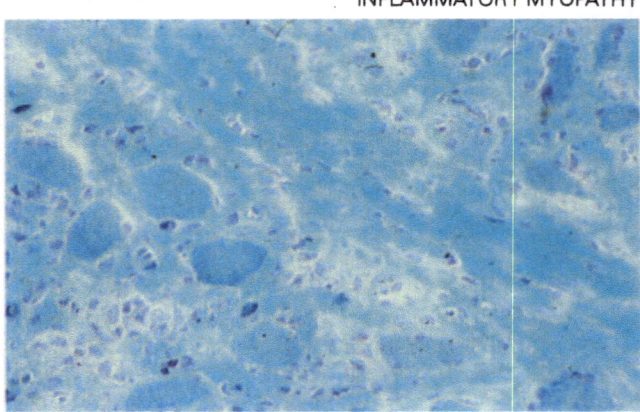

Figure 13.26 Fibrosis in chronic polymyositis. Interstitial connective tissue is well demonstrated by the trichrome stain. There is an increase in both endomysial and perimysial collagen. Gomori's trichrome × 180

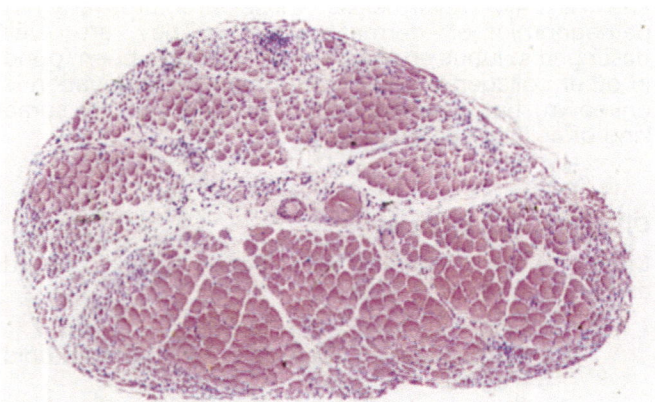

Figure 13.27 Perifascicular fibre atrophy in deltoid muscle of 62-year-old man with polymyositis and carcinoma of the bronchus. (Same case shown in Figure 13.28, also 13.3 and 13.9–13.11.) H & E × 7.5

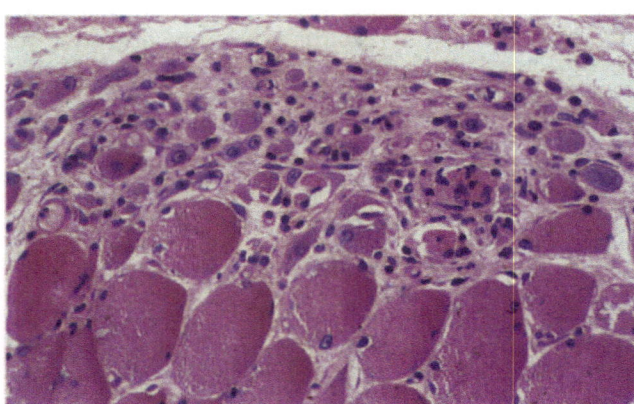

Figure 13.28 Perifascicular fibre atrophy in polymyositis. Severely atrophic peripheral fibres and endomysial fibrosis. This zonal atrophy, in the absence of inflammation, suggests an ischaemic mechanism. H & E × 180

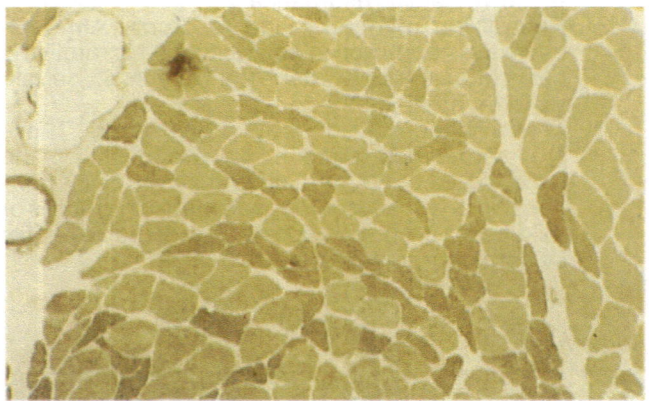

Figure 13.29 Selective type 2 fibre atrophy in polymyositis. Type 2 fibres (dark) show preferential atrophy. (Same case shown in Figure 13.30.) ATP-ase pH 9.4 × 75

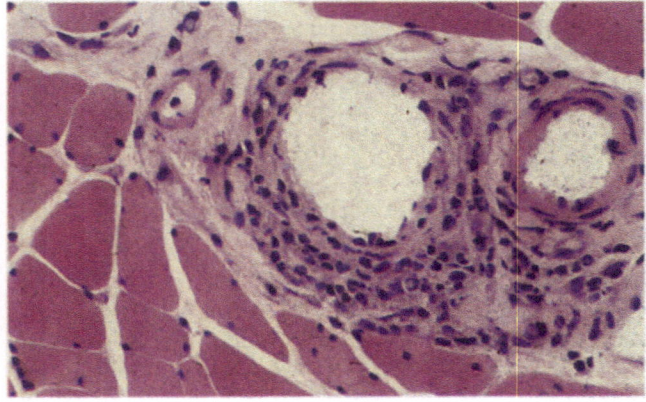

Figure 13.30 Perivascular chronic inflammatory cells, lymphocytes and plasma cells, in a case of polymyositis showing selective type 2 fibre atrophy. H & E × 180

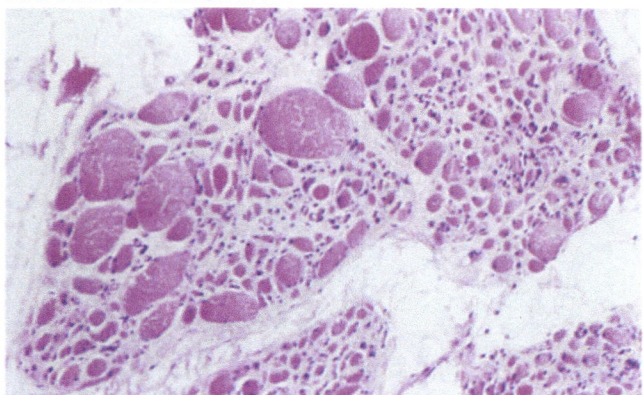

Figure 13.31 Chronic polymyositis with fibre hypertrophy, in 73-year-old man with 5-year history and no treatment. A few grossly hypertrophied fibres contrast with the severely atrophic fibres. Fibre hypertrophy is unusual in poly-myositis, but may appear in chronic disease. Perhaps, as the disease begins to burn out, so surviving fibres undergo compensatory hypertrophy. However, active inflammation was present elsewhere in this biopsy. (Same case shown in Figure 13.32, also in 13.15 and 13.19–13.22. H & E × 75

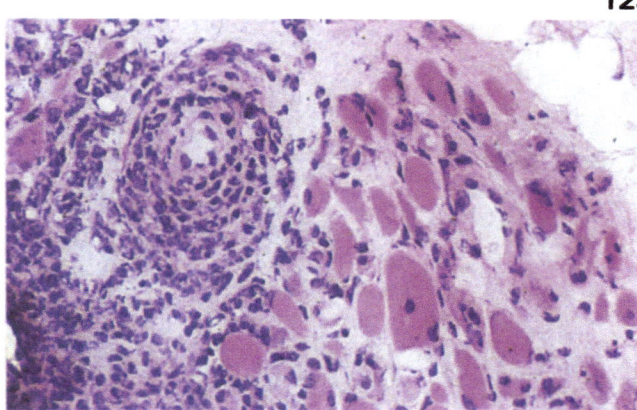

Figure 13.32 Perivascular chronic inflammatory cells in the septum and encroaching upon the fascicle in chronic polymyositis. Active inflammation is still present in this muscle, despite a 5-year clinical history. H & E × 180

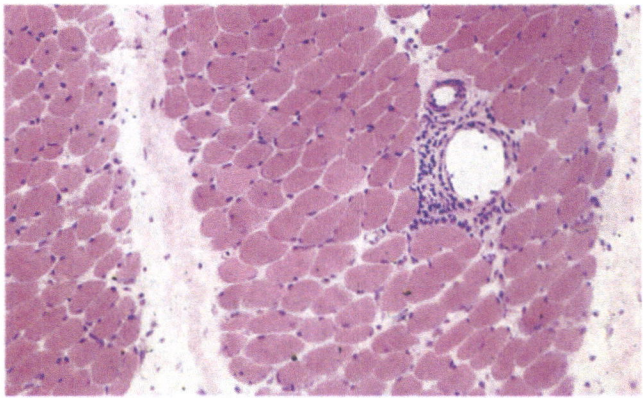

Figure 13.33 Juvenile dermatomyositis. 6-year-old boy with typical clinical picture of dermatomyositis. A miserable child with a skin rash and proximal muscle weakness. Biopsy of quadriceps muscle shows septal, perivascular chronic inflammation and perifascicular fibre atrophy. This histological pattern is commonly seen in juvenile dermatomyositis. H & E × 75

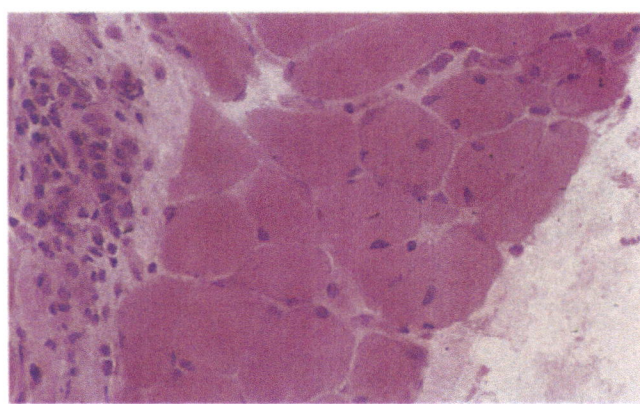

Figure 13.34 Juvenile dermatomyositis. Cluster of atrophic, peripheral fibres with central nuclei. The zonal distribution supports an ischaemic mechanism. H & E × 300

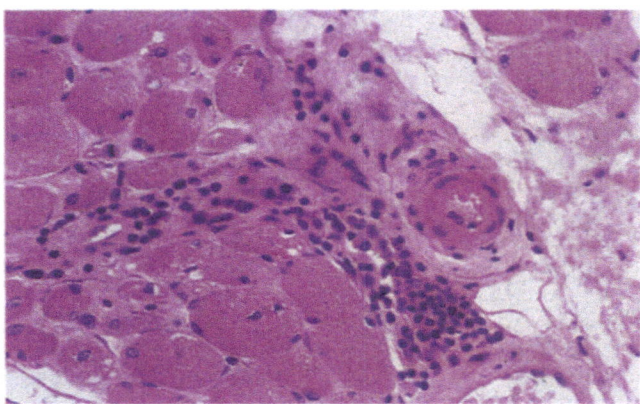

Figure 13.35 Adult dermatomyositis. 37-year-old woman with malaise, purplish discolouration of eyelids, rash on backs of hands and proximal muscle weakness of 5 weeks' duration. Deltoid muscle biopsy shows chronic inflam-matory cells surrounding venules in the septum and also sheathing capillaries as they enter the fascicle. There is fibre atrophy alongside these vessels. The arteriole in the septum appears thickwalled, with a narrow lumen. Elsewhere in this biopsy there is fibrinoid necrosis of small septal arteries. (Same case is shown in Figure 13.36.) H & E × 180

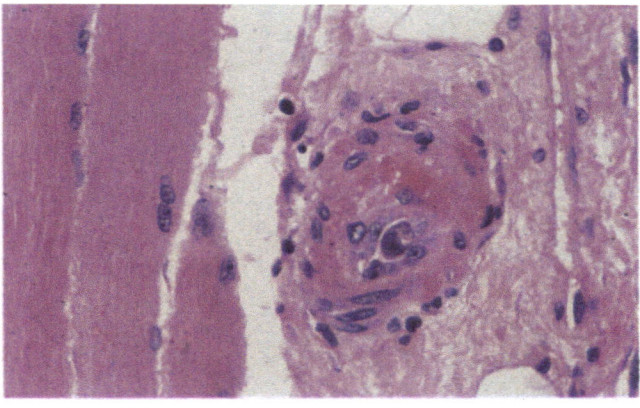

Figure 13.36 Adult dermatomyositis with vasculitis. Small septal artery shows eosinophilic fibrinoid necrosis of the wall and swelling of the endothelial cells virtually occluding the lumen. H & E × 300

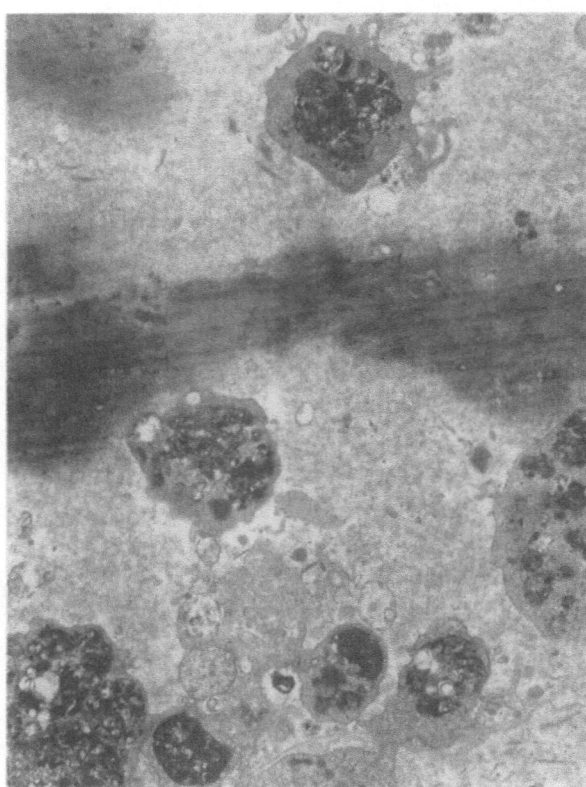

Figure 13.37 Necrotic fibre showing amorphous degenerate cytoplasm invaded by phagocytes. The electron-dense band in the centre is a clump of disintegrating myofilaments. The macrophages contain large secondary lysosomes.   EM × 4500

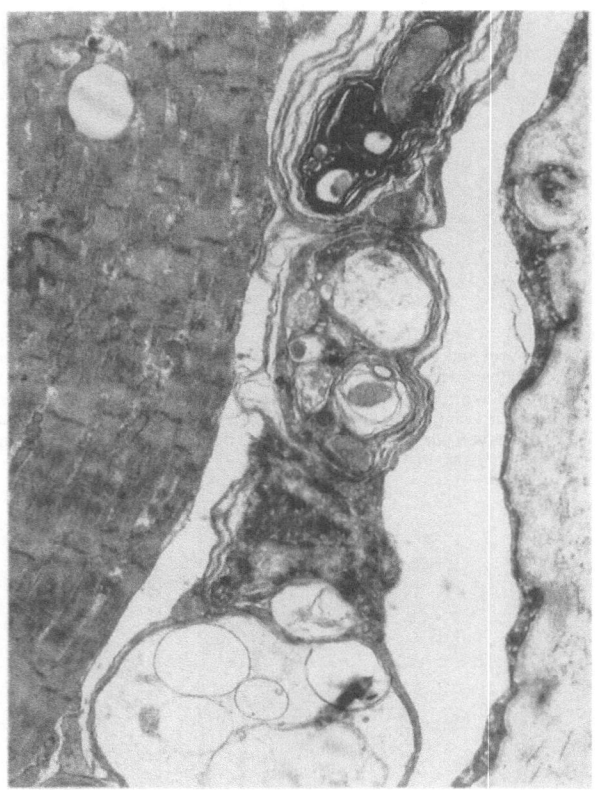

Figure 13.38 Large subsarcolemmal membranous whorls in adult polymyositis. These probably represent lysosomal structures derived from the sarcoplasmic reticulum. They are found in many conditions where there is gradual cell degradation.   EM × 5700

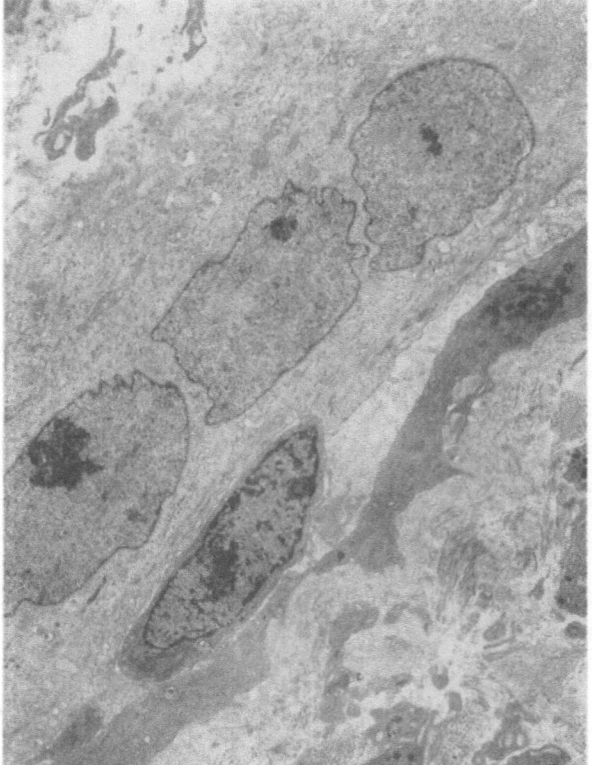

Figure 13.39 Regeneration in polymyositis. A row of large central nuclei in a myotube, formed by fusion of myoblasts. The cytoplasm contains only scanty myofilaments at this stage.   EM × 1900

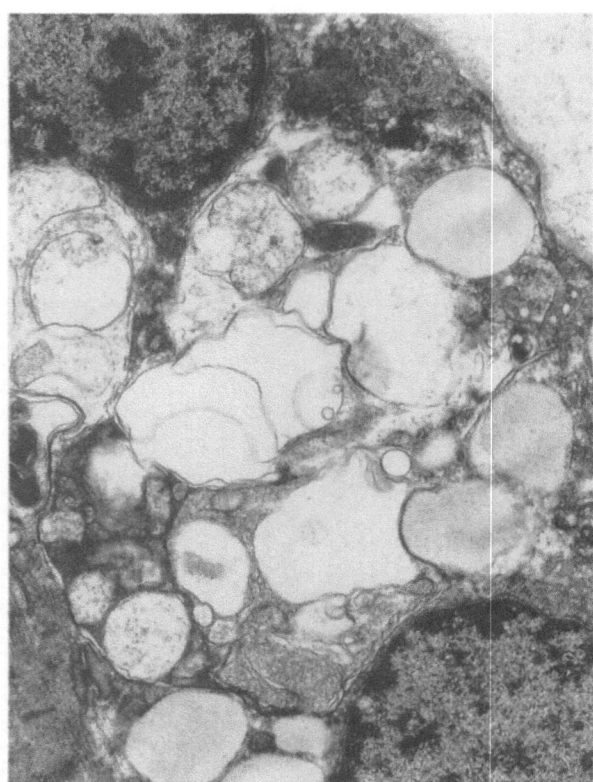

Figure 13.40 Large subsarcolemmal and perinuclear vacuoles in adult polymyositis. These are probably derived from sarcoplasmic reticulum and the forerunner of the more complex membranous whorls shown in Figure 13.38.   EM × 11000

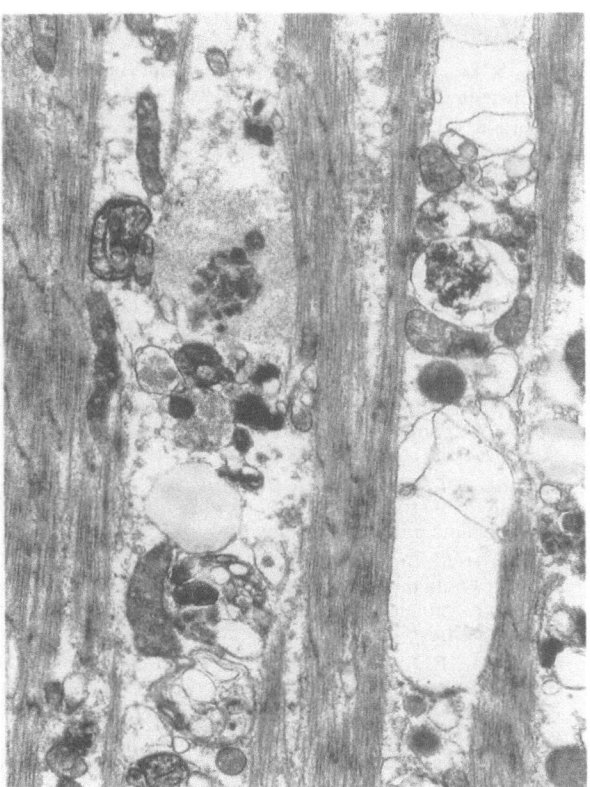

Figure 13.41 Numerous electron-dense membrane bodies, lysosomes, separating the myofibrils. Degenerating cell in adult polymyositis. EM × 7100

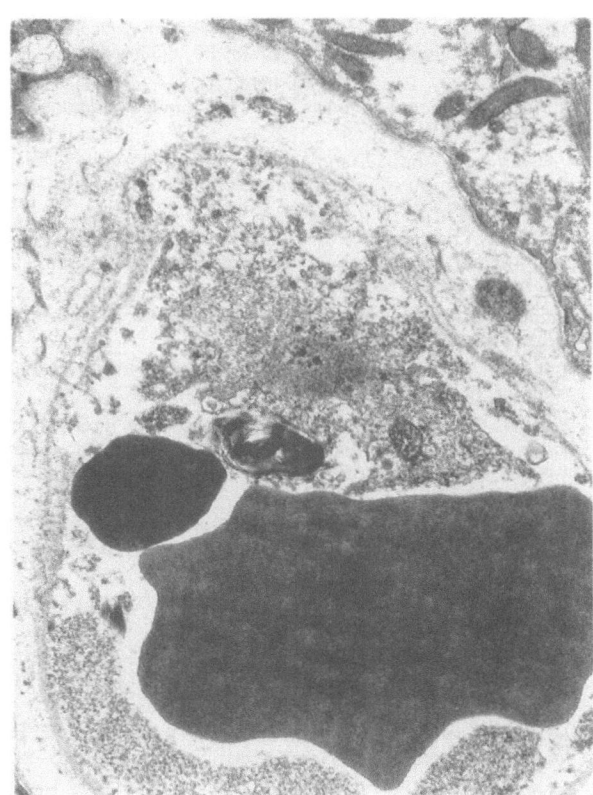

Figure 13.42 Endothelial cell necrosis in juvenile dermatomyositis. The endothelial cell membranes have disappeared and the cytoplasm is granular, with an occasional lysosome. There is also basement membrane reduplication. EM × 7100

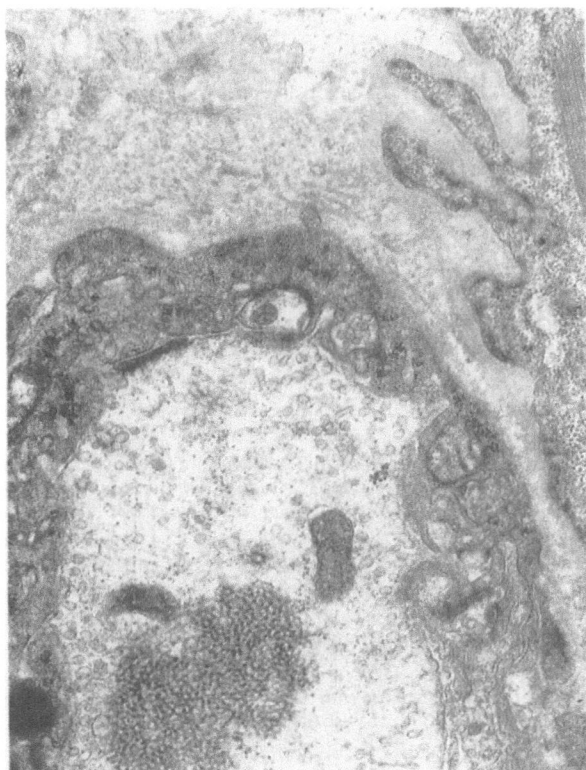

Figure 13.43 Tubular arrays in capillary endothelium in juvenile dermatomyositis. Large, pale endothelial cell containing structured electron-dense inclusion body. EM × 15 000

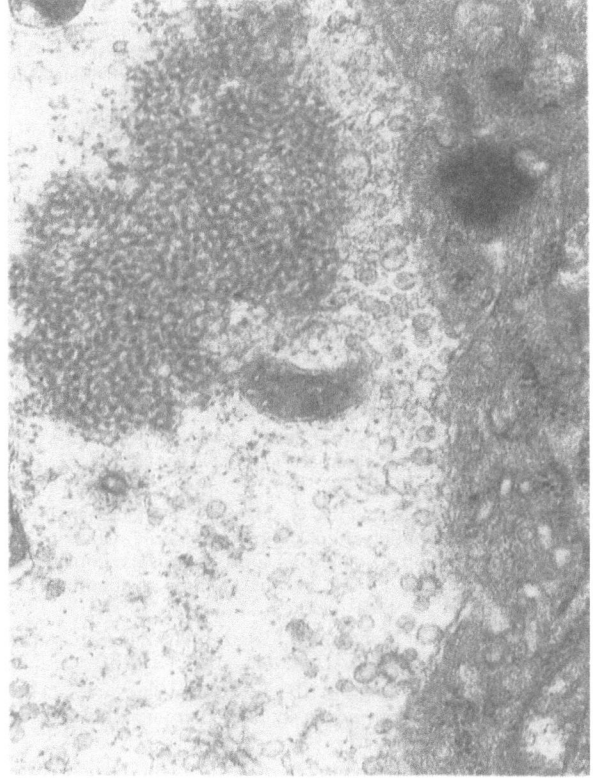

Figure 13.44 Tubular arrays in capillary endothelial cell cytoplasm in juvenile dermatomyositis. Higher magnifications show the complex structure. There is no evidence to suggest these inclusions are viral. They are also found in lupus erythematosus and presumably reflect altered cellular metabolic activity. EM × 25 000

4. De Vere, R. and Bradley, W. G. (1975). Polymyositis: its presentation, morbidity and mortality. *Brain*, **98**, 637–66

5. Venables, G. S., Bates, D., Cartlidge, N. E. F. and Hudgson, P. (1982). Acute polymyositis with subcutaneous oedema. *J. Neurol. Sci.*, **55**, 161–4

6. Fukuyama, Y., Ando, T. and Yokoto, J. (1977). Acute fulminant myoglobinuric polymyositis with picornavirus-like crystals. *J. Neurol. Neurosurg. Psychiatry.*, **40**, 775–81

7. Munsat, T. L., Piper, D., Cancilla, P. and Mednick, J. (1972). Inflammatory myopathy with facioscapulohumeral distribution. *Neurology*, **22**, 335–47

8. Smith, C. A. and Pinals, R. S. (1981). Localised nodular myositis. *J. Rheumatol.*, **8**, 815–19

9. Heffner, R. R. and Baron, S. A. (1981). Polymyositis beginning as a focal process. *Arch. Neurol.*, **38**, 439–42

10. Venables, P. J. N., Mumford, P. A. and Maini, R. N. (1981). Antibodies to nuclear antigens in polymyositis: relationship to autoimmune 'overlap' syndromes and carcinoma. *Ann. Rheum. Dis.*, **40**, 217–23

11. Carpenter, S., Karpati, G., Rothman, S. and Watters, G. (1976). The childhood type of dermatomyositis. *Neurology*, **26**, 952–62

12. Thompson, C. E. (1982). Infantile myositis. *Devel. Med. Child Neurol.*, **24**, 307–13

13. Miller, G., Heckmatt, J. Z. and Dubowitz, V. (1983). Drug treatment of juvenile dermatomyositis. *Arch. Dis. Child.*, **58**, 445–50

14. Henriksson, K. G. and Sandstedt, P. (1982). Polymyositis: treatment and prognosis. *Acta Neurol. Scand.*, **65**, 280–300

15. Behan, W. M. H., Behan, P. O. and Dick, H. A. (1978). HLA B8 in polymyositis. *N. Engl. J. Med.*, **298**, 1260–1

16. Banker, B. Q. and Victor, M. (1966). Dermatomyositis (systemic angiopathy) of childhood. *Medicine*, **45**, 261–89

17. Carpenter, S., Karpati, G., Rothman, S. and Walters, G. (1976). The childhood type of dermatomyositis. *Neurology*, **26**, 952–62

18. Whitaker, J. N. and Engel, W. K. (1972). Vascular deposits of immunoglobulin and complement in idiopathic inflammatory myopathy. *N. Engl. J. Med.*, **286**, 333–8

19. Kamata, K., Kobayashi, Y., Shigematsu, H. and Saito, T. (1982). Childhood type polymyositis and rapidly progressive glomerulonephritis. *Acta Pathol. Jpn.*, **32**, 801–6

20. Mihas, A. A., Kirkby, J. D. and Kent, S. P. (1978). Hepatitis B antigen and polymyositis. *J. Am. Med. Assoc.*, **239**, 221–2

21. Damjanov, I., Moser, R. L., Moriber Katz, S. and Lyons, P. (1980). Immune complex myositis associated with viral hepatitis. *Human Pathol.*, **77**, 478–81

22. Esiri, M. M., MacLennan, I. C. M. and Hazleman, B. L. (1973). Lymphocyte sensitivity to skeletal muscle in patients with polymyositis and other disorders. *Clin. Exp. Immunol.*, **14**, 25–35

23. Rowe, D. J., Isenberg, D. A., McDougal, J. and Beverley, P. C. L. (1981). Characterisation of polymyositis infiltrates using monoclonal antibodies to human leucoctye antigens. *Clin. Exp. Immunol.*, **45**, 290–8

24. Arahata, K. and Engel, A. G. (1984). Monoclonal antibody analysis of mononuclear cells in myopathies. 1. Quantitation of subsets according to diagnosis and sites of accumulation and demonstration and counts of muscle fibres invaded by T cells. *Ann. Neurol.*, **16**, 193–208

25. Esiri, M. M. and MacLennne, I. C. M. (1974). Experimental myositis in rats. *Clin. Exp. Immunol.*, **17**, 139–50

26. Curtis, A. C., Heckaman, J. H. and Wheeler, A. H. (1961). Study of the auto-immune reaction in dermatomyositis. *J. Am. Med. Assoc.*, **178**, 571–3

27. Ducher, B. G. and Goodman, A. L. (1976). D penicillamine induced polymyositis in rheumatoid arthritis. *Ann. Intern. Med.*, **85**, 615–16

28. Medscer, T. A., Dawson, W. N. and Masi, A. T. (1970). The epidemiology of polymyositis. *Am. J. Med.*, **48**, 715–23

29. Landry, M. and Winkelman, R. K. (1972). Tubular cytoplasmic inclusion in dermatomyositis. *Mayo Clin. Proc.*, **47**, 479–92

30. Chou, S. M. and Gutmann, L. (1970). Picorna virus-like crystals in subacute polymyositis. *Neurology (Minneap.)*, **20**, 205–13

31. Mastaglia, F. L. and Walton, J. N. (1970). Virus-like particles in skeletal muscle from a case of polymyositis. *J. Neurol. Sci.*, **2**, 593–9

32. Gyorkey, F., Cabral, G. A., Gyorkey, P. K., Uribe Boero, G., Dreesman, G. T. and Melnick, J. L. (1978). Coxsackie-virus aggregates in muscle cells of a polymyositis patient. *Intervirology*, **10**, 69–77

33. Ry, C. G., Miinich, L. L. and Johnson, P. C. (1979). Selective polymyositis induced by Coxsackie virus B1 in mice. P.C. *J. Infect. Dis.*, **140**, 239–43

34. Tang, T. T., Sedmak, G. V., Siegesmund, K. A. and McCreadie, S. R. (1975). Chronic myopathy associated with Coxsackie virus type A9. A combined electron microscopical and viral isolation study. *N. Engl. J. Med.*, **292**, 608–11

35. Gamboa, E. T., Eastwood, A. B., Hays, A. P., Maxwell, J. and Penn, A. (1979). Isolation of influenza virus from muscle in myoglobinuric polymyositis. *Neurology*, **29**, 1323–35

36. Kessler, H. A., Trenholme, G. M., Harris, A. H. and Levin, S. (1980). Acute myopathy associated with influenza A infection: isolation of virus from a muscle biopsy specimen. *J. Am. Med. Assoc.*, **243**, 461–2

37. Middleton, R. J., Alexander, R. M. and Szymanski, M. T. (1970). Severe myositis during recovery from influenza. *Lancet*, **2**, 533–5

38. Bardelas, J. A., Winkelstein, J. A., Seto, D. S. Y., Tsai, T. and Rogol, A. D. (1977). Fatal Echo 24 infection in a patient with hypogammaglobulinaemia: relationship to dermatomyositis-like syndrome. *J. Pediatr.*, **90**, 396–9

39. Dawkins, R. L. and Zilko, P. J. (1975). Polymyositis and myasthenia; immunodeficiency disorders involving skeletal muscle. *Lancet*, **1**, 200

40. Karasawa, T., Takizawa, I., Morita, K., Ishibasi, H., Kanayama, S. and Shikata, T. (1981). Polymyositis and toxoplasmosis. *Acta Pathol. Jpn.*, **31**, 675–80

41. Pollock, J. L. (1979). Toxoplasmosis appearing to be dermatomyositis. *Arch. Dermatol.*, **115**, 736–7

42. Kagen, L. J., Kimball, A. C. and Christian, C. L. (1974). Serologic evidence of toxoplasmosis among patients with polymyositis. *Am. J. Med.*, **235**, 186–91

43. Samuels, B. S. and Rietschel, R. L. (1976). Polymyositis and toxoplasmosis. *J. Am. Med. Assoc.*, **235**, 60–1

44. Schwarz, H. A., Slavin, G., Ward, P. and Ansell, B. M. (1980). Muscle biopsy in polymyositis and dermatomyositis: a clinicopathological study. *Ann. Rheum. Dis.*, **39**, 500–7

45. Mashaly, R. *et al.* (1981). Polymyositis with infiltration by lymphoid follicles. *Arch. Neurol.*, **38**, 777–9

46. Stark, R. J. (1979). Eosinophilic polymyositis. *Arch. Neurol.*, **36**, 721–2

47. Paljarvi, L. and Snall, E. V. (1984). Morphometric approaches to perifascicular atrophy in muscle biopsy: Do they help to diagnose polymyositis? *Neuropathol. Appl. Neurobiol.*, **10**, 331–41

48. Banker, B. Q. (1975). Dermatomyositis of childhood: ultrastructural alterations of muscle and intramuscular blood vessels. *J. Neuropathol. Exp. Neurol.*, **34**, 46–74

49. Hughes, J. T. and Esiri, M. M. (1975). Ultrastructural studies in human polymyositis. *J. Neurol. Sci.*, **25**, 347–60

50. Chou, S. M., Nonaka, I. and Voice, G. F. (1980). Anastomoses of transverse tubules with terminal cisternae in polymyositis. *Arch. Neurol.*, **37**, 257–66

51. Oshima, Y., Becker, L. E. and Armstrong, D. L. (1979). An electron microscope study of childhood dermatomyositis. *Acta Neuropathol (Berl.)*, **47**, 189–96

Minor inflammatory changes may be found in muscle in connective disease without the full clinical and pathological picture of polymyositis. It seems logical to consider polymyalgia rheumatica with this group, although genuine myositis is most unusual. Inclusion body myositis is also usually included with the inflammatory myopathies, but despite the name, its qualifications are rather slight.

Inclusion Body Myositis

Diagnosis of this disorder rests upon histological criteria: the inclusion bodies, which are filamentous nuclear inclusions and cytoplasmic membranous whorls. As morphological abnormalities are rarely pathognomonic of a single disorder and the clinical picture is quite variable, it seems unlikely that inclusion body myositis is a single entity. Initial reports of distal wasting in elderly patients, chiefly males[1], have been superseded by finding the same histology in younger patients, occasionally in siblings[2], frequently in females and in patients with proximal weakness[3]. However, common to many, there seems to be a slowly progressive, painless muscular weakness, which does not respond to steroids. The CPK is normal or only slightly elevated and the EMG shows a mixed myopathic-denervating pattern. Of considerable interest is a recent report of isolation of an adenovirus from the muscle of one patient with inclusion body myositis[4]. All other attempts to prove the inclusions are viral have been unsuccessful and the possibility of a passenger virus cannot be denied. Although the nuclear inclusions have been regarded as specific, they are occasionally found in other disorders and quite similar filaments have been identified in oculopharyngeal dystrophy. The cytoplasmic whorls are seen in several different conditions, including distal myopathy, chloroquine myopathy and sometimes polymyositis. At present it seems that the histological abnormalities are indicative of a mild chronic degenerative process, but a unifying cause is doubtful.

Muscle Biopsy

By light microscopy cytoplasmic vacuoles draw attention to this condition[1] (Figure 14.1). Beside these, there are usually fairly minor, non-specific myopathic changes, or a hint of denervation atrophy. The vacuoles are small and irregular and may be single or multiple. Numerous fibres or only a few may be affected. With H & E the vacuoles have a basophilic rim. This is red with the trichrome stain. Vacuoles often appear empty but some contain darkly staining granular material.

There may be a weak acid phosphatase activity at the edge, suggesting lysosomal origin. The vacuoles are devoid of all other enzyme activity. Some degree of fibre atrophy is usual. This may be grouped atrophy, with small angular fibres, or scattered atrophic fibres[1]. Some fibres may show compensatory hypertrophy. Inflammation is very variable and often completely absent. There may be small patchy foci of endomysial lymphocytes. A few necrotic fibres may be found. Occasionally large sarcolemmal nuclei contain homogeneous eosinophilic nuclear inclusions[3].

Electron Microscopy

The cytoplasmic vacuoles are identified as osmiophilic membranous whorls (Figure 14.2). These may also contain glycogen granules and fragments of cell organelles. The distinctive finding in inclusion body myositis is masses of filaments, commonly within the cytoplasm and often within nuclei[5] (Figure 14.3). The filaments are around 15–20 nm wide and frequently in parallel array[2]. Their nature is unknown, but comparable size and arrangement have prompted the suggestion that they are derived from myosin, rather than viruses[6]. Large, abnormal mitochondria are also described.

Connective Tissue Disease – Rheumatoid Arthritis, SLE, Polyarteritis Nodosa, Scleroderma, MCTD

Muscle symptoms are not uncommon in these disorders, particularly in rheumatoid disease. All may co-exist with a muscle disorder, clinically and pathologically indistinguishable from idiopathic polymyositis, but this diagnosis should not be accepted without proper investigation. Vague, non-specific symptoms may be associated with minimal and equally non-specific pathology. A few lymphocytes and isolated atrophic fibres are quite common, but do not warrant the additional diagnosis of polymyositis. Patients with genuine muscle weakness are likely to have demonstrable pathology, for which there are several possible causes. Vasculitis is a common denominator of the connective diseases and occasionally may appear in muscle in any one of them.

Rheumatoid Arthritis

Localized muscle weakness, related to severely arthritic joints, is very common. In addition, about one-third of patients have diffuse muscle weakness[7]. Joint pains and immobility, cachexia, neuropathy and steroid

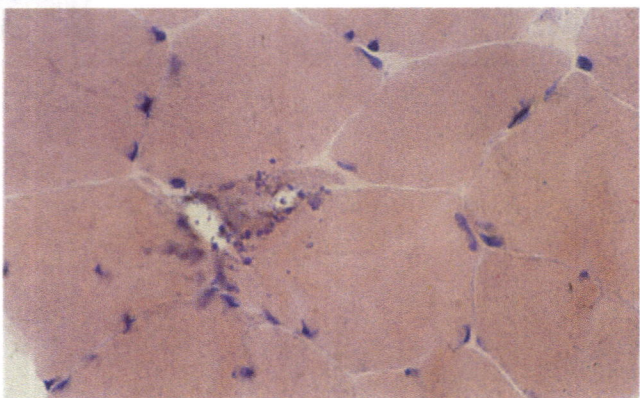

Figure 14.1 Probable inclusion body myositis. 82-year-old man. Well controlled, maturity onset diabetic, with mild, slowly progressive weakness of legs and cramps in one foot. Reflexes depressed but no sensory loss. The biopsy shows an atrophic fibre containing small vacuoles filled with basophilic debris. The biopsy contained scattered atrophic fibres, but only small numbers of vacuoles. (Same case shown in Figure 14.3.)   H & E × 450

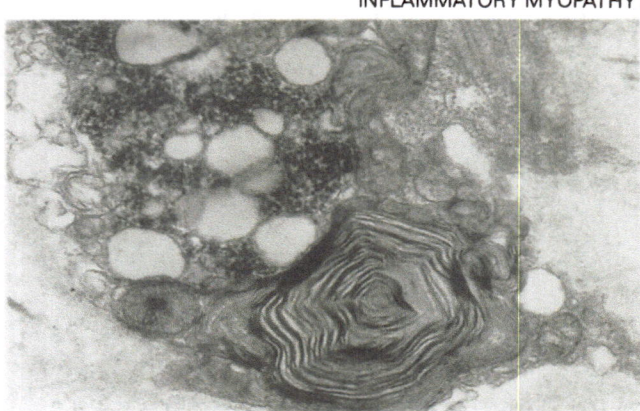

Figure 14.2 Cytoplasmic whorls. These whorls of membranous material, which probably represent lysosomes, were found to be quite numerous by electron microscopy. They are a characteristic feature, but not specific to inclusion body myositis. Filamentous inclusions were not demonstrated in this case.   EM × 25 000

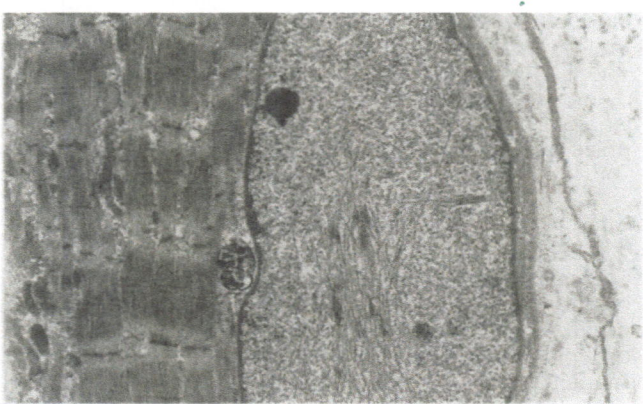

Figure 14.3 Nuclear filamentous inclusions. These are a characteristic finding, but are not unique to inclusion body myositis. The filaments shown here were found in the biopsy of a patient with a typical picture of polymyositis. The light microscopic findings of the case are illustrated in Figures 13.15, 13.19–13.22, 13.31 and 13.32.   EM × 7100

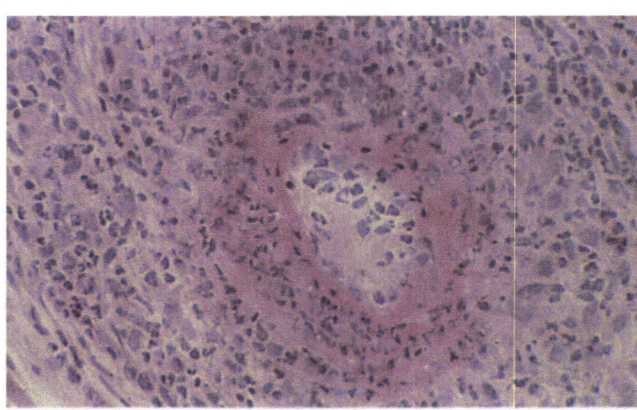

Figure 14.4 Polyarteritis nodosa. Quadriceps biopsy from a 52-year-old woman with asthma, eosinophilia, raised ESR and 4-month history of proximal muscle weakness. The biopsy contains a medium-size artery, which shows acute fibrinoid necrosis. In conjunction with the clinical picture, this histology confirms the diagnosis of polyarteritis nodosa. (Same case shown in Figures 14.5 and 14.6.)   H & E × 180

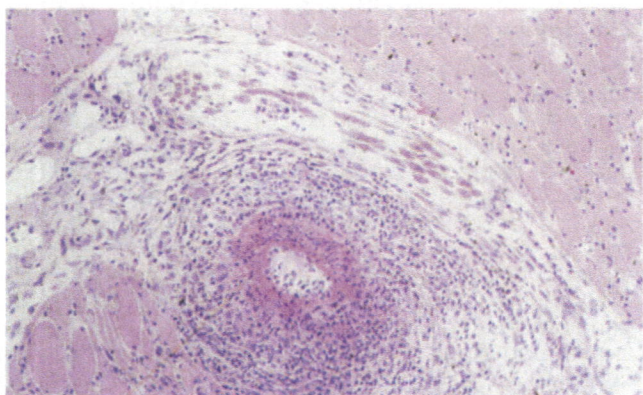

Figure 14.5 Polyarteritis nodosa. Atrophic muscle fibres in fascicles adjacent to the inflamed artery. A small myelinated nerve runs alongside the artery.   H & E × 75

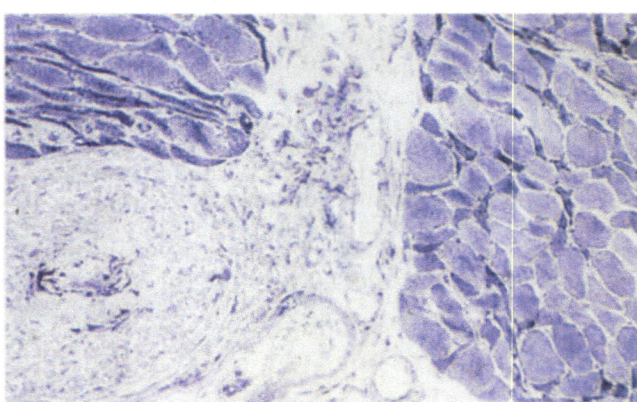

Figure 14.6 Polyarteritis nodosa. Atrophic fibres, adjacent to the inflamed, occluded artery. Fibre atrophy is not uniform and there are groups of angular darkly staining fibres. This pattern is probably due to ischaemia of the adjacent nerve, producing local denervation atrophy.   NADH-TR × 75

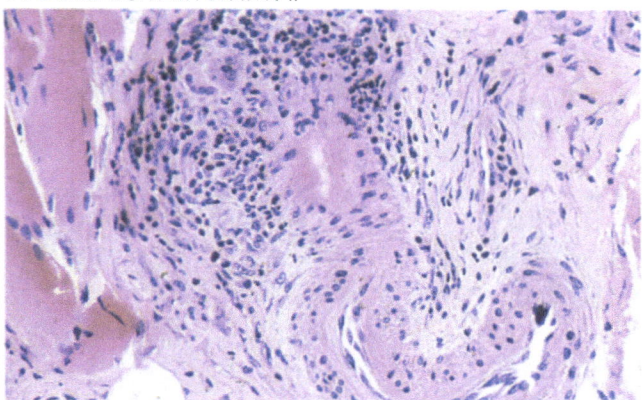

Figure 14.7 Polyarteritis nodosa. Quadriceps biopsy from a 65-year-old man with wasting and weakness of the right leg and slight weakness in the arms and sensory involvement suggesting a peripheral neuropathy. ESR – very high. CPK – normal. The biopsy shows fibrinoid necrosis in the wall of a medium-size muscular artery. The fibrinoid lesion is surrounded by lymphocytes, histiocytes and a solitary giant cell. This is a necrotizing vasculitis. A solitary giant cell does not make it giant cell-temporal arteritis. Together with the clinical picture, this histology is typical polyarteritis nodosa. (Same case shown in Figure 14.8.)   H & E × 180

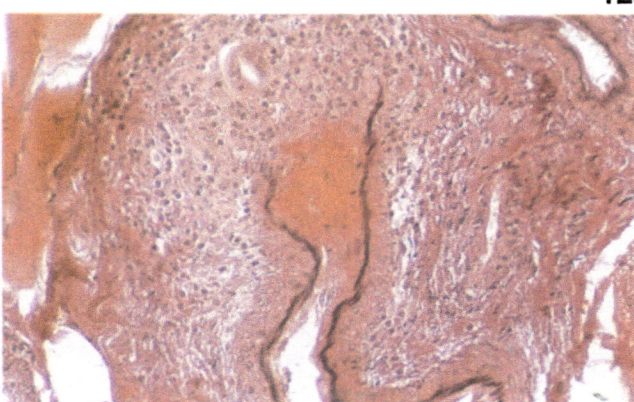

Figure 14.8 Polyarteritis nodosa. The elastic stain reveals complete interruption of the elastic lamina and muscle coat with fibrin thrombus filling the lumen. The clinical picture suggests muscle wasting is related to a peripheral neuropathy. This is almost certainly attributable to ischaemia of the nerves.   Elastic ponceau S × 180

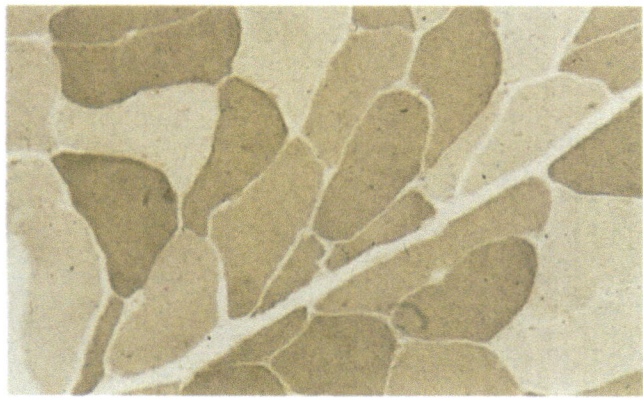

Figure 14.9 Polyarteritis nodosa. Several small angular fibres in fascicles adjacent to occluded artery, probably denervation atrophy.   ATP-ase pH 4.5 × 300

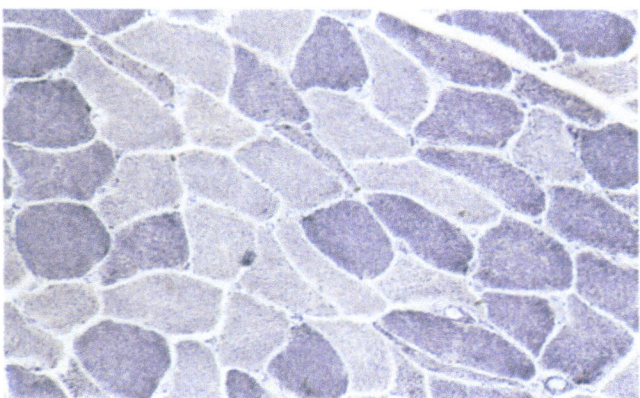

Figure 14.10 Polyarteritis nodosa. Scattered angular atrophic fibres in fascicles adjacent to the occluded artery. Unlike polymyositis, there are no necrotic or regenerating fibres and no epimysial inflammation.   NADH-TR × 180

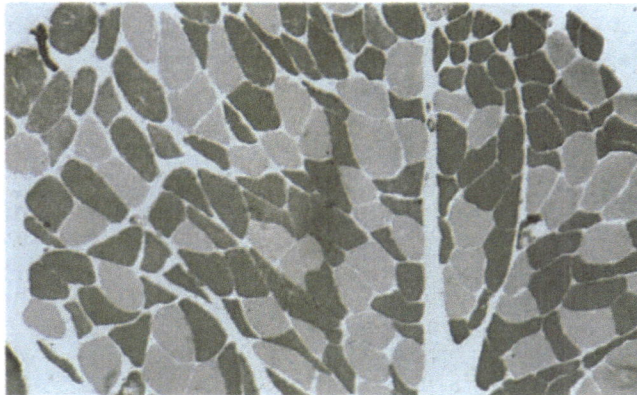

Figure 14.11 Polymyalgia rheumatica. Deltoid biopsy from a 62-year-old man with a 5-month history of pains around the shoulders, a stiff neck and scalp tenderness. He showed minimal weakness, but movements of the shoulder girdle musculature were limited by pain. No abnormality in lower limbs. ESR – raised. CPK – normal. A small dose of prednisone produced rapid alleviation of his symptoms. The biopsy shows a selective type 2 fibre atrophy. This is probably attributable to the limitation of movement imposed by pain. There are no inflammatory changes and no evidence of necrosis or regeneration. (Same case shown in Figure 14.12.)   ATP-ase pH 9.4 × 75

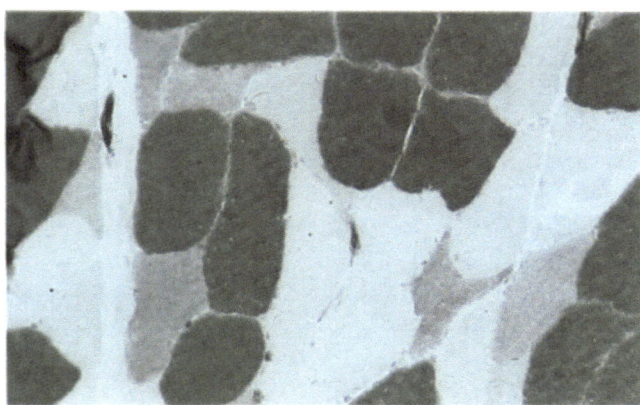

Figure 14.12 Polymyalgia rheumatica. Selective type 2B atrophy. Type 2A fibres are only slightly reduced in size. Type 1 are mostly of normal size. Type 2B fibres are invariably the most severely affected by immobility.   ATP-ase pH 4.5 × 300

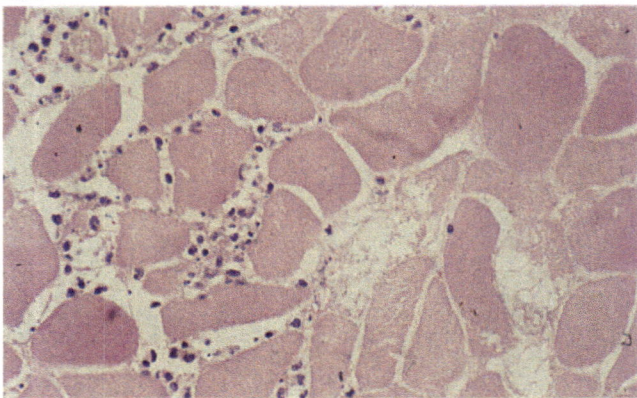

Figure 14.13 Gas gangrene. Black, soft rectus abdominis muscle, exuding foul smelling fluid, excised from a 40-year-old woman who had had abdominal surgery for intestinal obstruction 3 days previously. The muscle fibres are necrotic and pale staining, but there is only a scanty acute inflammatory exudate.   H & E × 180

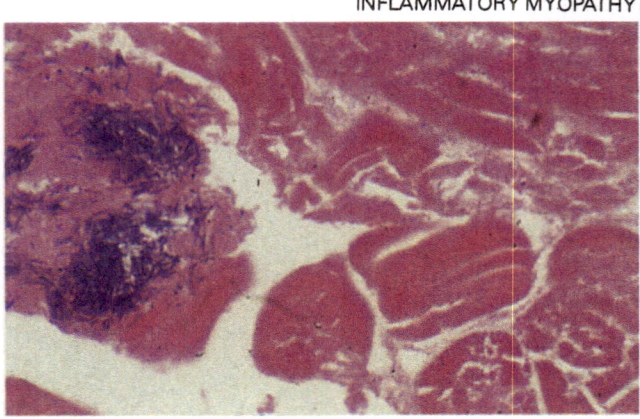

Figure 14.14 Gas gangrene. Clumped, necrotic and disintegrating muscle fibres around colonies of Clostridial bacilli, but no inflammatory response.   H & E × 300

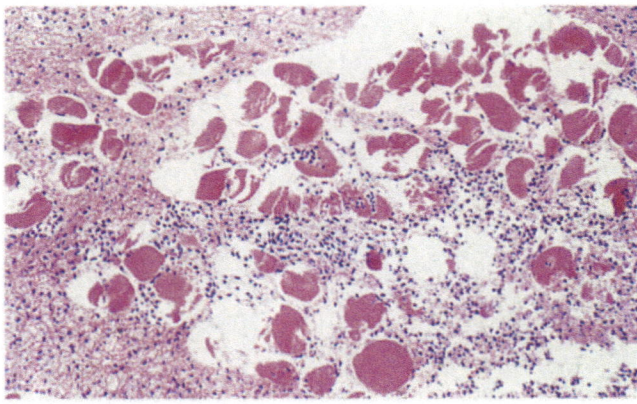

Figure 14.15 Streptococcal myositis. Forearm muscle from a 72-year-old woman with longstanding rheumatoid arthritis. She complained of pain and swelling in the arm, associated with a shivering attack. She collapsed and died 24 hours later. At postmortem the forearm muscles were soft, swollen and exuded watery purulent fluid, from which a haemolytic Group A Streptococcus was cultured. The muscle fibres are widely separated by fibrinopurulent exudate. (Same case shown in Figure 14.16.)   H & E × 75

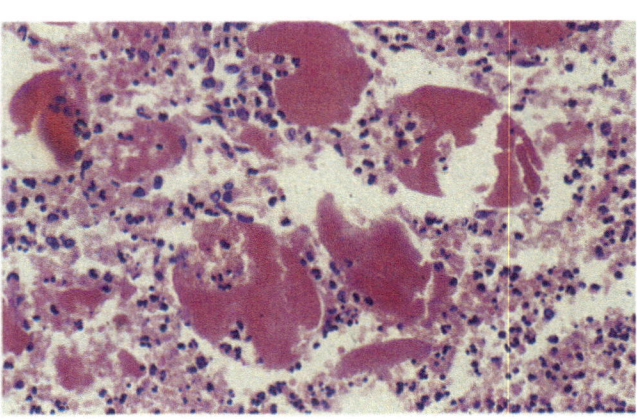

Figure 14.16 Streptococcal myositis. Disintegrating muscle fibres surrounded by polymorphoneutrophil leukocytes and fibrin.   H & E × 300

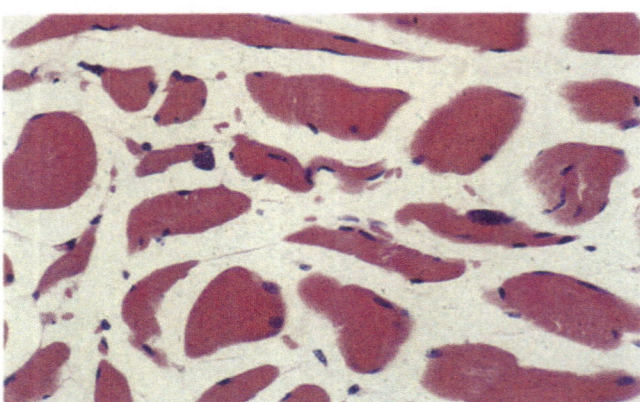

Figure 14.17 Toxoplasmosis. Postmortem skeletal muscle from an immunosuppressed cardiac transplant recipient. There is no inflammatory reaction and organisms are easily overlooked or mistaken for large nuclei. (Same case shown in Figure 14.18.)   H & E × 180

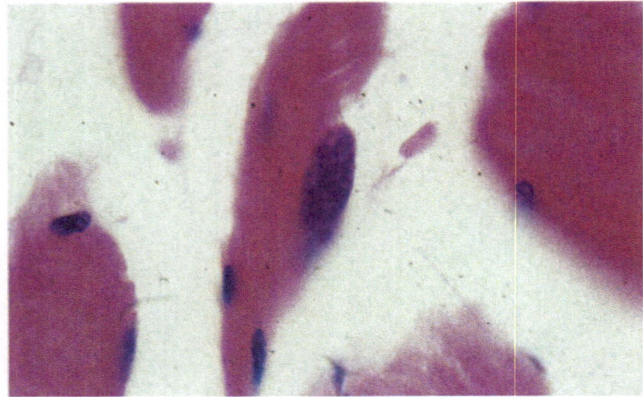

Figure 14.18 Toxoplasmosis. At higher magnification the rounded, encysted form of *Toxoplasma gondii* is seen within a muscle fibre, but apparently without harmful effect. There is no evidence of muscle necrosis or regeneration and no inflammation. The intracellular organisms are a mass of bradyzoites which occupy a cytoplasmic vacuole.   H & E × 750

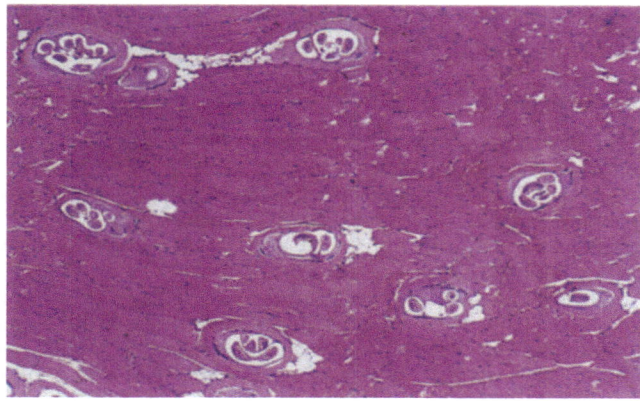

Figure 14.19 *Trichinella spiralis*. Numerous encysted larvae in skeletal muscle fibres. There is surprisingly little inflammatory response.   H & E × 30

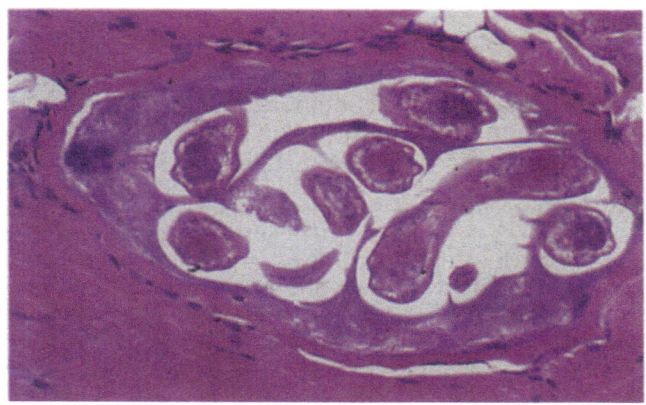

Figure 14.20 *Trichinella spiralis*. Encysted larva with hyaline cyst wall. Scanty surrounding inflammatory cells.   H & E × 180

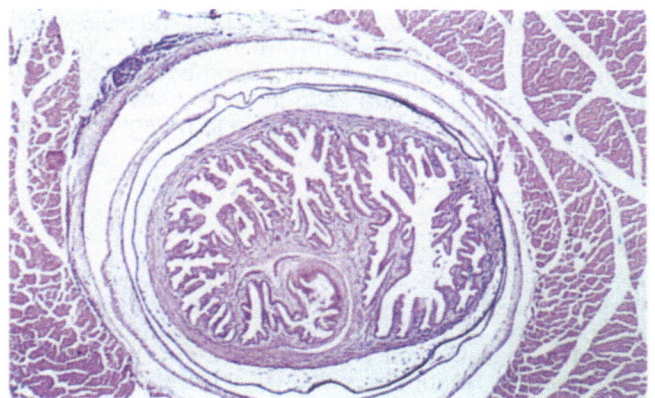

Figure 14.21 Cysticercosis. The larval form of the pork tapeworm, *Taenia solium*. Each cyst contains an invaginated scolex. There is a border of lymphocytes around the cyst.   H & E × 20

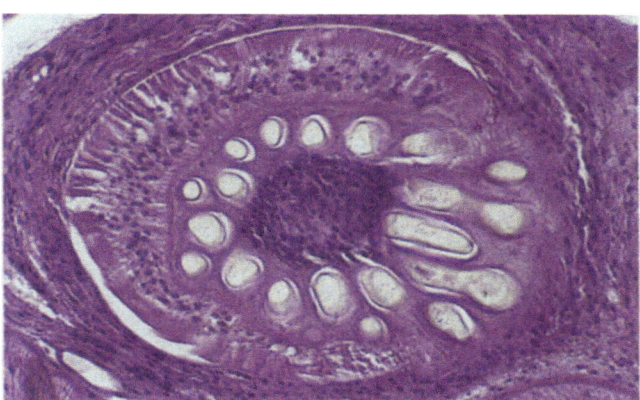

Figure 14.22 Cysticercosis. Ring of hooklets of the scolex, which are doubly refractile.   H & E × 180

therapy are all possible contributory factors. Evidence of peripheral neuropathy was found in 15% of patients in the series of Reza and Verity[7]. Thus in the muscle biopsy at times a mixed picture will be found. Small groups of angular atrophic fibres denote denervation. Isolated, interstitial aggregates of lymphocytes, without accompanying fibre necrosis, are quite a frequent finding, but on their own these are clinically insignificant[8]. However, large inflammatory aggregates or diffuse infiltration of the fascicles are usually associated with muscle fibre damage and these cases belong in the polymyositis overlap category. Vasculitis is an important feature of systemic rheumatoid disease. Microangiopathy is seen in the overlap group, but, apart from this, rheumatoid patients occasionally develop fibrinoid necrosis of medium-size muscular arteries, resembling polyarteritis nodosa[7]. Patients with rheumatoid myopathy may show a selective type 2 fibre atrophy without inflammation. This may be attributable to disuse and cachexia, but the possibility of steroid myopathy must be considered in patients receiving therapy.

Polyarteritis Nodosa

The typical pathological lesion of this systemic disease is fibrinoid necrosis of medium-sized, muscular arteries (Figures 14.4–14.8). The affected segment of vessel is occluded by thrombus, with resulting ischaemic lesions. Localized muscle weakness and tenderness is not uncommon, but generalized muscle wasting is unusual. Blind muscle biopsy is not a very fruitful way to attempt to prove this diagnosis, but biopsy of a clinically affected muscle may detect the characteristic lesion. An open biopsy is preferable, because a small needle biopsy is unlikely to pick up the larger blood vessels. The muscle fibres in fascicles around an affected artery are likely to show varying degrees of ischaemic injury, or denervation atrophy, due to peripheral nerve ischaemia, but there is usually no significant microangiopathy or epimysial inflammation (Figures 14.6, 14.9 and 14.10).

Polymyalgia Rheumatica

This is a disease in which pain and stiffness in proximal muscles, rather than weakness, is the main problem. It is a disorder of unknown aetiology, commoner in women and occurring in late middle age and old age. The CPK is usually normal, but the ESR is greatly increased. The muscle pain is not associated with any progressive pathology and a far more serious problem is the presence of temporal arteritis in approximately 20% of cases. Both arteritis and muscle symptoms respond rapidly to steroid therapy. The concurrence of temporal arteritis suggests a vasculitic basis for muscle symptoms but this does not appear to be the case. The muscle biopsy does not reveal either inflammatory or vasculitic lesions, but minor non-descript changes, which correlate with the minimal clinical signs. Mild type 2B atrophy may result from inactivity (Figures 14.11 and 14.12). There is no satisfactory explanation for the muscle pain in this condition. Possibly it is referred pain from ligaments or joints.

Sarcoidosis

Symptomatic muscle disease in patients with sarcoidosis is unusual[9]. Only a minority complain of muscle tenderness. A minority also have slightly raised muscle enzymes. However, random muscle biopsy has detected granulomata in a much larger proportion (approximately 50%)[10] and therefore has some use as a diagnostic test. The gastrocnemius muscle has been examined most often and a positive biopsy obtained most frequently in patients with acute sarcoid, with the triad of fever, erythema nodosum and hilar lymphadenopathy. The discrete, non-caseating epithelioid and giant cell granulomata, which characterize sarcoid at any site, are usually located in the connective tissue septa of skeletal muscle, only occasionally in the fascicles[10]. Serial sections are advocated to increase the diagnostic yield. The granulomata may be surrounded by a scanty rim of small lymphocytes, but there is no diffuse lymphocytic infiltrate. There may be a few atrophic fibres immediately adjacent to granulomata, but otherwise skeletal muscle fibres show no abnormalities. Other granulomatous diseases rarely affect muscle. Granulomata are rare histological components of polymyositis but are then accompanied by atrophic, necrotic and degenerative changes in muscle fascicles (see chapter 13).

Infective Myositis

All manner of organisms, viruses, bacteria, fungi and larger parasites occasionally invade muscle, with symptomatic effects. Postinfluenzal myositis is well recognized, but is not a clinical problem that requires investigation. Rhabdomyolysis is reported as an exceptionally rare complication of influenza[11]. Myositis due to the direct effects of bacterial or parasitic invasion of muscle are relatively uncommon in Britain and Western Europe, but well known in the tropics.

Gas Gangrene

Clostridial infection of devitalized, traumatized tissue is the most lethal form of myositis. It is manifest by severe pain and swelling with serosanguinous exudation from the wound, soon accompanied by systemic illness and prostration. Rapidly spreading muscle necrosis is due to Clostridial toxins, especially lecithinase, which breaks down cell membranes. Histology shows extensive muscle cell necrosis and disintegration, associated with masses of vegetative bacilli, but only scanty polymorphoneutrophil leukocytes (Figures 14.13 and 14.14).

Streptococcal Myositis

Acute Streptococcal myositis is fortunately rare, but frequently runs a very rapid fatal course and is not recognized until postmortem[12]. There is no history of trauma. Infection appears to be blood borne, but the portal of entry is invariably unknown. The affected muscles are swollen, soft and necrotic and sometimes haemorrhagic. Watery, purulent exudate, teeming with organisms, exudes from the cut surface. Group A haemolytic Streptococci are obtained by culture. Death is attributable to severe toxaemia, which is associated with intravascular coagulation[13]. Muscle histology shows necrotic muscle fibres, surrounded by abundant acute inflammatory exudate containing numerous polymorphoneutrophil leukocytes (Figures 14.15 and 14.16). Gram staining demonstrates numerous Gram-positive cocci.

Toxoplasmosis

Toxoplasma gondii is an obligate intracellular parasite, with worldwide distribution in man and many animals. Primary infection in man occasionally resembles glandular fever and myalgia may be present. However, the very common finding of Toxoplasma antibodies in the serum of the general population suggests acquired infection is usually asymptomatic[11]. A hypersensitivity response to Toxoplasma organisms is one postulated cause of 'idiopathic' polymyositis[14]. Organisms have been recovered at postmortem from brain and muscle of completely asymptomatic adults[15], indicating that a persistent infection can exist without tissue injury or significant host inflammatory response. Quite numerous, encysted organisms have been identified in both cardiac and skeletal muscle of the immuno-suppressed cardiac transplant patients, but are not a cause of skeletal muscle symptoms and are not associated with muscle cell necrosis or inflammation (Figures 14.17 and 14.18).

Trichinella

Trichinella is one of the better known skeletal muscle parasites. Even today it is not a rare disease in the USA[16]. Trichinosis is contracted by eating undercooked meat contaminated with the nematode – *Trichinella spiralis*. Fertilized worms in the small intestine release larvae, which enter the bloodstream and preferentially localize in muscle. Infection is often subclinical, but in severe infection, many muscles, including facial and extraocular muscles, may be involved and exquisitely painful[11]. Biopsy reveals encysted larvae within muscle fibres (Figures 14.19 and 14.20), associated with degenerative changes and a florid, local chronic inflammatory cell infiltrate, containing many eosinophils[17]. Heavy infestation may cause a peripheral blood eosinophilia.

Cysticercosis

Cysticercosis, due to infection with the larval stage of the pork tapeworm. *Taenia solium*, usually presents with epilepsy, but muscle involvement is also common[9]. Infection is acquired by eating undercooked pork. It is most common in Eastern Europe, Africa, Central America and parts of Asia. Patients may complain of generalized myalgia or focal tender nodules. Rarely there is diffuse swelling of all limbs, a pseudohypertrophic myopathy[16]. This is responsible for generalized pain and weakness and the skin appears

stretched over the swollen muscles. Biopsy reveals a focal chronic inflammatory response around the cysts, in which acid-fast birefrigent hooklets may be visible (Figures 14.21 and 14.22). In addition to this local reaction, there is sometimes a more generalized inflammatory myopathy, possibly an allergic phenomenon, as it shows some response to steroids[16].

References

1. Carpenter, S., Karpati, G., Heller, I. and Eisen, A. (1978). Inclusion body myositis: a distinct variety of idiopathic inflammatory myopathy. *Neurology*, **28**, 8–17

2. Eisen, A., Berry, K. and Gibson, G. (1983). Inclusion body myositis (IBM): myopathy or neuropathy? *Neurology*, **33**, 1109–14

3. Danon, M. J. *et al.* (1982). Inclusion body myositis. *Arch. Neurol.*, **39**, 760–4

4. Mikol, J. *et al.* (1982). Inclusion body myositis: clinicopathological studies and isolation of adenovirus type 2 from muscle biopsy specimen. *Ann. Neurol.*, **11**, 576–81

5. Julien, J. *et al.* (1982). Inclusion body myositis – clinical, biological and ultrastructural study. *J. Neurol. Sci.*, **55**, 15–24

6. Tome, F. M., Fardeau, M., Lebon, P. and Chevallay, M. (1981). Inclusion body myositis. *Acta Neuropathol. (Berl.)*, **Suppl. VII**, 287–91

7. Reza, M. J. and Verity, M. A. (1977). Neuromuscular manifestations of rheumatoid arthritis: a clinical and histomorphological analysis. *Clin. Rheum. Dis.*, **3**, 565–88

8. Haslock, D. I., Wright, V. and Harriman, D. G. F. (1970). Neuromuscular disorders in rheumatoid arthritis. *Q. J. Med.*, **39**, 335–58

9. Uddenfeldt, P., Bjelle, A., Olsson, T., Stjernberg, N. and Thunell, M. (1983). Musculo-skeletal symtpms in early sarcoidosis, 24 newly diagnosed patients and a 2-year follow up. *Acta. Med. Scand.*, **24**, 279–84

10. Stjernberg, N., Cajander, S., Truedsson, H. and Uddenfeltd, P. (1981). Muscle involvement in sarcoidosis. *Acta Med. Scand.*, **209**, 213–16

11. Kallen, P. S., James, S. L., Nies, K. M. and Bayer, A. S. (1982). Infectious myositis and related syndromes. *Sem. Arthritis Rheum.*, **11**, 421–39

12. Barret, A. M. and Gresham, G. A. (1958). Acute streptococcal myositis. *Lancet*, **1**, 347–51

13. Svane, S. (1971). Peracute spontaneous streptococcal myositis. A report on 2 fatal cases with review of literature. *Acta Chir. Scand.*, **137**, 155–63

14. Samuels, B. S. and Rietschel, R. L. (1976). Polymyositis and toxoplasmosis. *J. Am. Med. Assoc.*, **235**, 60–1

15. Remington, J. S. and Cavanaugh, E. N. (1965). Isolation of the encysted form of Toxoplasma gondii from human skeletal muscle and brain. *N. Engl. J. Med.*, **273**, 1308–10

16. Most, H. (1978). Trichinosis – preventable but still with us. *N. Engl. J. Med.*, **298**, 1178–80

17. Davis, M. J., Cilo, M., Plaitkis, A. and Yahr, M. D. (1976). Trichinosis: Severe myopathic involvement with recovery. *Neurology*, **26**, 37–40

18. Sawney, B. B., Chopra, J. S., Banerji, A. K. and Wahi, P. L. (1976). Pseudohypertrophic myopathy in cysticercosis. *Neurology*, **26**, 270–2

Many different myopathies probably result from a metabolic disturbance in the muscle cell. At present the biochemical events responsible for changes, such as the abnormal permeability of the cell membrane in Duchenne dystrophy, are unknown. The mode of action of various drugs and hormones is not well defined. There is, however, a sizeable group of myopathies where a fundamental biochemical defect, often a specific enzyme deficiency, has been identified. These disorders can justifiably be referred to as metabolic myopathies. Undoubtedly there will be many additions as further biochemical lesions are detected.

Myopathies with Known or Suspected Enzyme Defects

Enzyme defects are frequently inherited and the effects depend on the particular biochemical pathways involved. Altered metabolism can induce morphological changes in the muscle cell. Thus absence of an enzyme may lead to accumulation of its substrate and provide a visible clue to the metabolic defect. Substrate deposition may disrupt cell organelles eventually causing cell death, manifest clinically as a progressive myopathy. Interruption of pathways of energy production can cause severe exercise intolerance. The major energy sources of the muscle cell are glycogen, glucose and free fatty acids and enzyme defects have been identified at many points in their biochemical pathways[1].

Defects in Glycogen Metabolism

Glycogen is stored in the cell under resting conditions and utilized in the initial stage of moderate, dynamic exercise, after which fuel stores are replenished by blood-borne glucose and fatty acids. Glycogen is the obligate substrate in high intensity or sustained, isometric exercise when the muscle is contracting under anaerobic conditions. In moderate exercise type 1 fibres are recruited first and show glycogen depletion before type 2 fibres[2]. The latter are preferentially recruited for short bursts of high intensity exercise dependent upon anaerobic glycolysis. Metabolism of glycogen takes place mainly in the cytosol. Glycogen is normally broken down to pyruvate and under aerobic conditions metabolized further within the mitochondrion. During anaerobic metabolism pyruvate is converted to lactate. Defects of glycolysis prevent the rise of venous lactate that normally occurs in ischaemic exercise.

Myophosphorylase Deficiency (McArdle's Disease)

This disorder usually becomes apparent in late childhood or adolescence, characteristically through muscle stiffness, induced by vigorous exercise[1]. If patients reduce the level of exercise at the onset of symptoms, they may experience a 'second wind' and be able to continue with mild exercise. This phenomenon is probably attributable to increased muscle blood flow providing additional energy substrates of glucose and free fatty acids. Continued, vigorous exercise may induce painful, cramp-like contractions, occasionally followed by myoglobinuria[3]. The serum CPK is usually mildly elevated, but reaches transient, very high levels if there is myoglobinuria. In approximately 50% of cases myophosphorylase deficiency is an inherited, autosomal recessive condition, but in this and the clinically similar phosphofructokinase deficiency there is a higher incidence in males. There is selective involvement of skeletal muscle. Cardiac muscle and other tissues are spared by the presence of tissue specific isoenzymes. Thus, this is rarely a fatal disorder. Mild proximal weakness is usually non-progressive and the disorder is not serious, unless repeated episodes of myoglobinuria cause renal tubular dysfunction. Unusual clinical variants include an infantile and late onset progressive myopathy. Subtypes of myophosphorylase deficiency, with different molecular abnormalities, have been described[3].

Biopsy

Muscle biopsy shows multiple, large, clear, subsarcolemmal blebs, which stain positively with PAS. Occasionally there is a more diffuse vacuolar change within the fibres. The histochemical reaction for phosphorylase is negative in the cytoplasm of the muscle fibres, but the enzyme is present in the walls of intramuscular blood vessels.

Electron microscopy shows subsarcolemmal accumulation of glycogen granules, also between the myofibrils and sometimes within the mitochondria. In contrast to acid maltase deficiency, the excess glycogen lies free and is not membrane bound.

In biochemical analysis the phosphorylase isoenzyme normally present in skeletal muscle is completely absent in some patients, whereas in others an inactive form can be detected. A biopsy taken shortly after an episode of myoglobinuria contains both necrotic and regenerating fibres and a transient positive histochemical reaction appears because regenerating myotubes contain a fetal iso-enzyme, which is absent from mature fibres.

Phosphofructokinase Deficiency (PFK)

The clinical picture of the less common enzyme defect, PFK deficiency, is very similar to McArdle's disease, including episodes of myoglobinuria triggered by intensive exercise. In addition, PFK deficiency may be associated with a mild haemolytic anaemia, because the muscle iso-enzyme is also present in erythrocytes. It is usually an autosomal recessive condition.

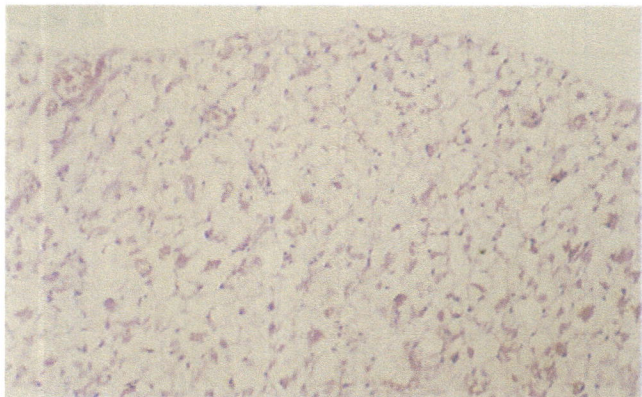

Figure 15.1 Infantile acid maltase deficiency. Pompe's disease. Skeletal muscle in child dying at 2 years with the generalized disorder. Widespread vacuolar myopathy. The change is so severe that at low magnification skeletal muscle resembles adipose tissue. The vacuoles contain glycogen, not lipid. H & E × 180

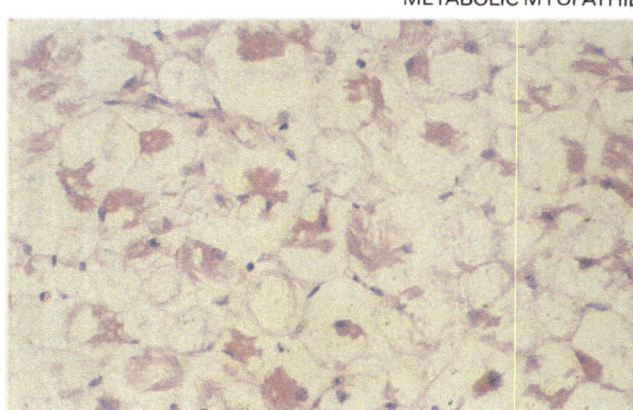

Figure 15.2 Infantile acid maltase deficiency. Large vacuoles, which appear empty by H & E stain, but in fact contain glycogen which displaces the myofibrils. H & E × 300

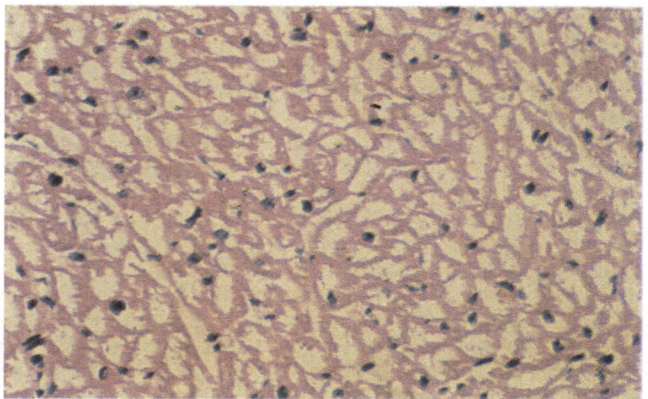

Figure 15.3 Infantile acid maltase deficiency. Cardiac muscle. In this severe form, cardiac muscle involvement is responsible for early death. Every fibre is vacuolated. H & E × 300

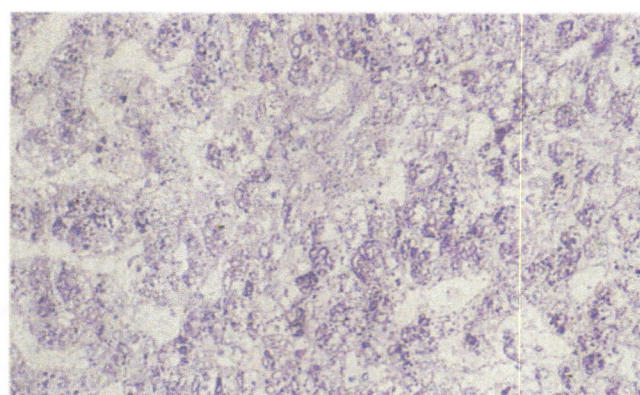

Figure 15.4 Infantile acid maltase deficiency, showing excess glycogen in the liver cells. Clinically the liver was greatly enlarged. PAS × 300

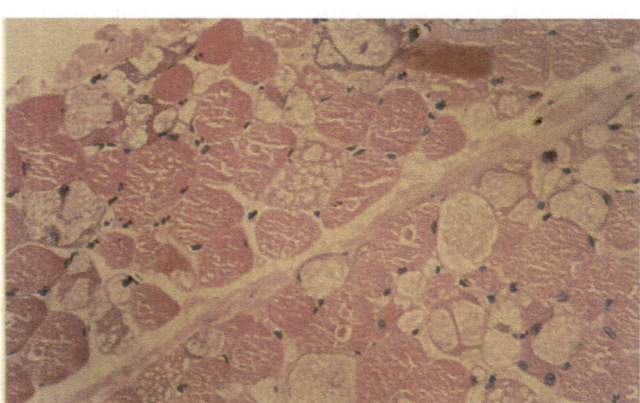

Figure 15.5 Acid maltase deficiency presenting in childhood. Quadriceps biopsy from a 7-year-old boy with a proximal myopathy and clinical diagnosis of Duchenne dystrophy. There is a severe vacuolar myopathy. (Same case shown in Figure 15.6.) H & E × 180

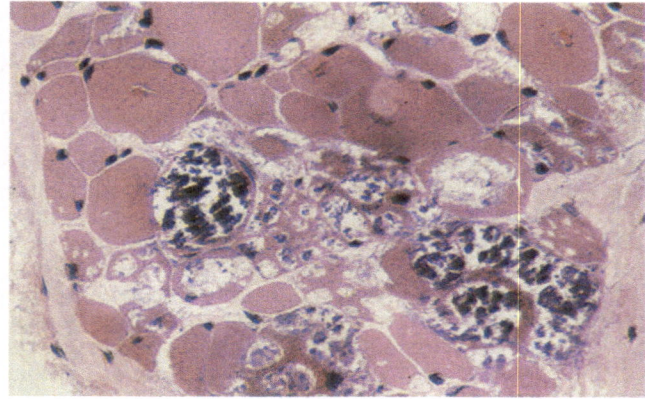

Figure 15.6 Acid maltase deficiency. The vacuoles contain large PAS positive granules, which are composed of glycogen. Glycogen is best demonstrated in frozen sections as much is dissolved out of formalin fixed tissue. H & E × 300

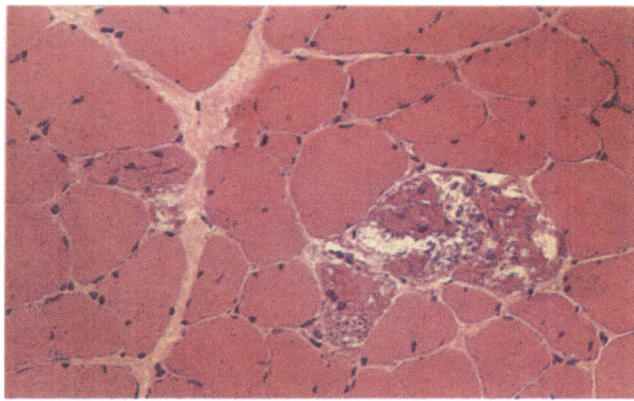

Figure 15.7 Acid maltase deficiency of adult onset. 48-year-old woman with a slowly progressive, proximal myopathy. There is variation in fibre size and fewer vacuolated fibres than in the previous case of childhood onset. (Same case shown in Figures 15.8–15.12.) H & E × 180

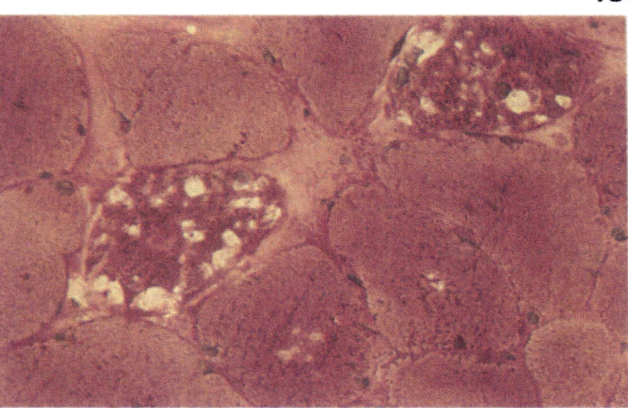

Figure 15.8 Acid maltase deficiency. Granular PAS positive staining is most obvious in the vacuolated fibres. PAS × 300

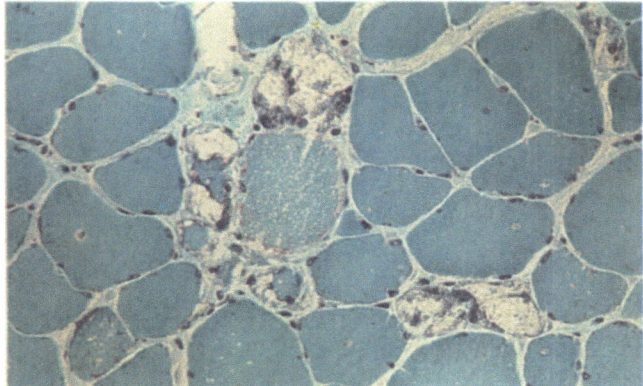

Figure 15.9 Acid maltase deficiency. The disruption of fibre architecture by the excess glycogen is quite well demonstrated with the trichrome reaction. Gomori's trichrome × 180

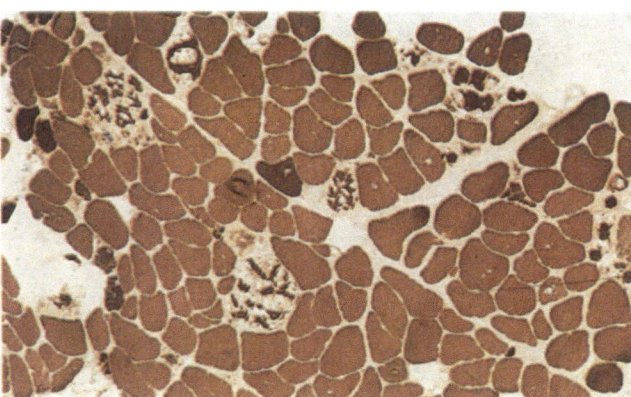

Figure 15.10 Acid maltase deficiency. There is a type 1 predominance in this muscle, but vacuoles are present in type 1 and type 2 fibres. ATP-ase pH 9.4 × 75

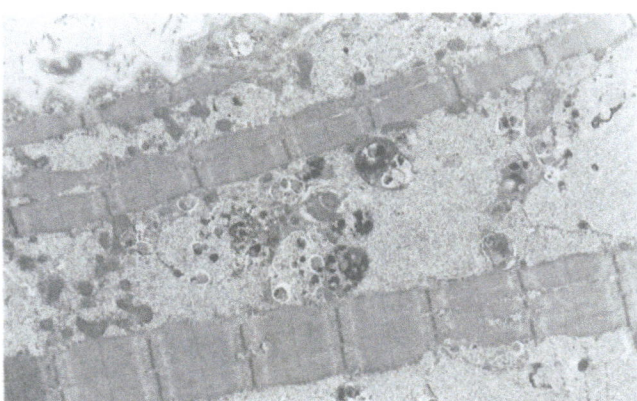

Figure 15.11 Acid maltase deficiency. The myofibrils are widely separated by the excess cytoplasmic glycogen. EM × 5700

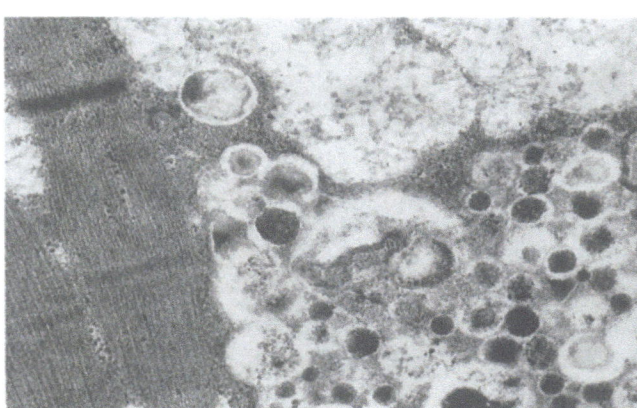

Figure 15.12 Acid maltase deficiency. The excess glycogen is partly membrane bound, within lysosomes and also lying free within the cytoplasm. Acid maltase is a lysosomal enzyme and numerous glycogen-filled lysosomes are characteristic of the enzyme deficiency. They are not seen in other glycogen storage diseases. EM × 22 500

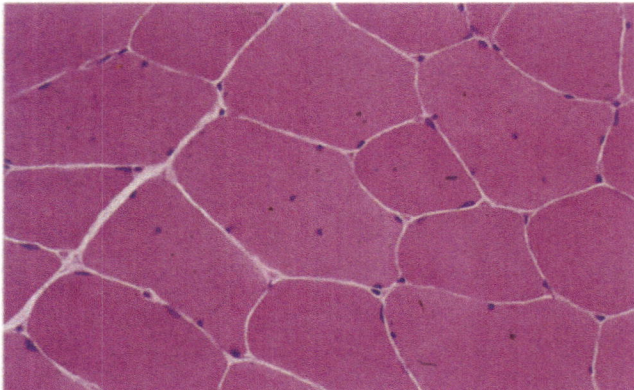

Figure 15.13 Debrancher enzyme deficiency. Quadriceps muscle from a 22-year-old man who had an episode of myoglobinuria causing temporary renal failure after modest, but unaccustomed exercise. Prior to this he experienced no symptoms of a muscle disorder. He does, however, have a history of asymptomatic hepatomegaly in childhood, as does his brother. Review of his liver biopsy showed glycogen storage. After recovery from renal failure, he has no clinically demonstrable weakness but his serum CPK has remained moderately elevated. The quadriceps muscle does not show a vacuolar myopathy. There is only slight variation in fibre size with an excess of central nuclei. Debrancher enzyme deficiency was demonstrated in his muscle and white cells. (Same case shown in Figures 15.14 and 15.15.) H & E × 180

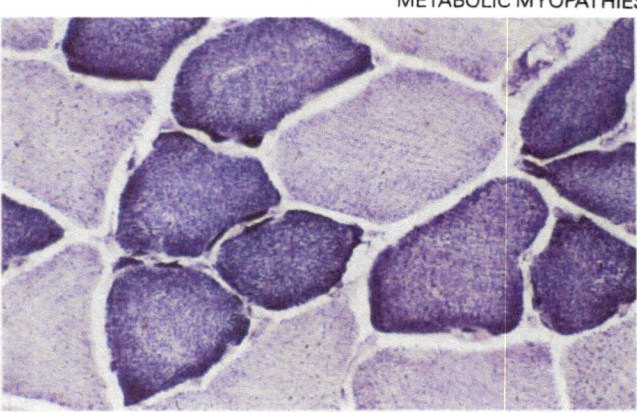

Figure 15.14 Debrancher enzyme deficiency. Vacuolar myopathy and excess glycogen was not demonstrable by light microscopy. However, the biopsy is not entirely normal. There are scattered small fibres and some type 1 fibres have a narrow, darkly stained border with the oxidative enzyme reaction. A prolonged search under the electron microscope did reveal occasional fibres with peripheral cytoplasmic blebs filled with glycogen granules and mitochondria. NADH-TR × 300

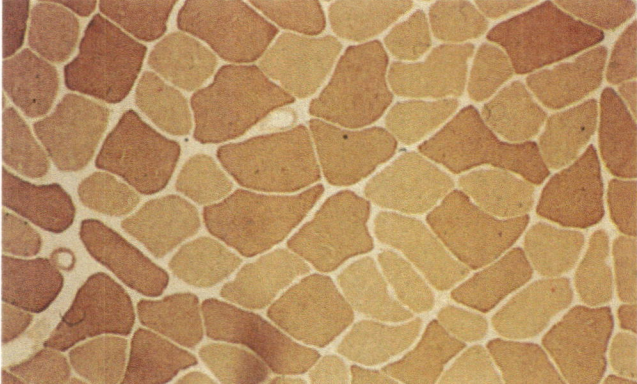

Figure 15.15 Debrancher enzyme deficiency. There is mild type 1 fibre atrophy. ATP-ase pH 9.4 × 180

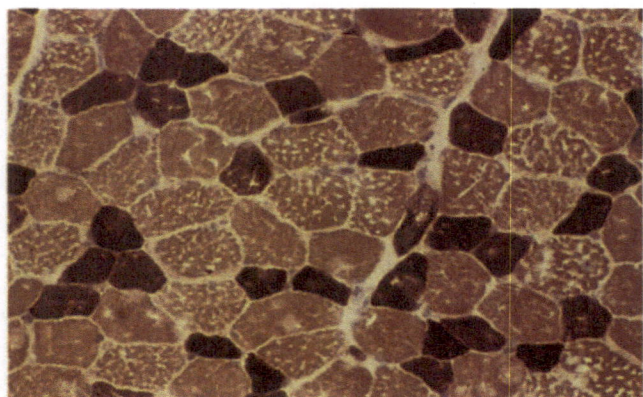

Figure 15.16 Muscle carnitine deficiency in a 9-year-old boy. The biopsy shows mild type 2 fibre atrophy. The myosin ATP-ase reaction has a spotty appearance. The tiny, unstained dots are due to large lipid droplets in the cytoplasm. (Same case shown in Figures 15.17 and 15.18.) ATP-ase pH 9.4 × 180

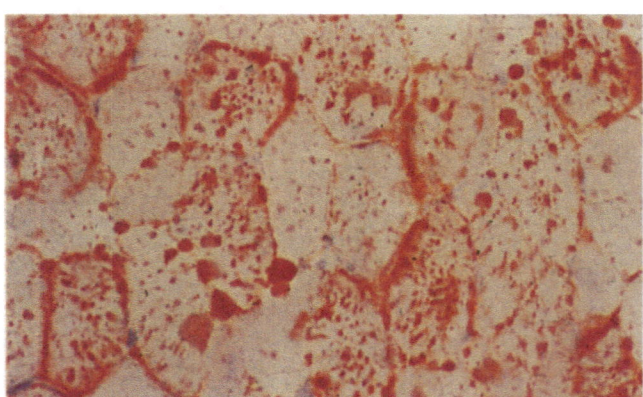

Figure 15.17 Carnitine deficiency. The fibres contain numerous large lipid droplets. The lipid is most conspicuous in the larger, type 1 fibres. Oil red O × 300

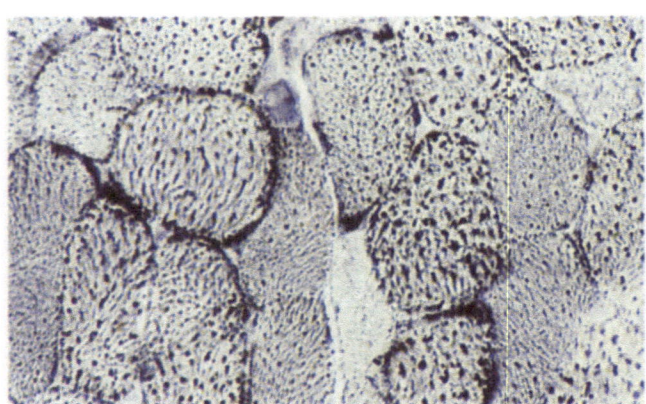

Figure 15.18 Carnitine deficiency. The oxidative enzyme reaction demonstrates large mitochondria – the positive dots – in type 1 fibres. NADH-TR × 300

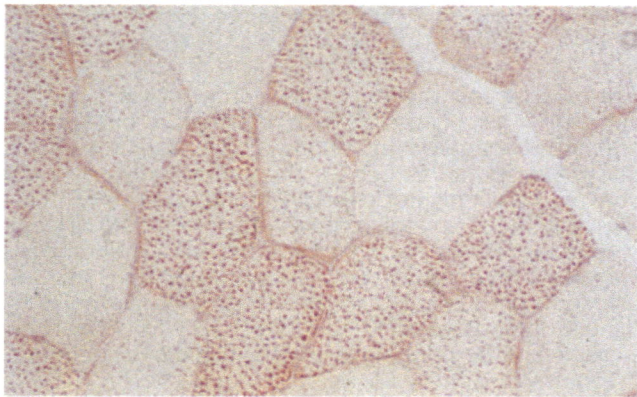

Figure 15.19 Lipid myopathy. This patient did not complain of fatigue, but simply collapsed when taken for a walk. The biopsy is from a Clumber spaniel and shows conspicuous lipid droplets in type 1 fibres. A deficiency of pyruvate dehydrogenase was identified. This enzyme, located in the mitochondrial matrix, catalyses the conversion of pyruvate to acetyl CoA. (Same biopsy shown in Figure 15.20.) Oil red O × 300

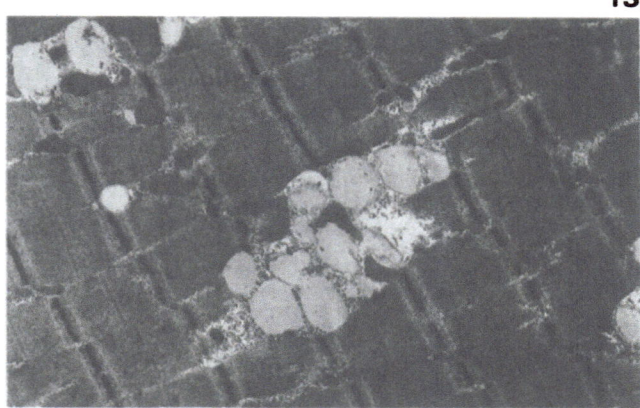

Figure 15.20 Lipid myopathy. Large lipid droplets are present between the myofibrils. The cells also contained large collections of mitochondria. EM × 7100

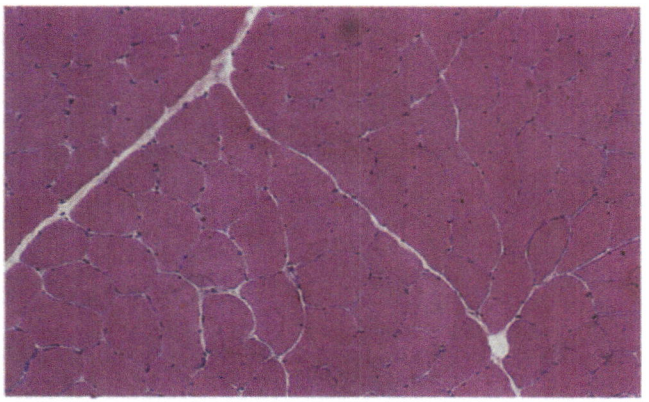

Figure 15.21 Carnitine palmitoyl transferase deficiency. Deltoid muscle biopsy from a 25-year-old woman with a history of recurrent episodes of muscle stiffness since childhood. Attacks precipitated by exercise, cold or if she missed a meal. A severe attack after exercise was followed by myoglobinuria and acute renal failure. Muscle biopsy taken several weeks later, when she had fully recovered, is entirely normal, by light and electron microscopy. CPT deficiency was demonstrated in the muscle by biochemical estimation. A normal muscle biopsy is usual in CPT deficiency, except after a severe attack. There is no progressive myopathy. (Same case shown in Figures 15.22–15.24.) H & E × 75

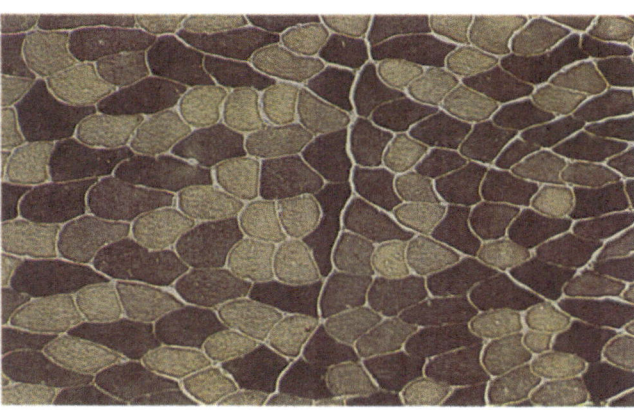

Figure 15.22 Carnitine palmitoyl transferase deficiency. Normal biopsy. Myophosphorylase × 75

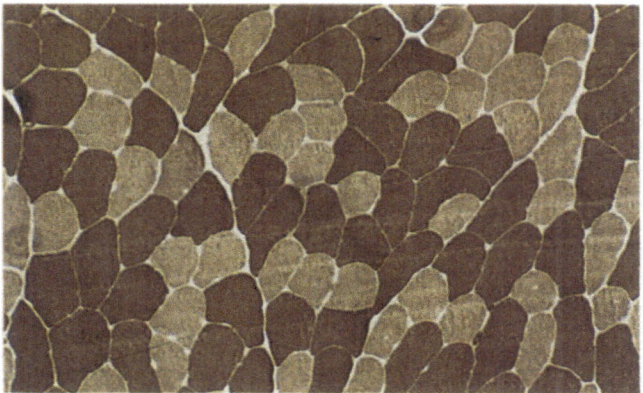

Figure 15.23 Carnitine palmitoyl transferase deficiency. Normal biopsy. Myosin ATP-ase pH 9.4 × 75

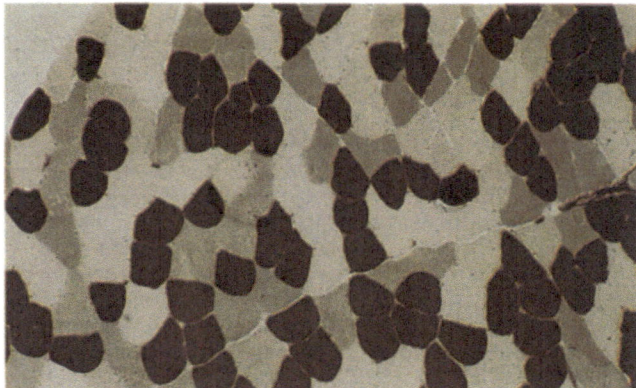

Figure 15.24 Carnitine palmitoyl transferase deficiency. This normal biopsy is shown to emphasize the need to freeze a sample of muscle for biochemical analysis, whenever an enzyme deficiency is suspected. Myosin ATP-ase pH 4.5 × 75

Biopsy

The muscle biopsy shows a vacuolar myopathy due to glycogen accumulation similar to myophosphorylase deficiency. A histochemical method is also available for demonstration of phosphofructokinase[4].

Acid Maltase Deficiency

Acid maltase deficiency is a lysosomal storage disease. Excess intracellular glycogen is normally taken up into lysosomal vacuoles and degraded by acid maltase-(α-1-glucosidase). Deficiency of the enzyme does not affect the pathway of energy production, but causes progressive accumulation of glycogen which disrupts normal cell structure and function. The disease may present in early infancy, childhood or adult life[6,7]. Infantile onset (Pompe's disease) is associated with a generalized enzyme defect, enlargement of liver, spleen and tongue and early death due to cardiac involvement (Figures 15.1–15.6). Disease of later onset is dominated by progressive weakness of limb girdle and truncal muscles, which may resemble a muscular dystrophy. Cardiac muscle is usually spared, but death due to respiratory muscle failure is not uncommon in childhood. Adult onset disease is generally mild and only slowly progressive. Variation in clinical severity shows no correlation with acid maltase levels, which are very low in all cases. Differences in the clinical picture may be attributable to the compensatory activity of neutral maltase[6]. Acid maltase deficiency is an autosomal recessive disorder. Heterozygotes have slightly reduced levels of the enzyme, but no evidence of clinical disease. The enzyme deficiency can be detected *in utero* by biochemical analysis of cultured amniotic fluid cells[7].

Biopsy

All three forms of acid maltase deficiency show a vacuolar myopathy[8] (Figures 15.1–15.6, 15.7 and 15.10). In infantile cases vacuoles fill the cytoplasm of almost every fibre, so that at low power in transverse section the biopsy resembles adipose tissue (Figures 15.1 and 15.2). In children and severely affected adults vacuolated fibres are also numerous, but in mild adult cases vacuoles may be sparse. The vacuoles appear empty with H & E staining, but the contents are PAS positive (Figures 15.6 and 15.8) and highly reactive for the lysosomal enzyme acid phosphatase. Acid phosphatase containing vacuoles are not entirely specific for acid maltase deficiency and can be found in chloroquine myopathy, occasionally in polymyositis and other myopathies. In childhood and adult cases vacuoles are found in all fibre types but seem to be most numerous in type 1 fibres[9,10]. Fibre type grouping has also been described in some adult cases, suggesting a neurogenic component.

Electron microscopy reveals a great excess of intracellular glycogen separating the myofibrils. The granules are present in membrane bound, lysosomal vacuoles and also lying free within the cytoplasm (Figures 15.11 and 15.12).

Although morphological changes may vary in different muscles and between individual cells, the enzyme deficiency in skeletal muscle is uniform and should be confirmed by biochemical analysis. In addition to muscle, isolated lymphocytes can be used for biochemical diagnosis[11].

Other Defects of the Glycolytic Pathway

Debrancher enzyme deficiency is probably the commonest of the glycolytic enzyme defects but although it may cause growth retardation, convulsions and hepatomegaly in childhood, these problems usually disappear spontaneously. If myopathy is present, it is very mild and only occasionally progressive[1,12,13]. It is a rare cause of myoglobinuria after exercise. Muscle biopsy in debrancher enzyme deficiency may show a vacuolar myopathy due to accumulation of free glycogen granules, but in other cases the changes are minor and non-specific (Figures 15.13–15.16). There is no clear correlation with the clinical evidence of myopathy.

Phosphoglycerate kinase deficiency has recently been identified as a cause of muscle cramps and myoglobinuria. Muscle biopsy showed a slight increase in glycogen[14]. Myoadenylate deaminase deficiency has been described in association with exertional myalgia, but is not a cause of progressive myopathy[15]. In some cases it has been an incidental discovery[1] and muscle biopsy is entirely normal.

Defects in Mitochondrial Metabolism – Fatty Acid Metabolism

Fatty acid oxidation provides most of the energy requirements of resting muscle. In exercise, following initial utilization of stored glycogen, blood-borne fatty acids are the major energy substrate for any moderate activity and are particularly important in endurance exercise. Type 1 fibres which chiefly employ aerobic pathways of metabolism and show the greatest resistance to fatigue, are seen to increase in size with endurance training, such as marathon running[16].

· Fatty acid oxidation takes place in the mitochondrion. Essentially, long chain fatty acids are activated on the outer surface of the mitochondrion to fatty acyl CoA units which are then transported into the matrix space via specific carrier systems. Carnitine acts as the carrier molecule and on the external face of the inner mitochondrial membrane carnitine palmitoyl transferase 1 (CPT-1) catalyses conversion of fatty acyl CoA to fatty acyl carnitine. On the inner face the reaction is reversed by CPT-2 and fatty acyl CoA is released for B-oxidation. Acetyl CoA is produced from B-oxidation and enters the Kreb's cycle. From both processes hydrogen is transferred to the electron transport chain and finally to molecular oxygen. Under normal circumstances this mitochondrial respiration is closely coupled to phosphorylation of ADP.

Defects of mitochondrial respiration have been identified at several points along the metabolic pathways[1]. Some of these are disorders exclusive to skeletal muscle, others are multisystem disorders with widespread effects. Some present with exercise intolerance, whereas others give rise to a progressive myopathy. In several of these disorders involvement of external ocular muscles is responsible for ophthalmoplegia. Morphological changes in a muscle biopsy, which arouse suspicion of defective fatty acid metabolism, are widespread intracellular accumulation of the lipid substrate or a profusion of abnormal mitochondria, hence the term mitochondrial myopathy. Final diagnostic proof nearly always requires biochemical analysis. A biochemical defect has not been identified for every clinical form of myopathy with abnormal mitochondria. In these cases diagnosis of deficient mitochondrial metabolism is still speculative, awaiting identification of further enzyme defects. The importance of attempting to identify the specific biochemical abnormality is emphasized by the few disorders, such as carnitine deficiency, where dietary manipulation has had some success in overcoming the metabolic block and given rise to clinical improvement.

Carnitine Deficiency

Carnitine deficiency is a biochemically heterogeneous condition[17], which is either systemic, with multiple organ involvement, or restricted to skeletal muscle[18,19]. Systemic carnitine deficiency presents in childhood with recurrent episodes of nausea, vomiting and encephalopathy in addition to muscular weakness[1]. It is probably due to a defect in hepatic synthesis and the levels of carnitine are low in liver, serum and skeletal muscle. The localized, myopathic form also usually presents in childhood with proximal muscle weakness. Exercise intolerance, with undue fatigue and aching after exercise may occur. In other children severe progressive proximal muscle weakness and wasting can resemble a muscular dystrophy[18]. Muscle carnitine deficiency may be due to different biochemical mechanisms including impaired membrane transport or excessive leakage of carnitine from muscle cell[17]. Some patients have responded to treatment with oral carnitine[20,21], or prednisone[17]. However, whilst the myopathic form is usually a fairly benign disorder, the systemic disease is usually fatal due to cardiac involvement[19]. Carnitine deficiency is either sporadic or an autosomal recessive condition[1].

Muscle Biopsy

In both systemic and muscle carnitine deficiency the muscle biopsy shows a great accumulation of lipid droplets, especially in type 1 and 2A fibres (Figures 15.16 15.18). The majority of type 1 fibres are affected and in some cases are also atrophic[18,20]. The lipid appears as tiny empty vacuoles with H & E and stains positively with Oil red O for neutral lipid (Figure 15.17). In the systemic form lipid droplets are also present in cardiac muscle and liver[22].

Electron microscopy shows columns of non-membrane bound lipid vacuoles in parallel rows between the myofibrils. The mitochondria are of normal size, but may be increased in number and show structural abnormalities such as densely packed cristae or 'paracrystalline' inclusions.

Biochemical analysis shows a severe reduction in muscle carnitine, between 5 and 32% of normal. A moderate number of lipid vacuoles and mild reduction in muscle carnitine has also been described in the heterozygote. Clinical improvement with either steroid or oral carnitine therapy is associated with a decrease in lipid droplets although muscle carnitine content remains low[20].

Carnitine Palmitoyl Transferase Deficiency (CPT)

Carnitine palmitoyl deficiency characteristically presents in childhood or adolescence with episodes of muscle pain and myoglobinuria triggered by prolonged exercise or fasting. It is probably the most common cause of hereditary recurrent myoglobinuria. CPT deficiency is usually confined to skeletal muscle, or occasionally to liver and muscle, as other tissue specific iso-enzymes are under separate genetic control. The enzyme defect may be CPT-1 or CPT-2 or a combined deficiency[23]. In contrast to carnitine deficiency, this is not a progressive muscle disorder and there is complete recovery between attacks. The serum CPK rises rapidly to high levels during an attack, but returns to normal at rest. The only serious consequence is renal tubular dysfunction due to repeated episodes of myoglobinuria. Nevertheless, the prognosis is good, provided strenuous exercise and other precipitating factors are avoided. A low fat, high carbohydrate diet is also beneficial.

Biopsy

Muscle biopsy taken immediately after an episode of rhabdomyolysis shows fibre necrosis, particularly of type 1 fibres and also there may be an accumulation of lipid droplets in the type 1 fibres. Following an attack, regeneration and restoration of normal structure is complete and biopsy in the symptom-free period is usually normal by both light and electron microscopy[24] (Figures 15.21–15.24).

Biochemical analysis reveals very low CPT in muscle, usually less than 10% of normal[1]. The enzyme defect is also expressed in leukocytes.

Other Mitochondrial Myopathies with Known Enzyme Defects

Deficiencies of the respiratory electron chain have been identified. Cytochrome oxidase deficiency has been reported in association with a multisystem disorder, which includes progressive muscle weakness and is usually fatal in childhood[25]. Cytochrome b deficiency has been discovered in some patients with episodic weakness and excessive fatiguability[26]. Other metabolic disorders involving skeletal muscle that have been identified in just a few patients include respiratory chain defects[27–29] (Figures 15.19 and 15.20).

Mitochondrial Myopathies with Suspected Enzyme Defects

The clinical syndromes of external ophthalmoplegia combined with central nervous system and other systemic disorders are also thought to be due to defective mitochondria metabolism because abnormal mitochondria are readily identified in the skeletal muscle biopsy. Partial cytochrome c oxidase deficiency has been reported in a few patients with external ophthalmoplegia[30], but in the majority specific biochemical defects have not been identified. Confusing terminology for a variety of clinical subdivisions includes chronic progressive external ophthalmoplegia, ophthalmoplegia plus, Kearns–Sayre syndrome and oculo-cranio somatic neuromuscular disease. Hopefully, the classification of external ophthalmoplegia will be simplified when the biochemical basis is clarified.

Muscle Biopsy in Mitochondrial Myopathies – General Description

All these syndromes are characterized by mitochondrial abnormalities in skeletal muscle[31]. Mitochondria may be increased in size and number and sometimes have a bizarre structure. Electron microscopy is necessary to demonstrate these abnormalities, but certain light microscopic changes suggest their presence (Figures 15.25–15.28, 15.34–15.36). There is said to be a quantitative relationship between mitochondrial abnormalities and muscle weakness. Fibres containing numerous mitochondria may show a basophilic rim and granular cytoplasm with a routine H & E stain. The fibres also appear coarsely granular and heavily stained with the NADH-TR reaction. The Gomori's trichrome reveals patchy, irregular red staining of the cytoplasm, the so-called 'ragged red fibre' (Figures 15.27 and 15.33). Whilst occasional ragged red fibres may be

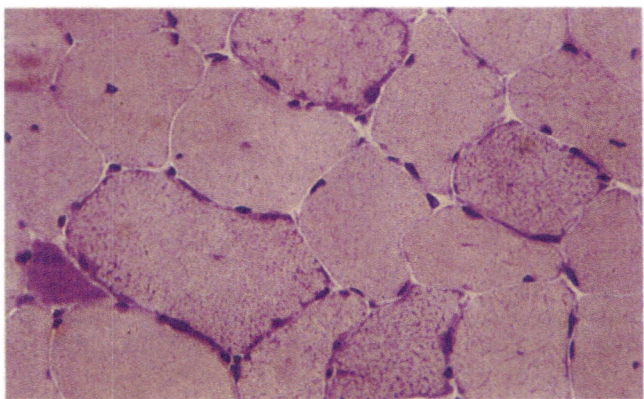

Figure 15.25 Mitochondrial myopathy. Deltoid biopsy from a 24-year-old woman with external ophthalmoplegia and mild proximal myopathy. A sister is similarly affected. The biopsy contains many fibres showing a rim of basophilia and faintly granular staining pattern. (Same case shown in Figures 15.26–15.30.) H & E × 300

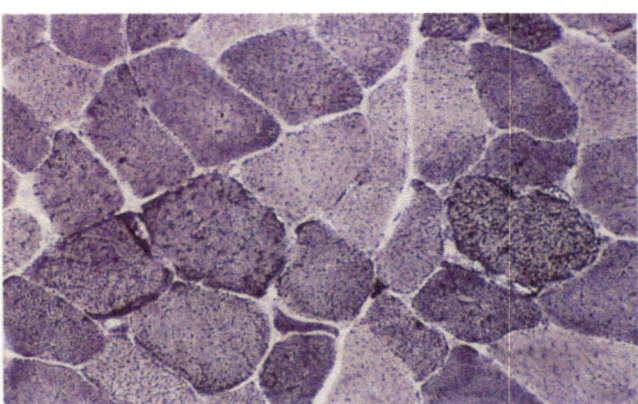

Figure 15.26 Mitochondrial myopathy. Several type 1 fibres show a coarse granular staining reaction and increased peripheral oxidative enzyme activity. NADH-TR × 180

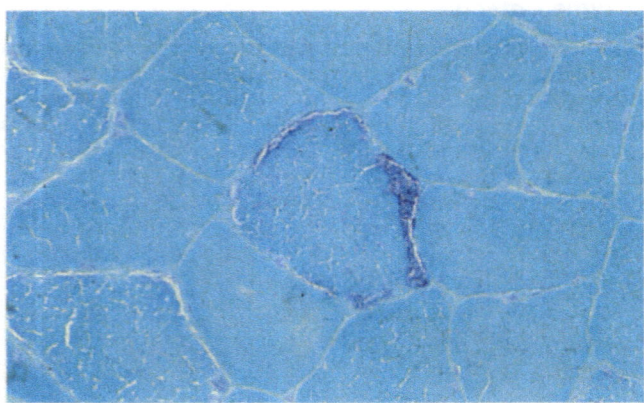

Figure 15.27 Mitochondrial myopathy. The trichrome reaction reveals a granular reddish border to many fibres. When numerous, these so-called 'ragged red' fibres strongly suggest a mitochondrial myopathy. Gomori's trichrome × 300

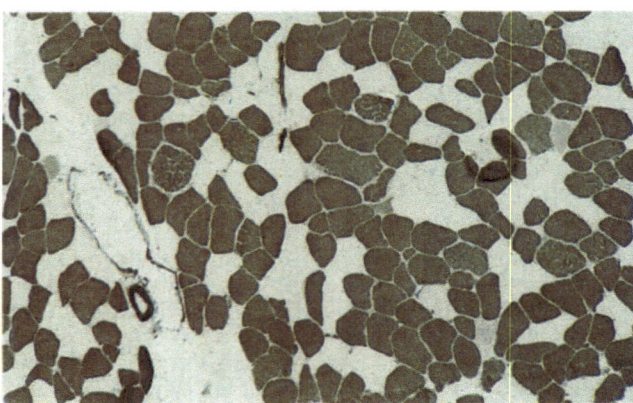

Figure 15.28 Mitochondrial myopathy. There is a mild type 1 predominance and a paucity of 2B fibres. There is slight variation in fibre size, but no severe atrophy. ATP-ase pH 4.5 × 75

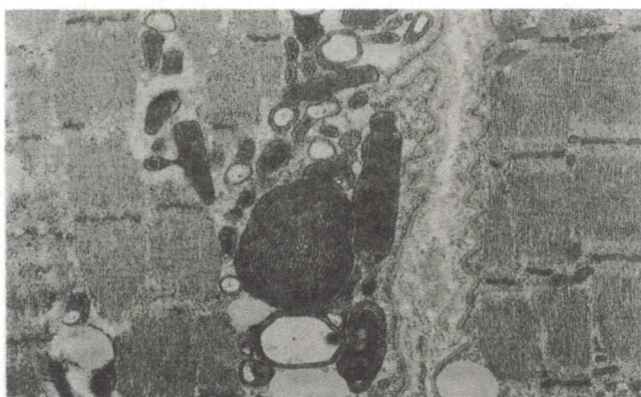

Figure 15.29 Mitochondrial myopathy. Electron microscopy reveals numerous abnormal mitochondria. Their presence was suggested by the light microscopic changes. Microscopic findings, a large mitochondrion shows a whorled arrangement of the cristae, another contains an inclusion. EM × 11 000

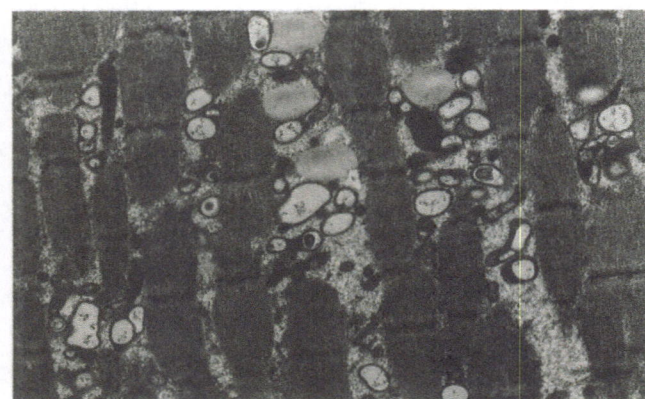

Figure 15.30 Mitochondrial myopathy. Large abnormal mitochondria, many of which appear vacuolated. There are also lipid droplets between the myofibrils. These findings suggest the myopathy is due to a defect in mitochondrial metabolism, but an enzyme deficiency has not been identified in this case. EM × 7100

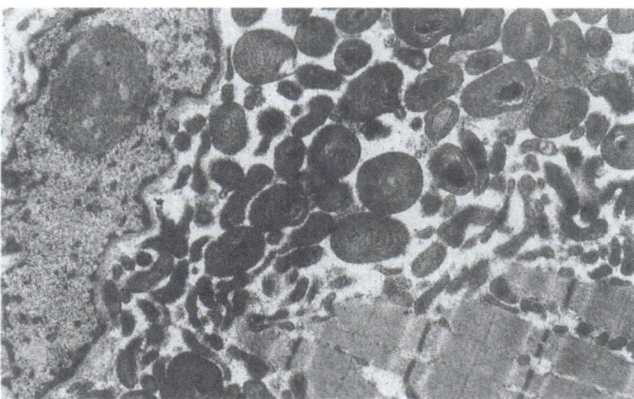

Figure 15.31 Mitochondrial myopathy. Collection of large abnormal mitochondria beneath the sarcolemma. The biopsy is from a strap muscle of a 66-year-old woman with several years history of mild proximal muscle weakness and more recently weakness of laryngeal muscles. Abnormal mitochondria were very numerous and a disorder of mitochondrial metabolism was suspected, but never proven. (Same case shown in Figures 15.32 and 15.33.)   EM × 7100

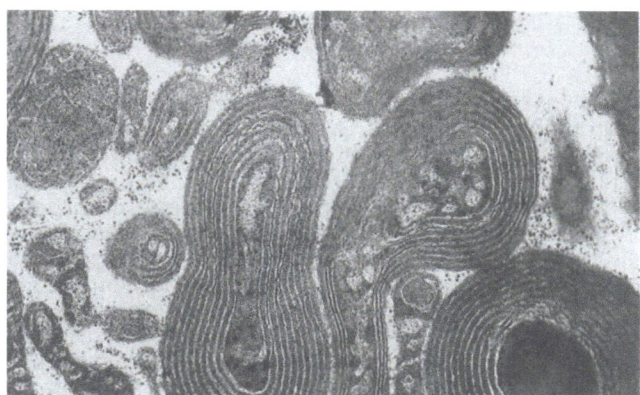

Figure 15.32 Abnormal mitochondria with concentric arrangement of the cristae   EM × 22 500

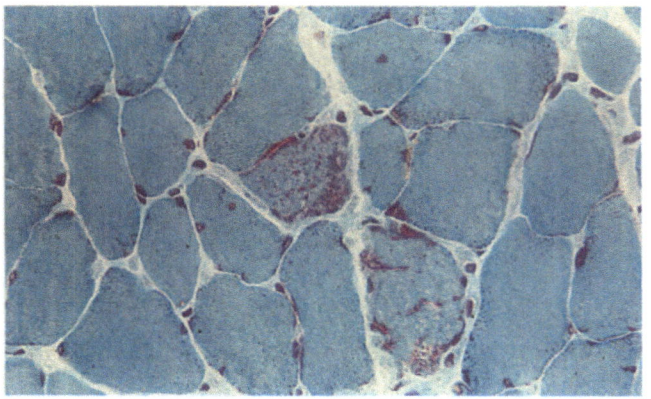

Figure 15.33 'Ragged red' fibres. These fibres, which show irregular, red staining with trichrome preparation, were numerous in the strap muscle from this patient. The abnormal staining pattern corresponds with the collections of large mitochondria.   Gomori's trichrome × 180

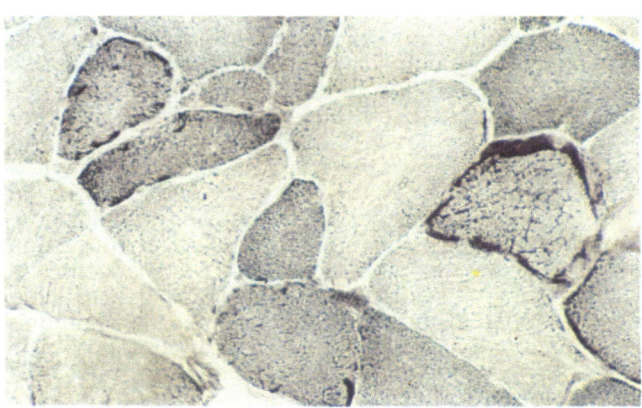

Figure 15.34 Ophthalmoplegia and proximal myopathy in 56-year-old man. Longstanding ptosis and limitation of eye movement, but more recent development of proximal limb muscle weakness. The deltoid biopsy shows many fibres with a peripheral rim of increased oxidative enzyme activity. (Same case shown in Figures 15.35 and 15.36.)   NADH-TR × 300

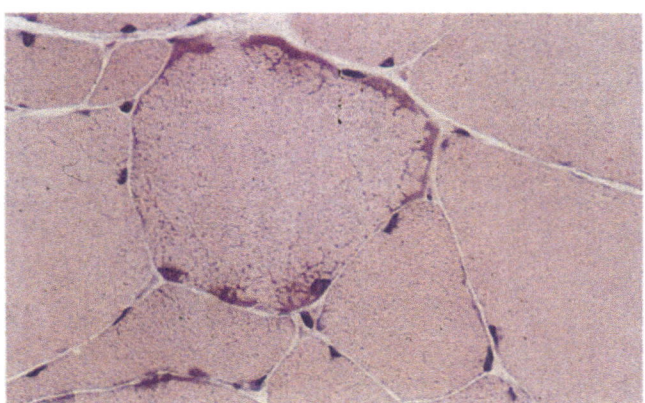

Figure 15.35 Basophilic granular peripheral staining reaction which corresponds with the 'ragged red' fibre.   H & E × 450

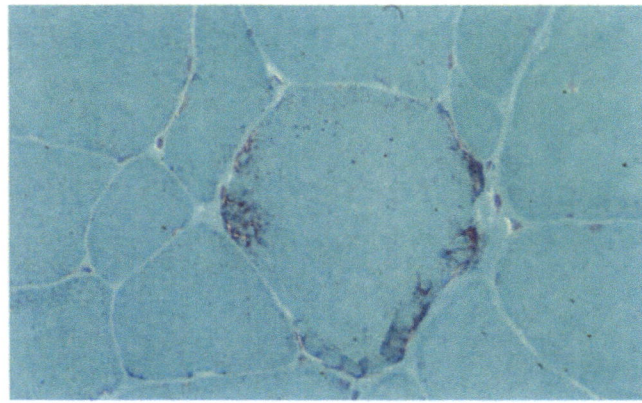

Figure 15.36 'Ragged red' fibre. Peripheral granular reddish stain. These fibres were quite numerous. Electron microscopy revealed collections of large, abnormally vacuolated mitochondria. A disorder of mitochondriac metabolism is suspected but unproven. Gomori's trichrome × 450

found in many different myopathies and sometimes neuropathic disorders[32], when numerous they should arouse strong suspicion of a mitochondrial myopathy.

Electron microscopy reveals a wide range of mitochondrial abnormalities, but none are disease specific. Large collections may be found beneath the sarcolemma. The mitochondria may be enlarged and contain concentric or branching cristae and sometimes electron-dense or paracrystalline inclusions (Figures 15.29–15.32). Abnormal mitochondria have been found in other organs in the multisystem disorders and occasionally in the external ocular muscles in cases with ophthalmoplegia. However, for obvious reasons eye muscles are unsuitable for biopsy and also pose difficulties in interpretation because the normal parameters differ from those of skeletal muscle. The abnormal mitochondria are frequently accompanied by an increase in cytoplasmic lipid.

Differential Diagnosis of Myoglobinuria

A single episode of myoglobinuria may be due to drug-induced muscle necrosis, rarely it may occur in normal untrained persons who undertake strenuous exercise. However, repeated episodes of myoglobinuria are almost certain evidence of a metabolic myopathy. The commonest cause is probably carnitine palmitoyl transferase deficiency but it may also occur in myophosphorylase or phosphofructokinase deficiency. Phosphoglycerate kinase deficiency has recently been identified as a cause and others may be discovered. In distinguishing these disorders it is probably best to avoid muscle biopsy in the acute stage when fibre necrosis and regeneration mask the basic histology and in the case of myophosphorylase deficiency a fetal iso-enzyme temporarily reappears.

References

1. Morgan-Hughes, J. A. (1982). Defects of the energy pathways of skeletal muscle. In Matthews, W. B. and Glaser, G. H. (eds.) *Recent Advances in Clinical Neurology*. pp. 1–46. (Edinburgh: Churchill Livingstone)

2. Gollnick, P. D., Piehl, K. and Saltin, B. (1974). Selective glycogen depletion pattern in human muscle fibres after exercise of varying intensity and at varying pedalling rates. *J. Physiol. (London)*, **241**, 45–57

3. Feit, H. and Brooke, M. H. (1976). Myophosphorylase deficiency: two different molecular etiologies. *Neurology*, **26**, 963–7

4. Bonilla, E. and Schotland, D. L. (1970). Histochemical diagnosis of muscle phosphofrucktokinase deficiency. *Arch. Neurol.*, **22**, 8–12

5. DiMauro, S. (1979). Metabolic myopathies. In Vinken, P. J. and Bruyn, G. W. (eds.) *Handbook of Clinical Neurology, 41*. pp. 175–224. (Amsterdam: North Holland)

6. Engel, A. G., Gomez, M. R., Seybold, M. E. and Lambert, E. H. (1973). Spectrum and diagnosis of acid maltase deficiency. *Neurology*, **23**, 95–106

7. Fensom, A. H., Benson, P. F., Blunt, S., Brown, S. P. and Coltart, T. M. (1976). Amniotic cell 4-methylumbelliferyl-alpha-glucosidase activity in prenatal diagnosis of Pompe's disease. *J. Med. Genet.*, **13**, 148–51

8. Hudgson, P. and Fulthorpe, J. J. (1975). The pathology of type 2 skeletal muscle glycogenosis. *J. Pathol.*, **116**, 139–47

9. Karpati, G. *et al.* (1977). The adult form of acid maltase deficiency. *Ann. Neurol.*, **1**, 276–80

10. Papapetroupoulos, T., Paschalis, C. and Manda, P. (1984). Myopathy due to juvenile acid maltase deficiency affecting exclusively the type I fibres. *J. Neurol. Neurosurg. Psychiatry*, **47**, 213–15

11. Shanske, S. and DiMauro, S. (1981). Late onset acid maltase deficiency. *J. Neurol. Sci.*, **50**, 57–62

12. Huijing, F. (1975). Glycogen metabolism and glycogen storage disease. *Physiol. Rev.*, **55**, 609–58

13. Cornelio, F., Bresolin, N., Singer, P. A., Di Mauro, S. and Rowland, L. P. (1984). Clinical varieties of Neuromuscular Disease in Debrancher Deficiency. *Arch. Neurol.*, **41**, 1027–32

14. DiMauro, S., Dalakas, M. and Miranda, A. F. (1981). Phosphoglycerate kinase deficiency: a new cause of recurrent myoglobinuria. *Ann. Neurol.*, **10**, 90

15. Keleman, J. *et al.* (1982). Familial myoadenylate deaminase deficiency and exertional myalgia. *Neurology*, **32**, 857–63

16. Prince, F. P. *et al.* (1981). A morphometric analysis of human muscle fibres with relation to fibre types and adaptation to exercise. *J. Neurol. Sci.*, **49**, 165–79

17. Willner, J. H. *et al.* (1979). Muscle carnitine deficiency: genetic heterogeneity. *J. Neurol. Sci.*, **41**, 235–46

18. Van Dyke, D. H. Griggs, R. C., Markesbery, W. and DiMauro, S. (1979). Hereditary carnitine deficiency of muscle. *Neurology*, **25**, 154–9

19. Hart, Z. H. *et al.* (1978). Muscle carnitine deficiency and fatal cardiomyopathy. *Neurology*, **28**, 147–51

20. Angelini, C., Lucke, S. and Cantarutti, F. (1976). Carnitine deficiency of muscle: report of a treated case. *Neurology*, **26**, 633–7

21. Hosking, G. P., Cavanagh, N. P. C. Smyth, D. P. L. and Wilson, J. (1977). Oral treatment of carnitine myopathy. *Lancet*, **1**, 853

22. Bourdin, G., Mikol, J., Guillard, A. and Engel, A. G. (1976). Fatal systemic carnitine deficiency with lipid storage in skeletal muscle, heart, liver and kidney. *J. Neurol. Sci.*, **30**, 313–25

23. DiDonato, S. *et al.* (1981). Heterogeneity of carnitine palmitoyl transferase deficiency. *J. Neurol. Sci.*, **50**, 207–15

24. Cumming, W. J. K., Hardy, M., Hudgson, P. and Wells, J. (1976). Carnitine palmitoyl transferase deficiency. *J. Neurol. Sci.*, **30**, 247–58

25. DiMauro, S. *et al.* (1980). Fatal infantile mitochondrial myopathy and renal dysfunction due to cytochrome C oxidase deficiency. *Neurology*, **30**, 795–804

26. Morgan-Hughes, J. A. *et al.* (1977). A mitochondrial myopathy characterised by deficiency in reducible cytochrome b. *Brain*, **100**, 617–40

27. Morgan-Hughes, J. A. *et al.* (1979). A mitochondrial myopathy with deficiency of respiratory chain NADH-CoQ reductase activity. *J. Neurol. Sci.*, **43**, 27–46

28. Morgan-Hughes, J. A. *et al.* (1982). Mitochondrial encephalo-myopathies. Biochemical studies in 2 cases revealing defects in the respiratory chain. *Brain*, **105**, 553–82

29. Hayes, D. J., Lecky, B. R. F., Landon, D. N., Morgan-Hughes, J. A. and Clark, J. B. (1984). A new mitochondrial myopathy. Biochemical studies revealing a deficiency in the cytochrome b-c_1 complex (complex III) of the respiratory chain. *Brain*, **107**, 1165–77

30. Johnson, M. A., Turnbull, D. M., Dick, D. J. and Sherratt, H. S. A. (1983). A partial deficiency of cytochrome C oxidase in chronic progressive external ophthalmoplegia. *J. Neurol. Sci.*, **60**, 31–53

31. Tassin, S. and Brucher, J. M. (1982). The mitochondrial disorders: pathogenesis and aetiological classification. *Neuropathol. Appl. Neurobiol.*, **8**, 251–63

32. Swash, M., Schwartz, M. S. and Seargeant, M. K. (1978). The significance of ragged red fibres in neuromuscular disease. *J. Neurol. Sci.*, **38**, 347–55

Drug-induced Myopathies

Steroid myopathy is probably the commonest iatrogenic muscle disorder, but many unrelated drugs can cause myopathies. Adverse reactions are often idiosyncratic and unpredictable. Clinical and histological findings are varied, but rarely unique and can resemble other neuromuscular diseases. The drug-induced myopathies described here are but a few well-recognized examples that illustrate the range of pathological reactions. Many other drugs have been incriminated and more will be added to the list. In clinical practice a high index of suspicion and careful note of all medication is needed to identify a drug-related myopathy.

Pathogenesis

There are many possible modes of action[1]. Drugs may interfere directly with pathways of muscle cell metabolism. Secondary effects are sometimes due to changes in serum ionic concentrations, to ischaemia, to a block in neuromuscular transmission or to the development of an autoimmune reaction. The most serious consequences result from systemic administration, but intramuscular injections occasionally have a local toxic effect and cause muscle cell necrosis. After a single injection the damaged muscle regenerates and the pain and swelling are short-lived. In drug addicts repeated injections in the same site, perhaps complicated by infection, occasionally cause permanent focal fibrosis.

Necrotizing Myopathy

Drugs which produce this reaction have a common clinical picture, ranging from mild myalgia to severe pain and profound weakness accompanied by myoglobinuria. This is exemplified by the myopathy of epsilon amino caproic acid (EACA – an inhibitor of plasmin synthesis). EACA myotoxicity represents an idiosyncratic response to a cumulative dose and the patient has usually been receiving the drug for several weeks before symptoms appear[2]. Respiratory muscle weakness may occur[3], but usually the most serious consequence is acute tubular necrosis due to myoglobinuria. The serum CPK may reach very high levels. Cessation of the drug is generally followed by complete recovery of both muscle and renal function. Clofibrate rarely causes a similar myopathy[4] and sometimes ECG abnormalities[5] within a week or two of starting treatment. A massive alcoholic binge is another cause, with very rapid onset.

Biopsy

At the onset biopsy shows a necrotizing myopathy[2,4]. Inflammation is absent and there are irregularly scattered necrotic fibres at approximately the same stage of breakdown. Necrosis is followed by phagocytic removal and complete regeneration. Repeat biopsies, after cessation of the drug, have shown no residual abnormalities in EACA myopathy. Relative preservation of type 2 fibres has been observed, suggesting a greater susceptibility of type 1 fibres[6].

(Alcoholic myopathy is described later in this chapter.)

Steroid Myopathy

Steroid myopathy, whether iatrogenic or due to Cushing's syndrome, is characterized by insidious onset of proximal weakness. The weakness is most severe in the pelvic girdle and less marked in the shoulder girdle and distal muscles[7,8]. There is no constant relationship with dose or duration of therapy, but the myopathy is most often a consequence of prolonged high dosage with fluorinated steroids[1]. However, cases have been reported with other steroid preparations and with low doses[8]. Patients who develop steroid-induced osteoporosis appear particularly prone to develop a myopathy. The EMG may reveal changes in patients on long-term steroids, even when they are asymptomatic. The serum CPK is not elevated, a point of distinction from an exacerbation of polymyositis during steroid therapy. The urinary creatine is increased and this measurement is advocated as a sensitive diagnostic test[7]. The metabolic basis of this myopathy is probably inhibition of protein synthesis, but it is not clear whether the selective vulnerability of type 2 fibres is due to metabolic differences between muscle cells or numbers of steroid receptors[1,9]. Exceptionally, a completely different pattern of acute, severe, generalized weakness, with greatly elevated CPK, follows high-dose intravenous hydrocortisone therapy[10].

Biopsy

In the common proximal myopathy the most obvious change is selective atrophy of type 2 fibres[7] (Figures 16.1 and 16.2). Atrophy involves both 2A and 2B fibres and can be severe. Fibre measurements have also revealed a lesser reduction in volume of type 1 fibres (Figure 16.3). Necrosis and inflammation are not present and by light microscopy there is generally a normal myofibrillar architecture. Excess lipid droplets are sometimes demonstrable with an oil red O preparation, particularly in type 1 fibres[11] (Figure 16.4).

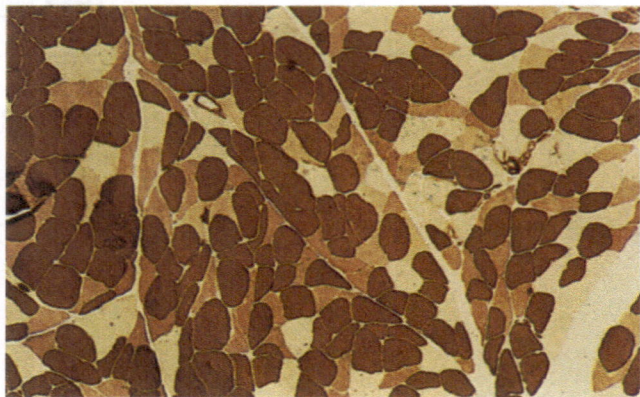

Figure 16.1 Steroid myopathy. Deltoid biopsy from a 71-year-old man who developed proximal muscle weakness whilst receiving steroid therapy for fibrosing alveolitis. The biopsy shows selective type 2 fibre atrophy and type 2B fibres are most severely affected. (Same case shown in Figures 16.2 and 16.3.)   Myosin ATP-ase pH 4.5 × 75

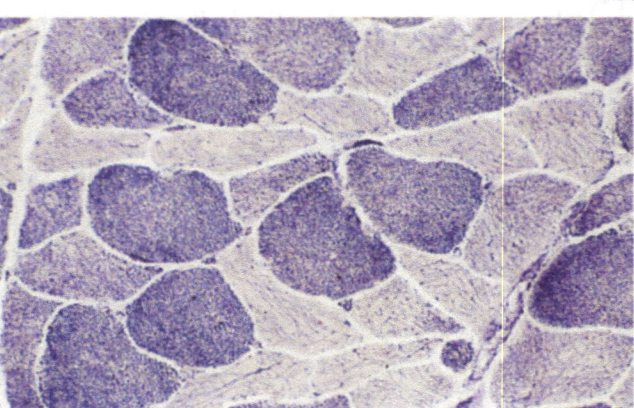

Figure 16.2 Steroid myopathy. Selective type 2 fibre atrophy, but essentially normal cytochemical architecture with the oxidative enzyme reaction.   NADH-TR × 180

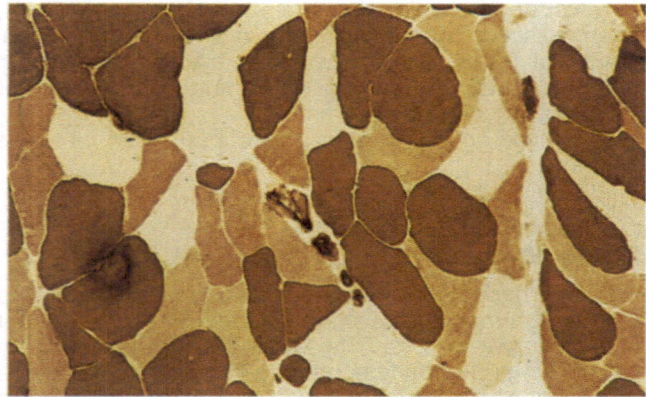

Figure 16.3 Steroid myopathy. Severe atrophy of type 2B fibres. Type 1 fibres are mostly of normal size, although there are occasional atrophic type 1 fibres.   Myosin ATP-ase pH 4.5 × 180

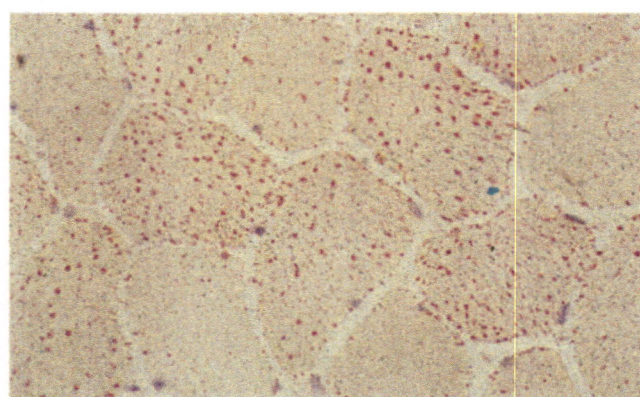

Figure 16.4 Lipid accumulation in a patient receiving steroid therapy. Deltoid biopsy from a 30-year-old woman who had received high-dose steroid therapy for 3 weeks for treatment of suspected polymyositis, although this was not confirmed by investigation. There is no significant fibre atrophy, but type 1 fibres contain conspicuous lipid droplets.   Oil Red O × 300

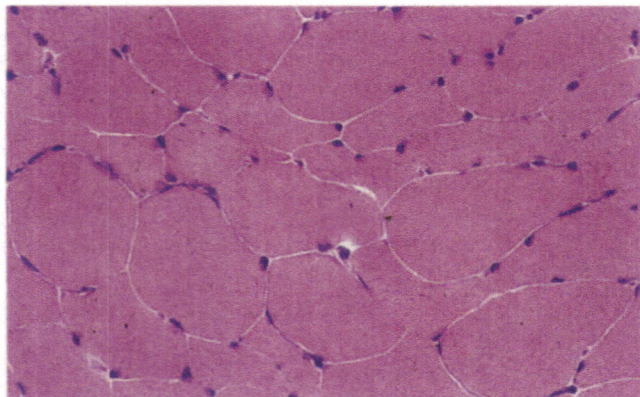

Figure 16.5 Alcoholic myopathy. Known chronic alcoholic with cirrhosis of the liver and a moderate degree of proximal muscle weakness. The biopsy shows variation in fibre size, with some normal-sized fibres and many quite severely atrophic fibres. (Same case shown in Figure 16.12.)   H & E × 180

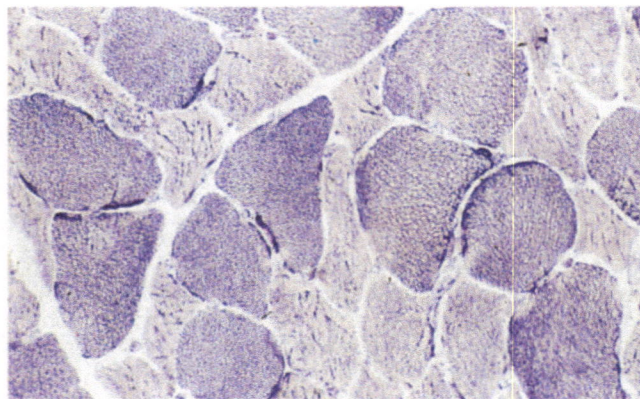

Figure 16.6 Alcoholic myopathy. There is selective type 2 fibre atrophy, which was found to be predominant 2B atrophy. Type 1 fibres are of normal size, but show slight patchy staining with the oxidative enzyme reaction.   NADH-TR × 180

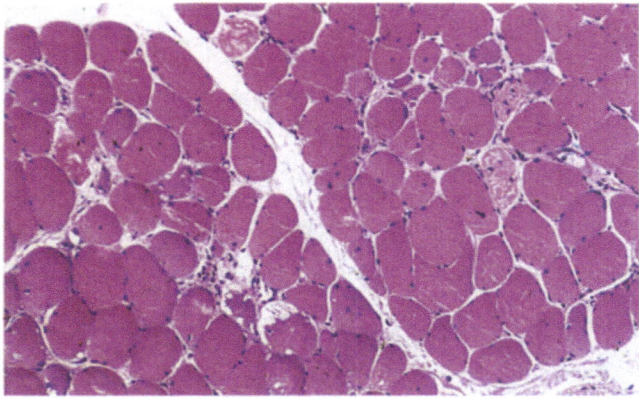

Figure 16.7 Polymyositis induced by penicillamine; 66-year-old man treated with penicillamine for seronegative arthritis for 1 year before onset of dysphagia and rapidly progressive proximal muscle weakness. The drug was stopped 10 weeks prior to the biopsy, which coincided with the first signs of improvement. There are no histological features that distinguish drug-induced from idiopathic polymyositis. This biopsy shows patchy fibre necrosis. (Same case shown in Figure 16.14.)   H & E × 75

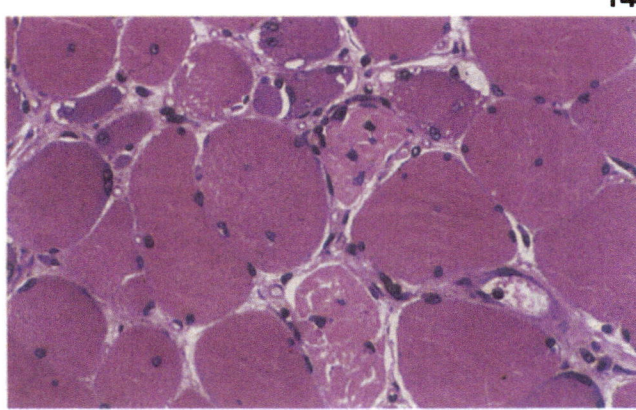

Figure 16.8 Polymyositis induced by penicillamine. Pale staining necrotic fibres and several small, faintly basophilic fibres, probably regenerating fibres.   H & E × 300

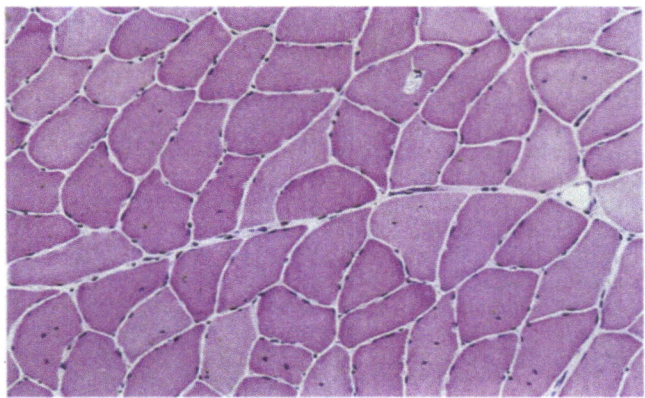

Figure 16.9 Malignant hyperpyrexia susceptibility. Muscle biopsy from a patient with a positive *in vitro* reaction. There is a moderate increase in central nuclei. (Other common, minor abnormalities are shown in Figures 16.6 and 16.7.)   H & E × 180

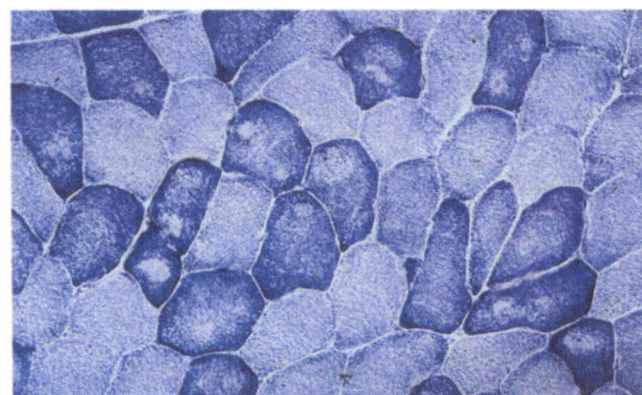

Figure 16.10 Malignant hyperpyrexia susceptibility. Muscle biopsy from a patient with a positive *in vitro* reaction. There is patchy staining, a moth-eaten appearance of type 1 fibres with the oxidative enzyme reaction and occasional fibres contain central cores.   NADH-TR × 180

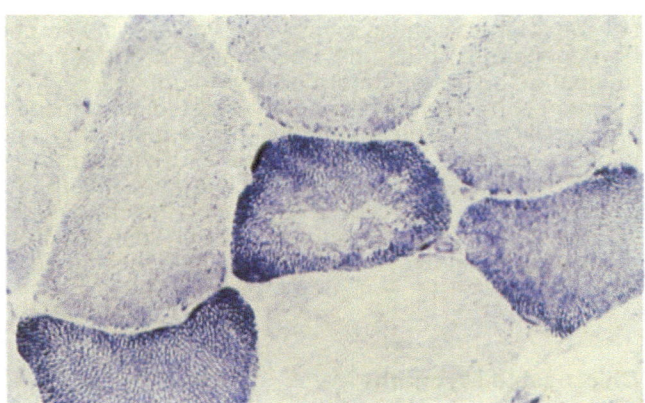

Figure 16.11 Malignant hyperpyrexia susceptibility. Muscle biopsy from a patient with a positive *in vitro* reaction. Irregular loss of staining from the centre of a type 1 fibre.   NADH-TR × 300

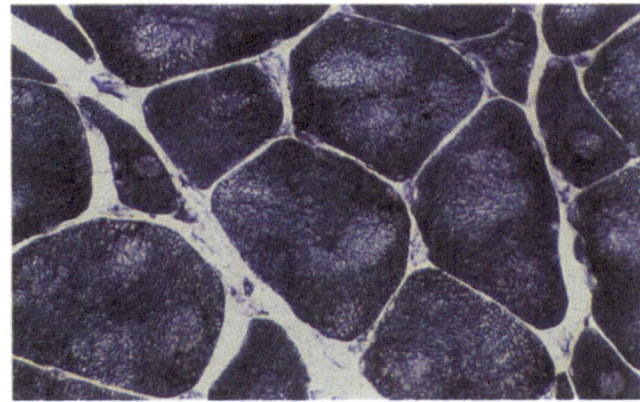

Figure 16.12 Central core disease. There is a rare association between this congenital myopathy and malignant hyperpyrexia. Although cores may be found in muscle of asymptomatic patients with MH susceptibility they are far more numerous in central core disease. This biopsy shows type 1 uniformity and one or more cores in every fibre. Type 1 uniformity or predominance is common in central core disease, but is not a feature of asymptomatic MH myopathy.   NADH-TR × 300

In my experience these may appear shortly after the onset of steroid therapy, but do not necessarily herald fibre atrophy, which is the most important correlate of symptomatic myopathy. Electron microscopy has shown excessive glycogen accumulation with myofilament loss, excess lipofuschin and large mitochondria[7].

The rare acute myopathy of intravenous hydrocortisone therapy is described as vacuolar change affecting all fibre types and regenerating fibres, presumably a consequence of acute necrosis[10]. Electron microscopy has shown excess glycogen lying free and within lysosomes[7].

Differential Diagnosis of Steroid Myopathy

The greatest difficulty is encountered in the patient with polymyositis, on steroid treatment, whose condition deteriorates. A raised CPK, together with persistent necrosis, regeneration and inflammation in the biopsy supports a flare-up of the original disease, rather than a steroid-induced myopathy. Selective type 2 atrophy in the absence of inflammation and with a normal CPK favours the steroid myopathy. However, this picture is not diagnostic because type 2 atrophy alone can occur in polymyositis[12]. Comparison with a pre-treatment biopsy is obviously valuable as it will show whether type 2 atrophy is a new event. However, if this is not available and the histology shows marked type 2 atrophy, despite an adequate dose of steroids, there is either steroid unresponsiveness or a deleterious effect, and a change in therapy is warranted.

Alcoholic Myopathy

Excess alcohol ingestion adversely affects both skeletal and cardiac muscle. Acute alcoholic myopathy is a consequence of a massive alcoholic binge and symptoms range from severe cramps to profound weakness associated with myoglobinuria[13]. Full recovery of muscle strength is possible if there is complete abstinence from alcohol. However, this can take several weeks and may be complicated by acute renal failure secondary to myoglobinuria[14]. Chronic alcoholic myopathy is characterized by weakness and wasting of proximal muscles, generally more severe in the legs than arms. These patients may also complain of muscle cramps and muscle tenderness[13]. In severe cases weakness may be diffuse and facial muscles are also involved. Some degree of proximal myopathy is a common complication of severe chronic alcoholism, that is in patients who have ingested 80–100 g ethanol daily for several years[15,16]. With this high alcohol intake, even those who do not have obvious muscle symptoms are likely to have a subclinical myopathy as revealed by an elevated CPK and abnormal EMG[14,17]. The incidence of mild chronic or subclinical myopathy in very heavy 'social' drinkers is unknown, but it is a condition to consider in adults who complain of vague cramps and show muscle tenderness on examination.

Alcoholic skeletal myopathy is likely to be accompanied by alcoholic liver disease. It is often associated with peripheral neuropathy and sometimes, but not invariably, with cardiomyopathy[18]. Experimental studies suggest that ethanol, or its metabolite acetaldehyde, has a direct toxic effect upon skeletal muscle cells. Alcohol has been shown to decrease muscle cell protein synthesis, to reduce mitochondrial fatty acid oxidation, to impair cell membrane transport and to

reduce contractility[15]. The summation of these effects in acute alcohol poisoning may lead to rhabdomyolysis and hence myoglobinuria. In chronic alcoholics the biochemical abnormalities may persist even after all the ingested alcohol has been metabolized. Recovery from chronic alcoholic myopathy is slow, but great improvement with reversal of morphologic abnormalities is possible if abstinence is maintained[14].

Biopsy

In severe acute alcoholic myopathy there is striking interstitial oedema and patchy muscle fibre necrosis, initially without inflammatory cell infiltration. Necrosis is followed by phagocytosis and regeneration. The changes are most florid in patients with myoglobinuria[14]. Acute alcoholic myopathy may well have a background of chronic changes.

Chronic alcoholic myopathy is characterized by selective type 2B fibre atrophy[19] (Figures 16.5 and 16.6). There is some correlation between the presence of atrophy and chronicity of alcoholism. Slavin et al. found no evidence of atrophy in a patient who had been ingesting more than 80 g ethanol daily for 6 months, but all patients exceeding this level for 2 years or more showed some degree of atrophy[17]. The change is reversible. Repeat biopsies have shown reversion of type 2B atrophy after several months of abstinence, but progression in alcoholics who continued to drink[19]. In addition the biopsy shows an accumulation of triglyceride, possibly the result of depressed fatty acid oxidation. An oil red O preparation reveals an increase in small lipid droplets often in both type 1 and type 2 fibres[20], sometimes preferentially in type 1 fibres. Almost inconspicuous fine droplets are a normal finding, particularly in type 1 fibres. The cytoplasmic lipid content is also increased in patients receiving corticosteroid therapy. The level of muscle triglyceride content shows good correlation with the level of recent daily alcohol intake, but does not relate to the degree of atrophy[20]. As with the fatty liver, the change appears to be a more sensitive indicator of recent high intake than of chronic damage. It was observed in normal volunteers given high daily alcohol intake for only 1 month[15]. It should be noted that there is no direct correlation between the severity of liver damage and the severity of the alcoholic myopathy. Occasional necrotic or degenerate fibres may be found in the chronic myopathy, but other abnormalities are unusual[19].

Electron microscopy has not revealed any specific abnormalities[15]. The myofibrils may appear thin and widely separated. There is an apparent excess of cytoplasmic glycogen. The lipid droplets lie beneath the sarcolemma and in rows between the myofibrils. Tubular aggregates, structures possibly derived from the sarcoplasmic reticulum, have been described in type 2 fibres[21].

Chloroquine Myopathy

The antimalarial chloroquine, also used as an antirheumatic drug, can produce a myopathy with fairly distinctive histological changes. Experimental evidence suggests that chloroquine both accelerates the formation of autophagic vacuoles and also inhibits their degradation by lysosomal enzymes[22,23]. Proximal muscle weakness is usually a complication of long-term administration. Biopsy reveals a vacuolar myopathy, principally involving type 1 fibres[24]. Electron microscopy shows that the change is due to many autophagic vacuoles (i.e. membrane-bound structures containing remnants of cell organelles) and membranous whorls. The latter, also called myeloid bodies, may be a type of autophagic vacuole, derived from the sarcoplasmic reticulum[22]. Sometimes the membrane-bound bodies contain unusual, closely packed, short, curved profiles[25]. These inclusions are particularly characteristic of chloroquine myopathy, but are also found in the central nervous system in Batten's disease. Chloroquine-induced inclusions may persist for a long time, apparently several years after cessation of therapy, and can be found when muscle function is clinically normal[25].

Penicillamine-induced Muscle Disorders

Long-term therapy with D-penicillamine is used in Wilson's disease and sometimes in rheumatoid arthritis. In genetically susceptible patients this drug has been shown to induce a wide spectrum of autoimmune diseases, including myasthenia gravis and polymyositis[26]. D-penicillamine reacts with many different tissue antigens and stimulates polyclonal B and T cell activity. The combined effects generate autoantibody formation and immune complex disease[27]. Myasthenia gravis can develop with elevated titres of acetylcholine receptor antibodies[28]. D-penicillamine has been shown to form covalent attachment to acetylcholine receptors and alter the binding properties[29]. This linkage is probably responsible for the antigenic modification that stimulates autoantibody production.

A rapidly progressive proximal muscle weakness, indistinguishable from idiopathic polymyositis, is also described[30], and the rash of dermatomyositis may develop. Onset has been reported from between 4 weeks and 2 years after commencing penicillamine therapy and is seemingly rather more sudden and rapidly progressive than the usual insidious presentation of the idiopathic disorder. In most cases there has been full recovery after withdrawal of the drug, but it may be several weeks before any clinical improvement is observed. There have been at least two fatal cases, where polymyositis has been associated with fulminant myocarditis[30].

Muscle Biopsy

The changes are those of a florid inflammatory myopathy, with fibre necrosis and phagocytosis, regenerating fibres and interstitial chronic inflammatory cell infiltration (Figures 16.7 and 16.8). Nevertheless, this picture is indistinguishable from idiopathic polymyositis or dermatomyositis. Autopsy of a fatal case has shown necrosis and inflammation in the myocardium[30].

Malignant Hyperthermia (Malignant Hyperpyrexia)

A remarkable number of people from the same kindred died as a direct result of general anaesthesia before the condition malignant hyperthermia was recognized[31]. Malignant hyperthermia is a rare, inherited, abnormal susceptibility to certain drugs, mostly inhalational anaesthetics. Under the influence of general anaesthesia susceptible individuals exhibit profound, generalized muscular rigidity and a rapid rise in body temperature, which is fatal unless promptly reversed. It is a completely avoidable, iatrogenic cause of death, but many people who carry this trait do not have obvious muscular disease[32]. The identification of patients at risk, prior to surgery, depends largely upon a detailed family history. Autosomal dominance is usual, but recessive inheritance and sporadic cases have been described. Other susceptible individuals do exhibit minor and non-specific musculo-skeletal abnormalities[33]. In addition malignant hyperthermia has been reported in association with central core disease[33] (see Chapter 12) and in a very small number of boys with Duchenne dystrophy[34,35], thus although the risk may be small, the potential hazard of malignant hyperthermia must be seriously considered in patients to be anaesthetized, who have any type of muscle disorder. Malignant hyperthermia has also recently been incriminated as a possible cause of the sudden infant death syndrome[37].

The serum CPK is mildly elevated in at least 70% of affected individuals whether or not there is overt muscle disease. Any patient suspected of malignant hyperthermia susceptibility by virtue of family history or previous anaesthetic complication should be fully investigated. When positive results are obtained, not only must the patient be fully alerted to the dangers of anaesthesia, but other members of the family should also be examined. Malignant hyperthermia cannot be confidently diagnosed by microscopy, by any biochemical test or EMG It requires muscle biopsy and exposure of the fresh specimens to known trigger drugs, which elicit the abnormal contraction *in vitro*[38,39]. Halothane, succinyl choline and caffeine are provocative agents. The *in vitro* test is not a routine laboratory procedure and biopsy should not be undertaken unless the specialist facilities are available. The contracture response is the only reliable diagnostic test, but even here there is uncertainty as to whether a positive *in vitro* response always signifies *in vivo* susceptibility[40]. At present if the test is positive it must be assumed to indicate susceptibility and the patient and family duly warned.

The pathogenesis is complex. Normal contraction involves the transient release and binding of calcium ions by the sarcoplasmic reticulum. Calcium ions activate the enzyme myosin ATP-ase. In malignant hyperthermia the anaesthetic agent in some way triggers an acute prolonged rise in intracellular calcium ion concentration, leading to sustained contracture, increased muscle cell metabolism and heat production. Initially there is increased aerobic metabolism, with high oxygen consumption and ATP depletion. The balance shifts towards anaerobic metabolism, accompanied by lactate production and a metabolic acidosis. Increased cell membrane permeability leads to hyperkalaemia and ultimately there may be muscle cell necrosis. The sequence suggests defective calcium binding by the sarcoplasmic reticulum, but a more generalized cell membrane abnormality may exist[31].

Malignant hyperthermia is nearly always associated with muscular rigidity, but a small proportion of patients develop the pyrexia without contracture. In these cases it is suggested that muscle metabolism is increased, but the level is insufficient to activate the contractile mechanism to the extent of rigidity[31]. Cardiomyopathy has been described in association with malignant hyperthermia myopathy, but specific pathological changes have not been identified. It seems likely that cardiac arrhythmias occurring during an episode of hyperthermia are more often secondary to the hyperkalaemia.

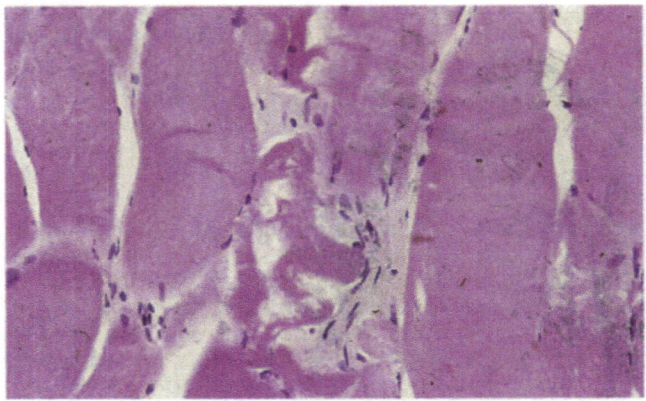

Figure 16.13 Fatal malignant hyperpyrexia. Post-mortem muscle from a young girl who died during an appendicectomy operation, in which she developed generalized rigidity and rise in temperature. Subsequent investigation revealed a family history of adverse reaction to anaesthesia. Hypercontracted fibres, with disruption of the cell architecture were quite numerous at postmortem. (Same case shown in Figure 16.10.) H & E × 300

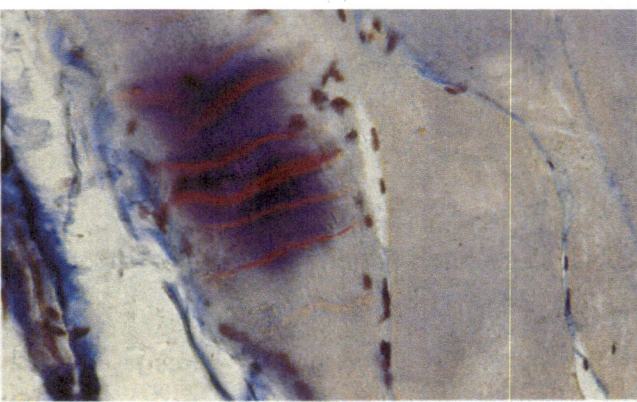

Figure 16.14 Fatal malignant hyperpyrexia. Postmortem muscle showing conspicuous contraction bands. These are not a feature of rigor mortis and indicate hypercontraction present at the time of death. Masson's trichrome × 300

Biopsy

No consistent or diagnostic abnormalities have been identified by either light or electron microscopy. Apart from the minority, who have histological evidence of another defined muscle disease, such as central core disease, biopsies from patients with a positive contracture test generally show fairly minor histologic abnormalities (Figures 16.9–16.12). Central nuclei are frequently increased. There may be isolated necrotic fibres or regenerating foci and scattered core-targetoid fibres[42,43]. Biopsies from patients with proven susceptibility may be entirely normal, particularly in childhood[43]. It is quite likely that many observed morphological abnormalities are acquired and secondary to subclinical episodes of altered muscle cell metabolism. In fatal cases postmortem examination may reveal contraction bands and widespread muscle necrosis (Figures 16.13 and 16.14).

References

1. Mastaglia, F. L. (1982). Adverse effects of drugs on muscle. *Drugs*, **24**, 304–21

2. Brown, J. A., Wollman, R. L. and Mullan, S. (1982). Myopathy induced by epsilon-aminocaproic acid. *J. Neurosurg.*, **57**, 130–4

3. Biswas, C. K., Reid Milligan, D. A., Agte, S. D. and Tilley, P. J. B. (1980). Acute renal failure and myopathy after treatment with aminocaproic acid. *Br. Med. J.*, **281**, 115–16

4. Abourizk, N., Khalil, B. A., Bahath, N. and Afifi, A. K. (1979). Clofibrate-induced muscular syndrome. *J. Neurol. Sci.*, **42**, 1–9

5. Smals, A. G. H., Beex, L. V. A. M. and Kloppenborg, P. W. C. (1977). Clofibrate-induced muscle damage with myoglobinuria and cardiomyopathy. *N. Engl. J. Med.*, **296**, 942

6. Britt, C. W., Light, R. R., Peters, B. H. and Schochet, S. S. (1980). Rhabdomyolysis during treatment with epsilon-amino-caproic acid. *Arch. Neurol.*, **37**, 187–8

7. Khaleeli, A. A., Edwards, R. H. T., Gohil, K., McPhail, G., Rennie, M. J., Round, J. and Ross, E. J. (1983). Corticosteroid myopathy: a clinical and pathological study. *Clin. Endocrinol.*, **18**, 155–66

8. Askari, A., Vignos, P. J. and Moskowitz, R. W. (1976). Steroid myopathy in connective tissue disease. *Am. J. Med.*, **61**, 485–92

9. Braunstein, P. W. and De Girolami, U. (1981). Experimental corticosteroid myopathy. *Acta Neuropathol.*, **55**, 167–72

10. Van Marle, W. and Woods, K. L. (1980). Acute hydrocortisone myopathy. *Br. Med. J.*, **281**, 271–2

11. Harriman, D. G. F. (1971). The fine structure of intramuscular lipids in human skeletal muscle. In *Basic Research in Myology*. International congress series No. 294. Excerpta Medica, Amsterdam.

12. Schwartz, H. A., Slavin, G., Ward, P. and Ansell, B. A. (1980). Muscle biopsy in polymyositis and dermatomyositis; a clinico-pathological study. *Ann. Rheum. Dis.*, **39**, 500–7

13. Perkoff, G. T., Dioso, M. M., Bleisch, V. and Klinkerfuss, G. (1967). Spectrum of myopathy associated with alcoholism. I. Clinical and laboratory features. *Ann. Intern. Med.*, **67**, 481–92

14. Klinkerfuss, G., Bleisch, V., Dioso, M. M. and Perkoff, G. T. (1967). A spectrum of myopathy associated with alcoholism. II. Light and electron microscopic observations. *Ann. Intern. Med.*, **67**, 493–510

15. Rubin, E. (1979). Alcoholic myopathy in heart and skeletal muscle. *N. Engl. J. Med.*, **301**, 28–33

16. Puszkin, S. and Rubin, E. (1975). Adenosine diphosphate effect on contractility of human muscle actomyosin: inhibition by ethanol and acetaldehyde. *Science*, **188**, 1319–20

17. Hanid, A., Slavin, G., Mair, W., Sowter, C., Ward, P., Webb, J. and Levi, A. J. (1981). Fibres type changes in striated muscles of alcoholics. *J. Clin. Pathol.*, **34**, 991–5

18. Perkoff, G. T. (1971). Alcoholic myopathy. *Ann. Rev. Med.*, **22**, 125–31

19. Slavin, G., Martin, F., Levi, J. and Peters, T. (1983). Chronic alcohol excess is associated with selective but reversible injury to type 2B muscle fibres. *J. Clin. Pathol.*, **36**, 772–7

20. Sunnasy, D., Cairns, S. R., Martin, F., Slavin, G., Peters, T. J. (1983). Chronic alcoholic skeletal muscle myopathy: a clinical, histological and biochemical assessment of muscle lipid. *J. Clin. Pathol.*, **36**, 778–84

21. Del Villar Negro, A., Merino Angulo, J., Rivera Pomar, J. M. and Aguirre Errasti, C. (1982). Tubular aggregates in skeletal muscle of chronic alcoholic patients. *Acta Neuropathol.*, **56**, 250–4

22. Trout, J. J., Stauber, W. T. and Schottelius, B. A. (1981). Increased autophagy in chloroquine-treated tonic and phasic muscles; an alternative view. *Tissue and Cell*, **13**, 393–401

23. Schmalbruch, H. (1980). The early changes in experimental myopathy induced by chloroquine and chlorphentermine. *J. Neuropathol. Exp. Neurol.*, **39**, 65–81

24. Mastaglia, F. L., Papadimitriou, J. M., Dawkins, R. L. and Beveridge, B. (1977). Vacuolar myopathy associated with chloroquine, lupus erythematosus and thymoma. *J. Neurol. Sci.*, **34**, 315–28

25. Neville, H. E., Maunder-Sewry, C. A., McDougall, J., Sewell, J. R. and Dubowitz, V. (1979). Chloroquine-induced cytosomes with curvilinear profiles in muscle. *Muscle and Nerve*, **2**, 376-81

26. Garlepp, M. J., Dawkins, R. L. and Christiansen, F. T. (1983). HLA antigens and acetylcholine receptor antibodies in penicillamine induced myasthenia gravis. *Br. Med. J.*, **286**, 338-40

27. Donker, A. J., Venuto, R. C., Vladutiu, A. O., Brentjens, J. R. and Andres, G. A. (1984). Effects of prolonged administration of D-penicillamine or Captopril in various strains of rats. Brown Norway rats treated with D-penicillamine develop auto-antibodies, circulating immune complexes and disseminated intravascular coagulation. *Clin. Immunol. Immunopathol.*, **30**, 142-55

28. Burres, S. A., Kanter, M. E., Richman, D. P. and Arnason, B. G. W. (1981). Studies on the pathophysiology of chronic D-penicillamine-induced myasthenia. *Ann. NY Acad. Sci.*, **377**, 640-51

29. Bever, C. T. *et al.* (1982). Penicillamine induced myasthenia gravis: effects of penicillamine on acetylcholine receptor. *Neurology*, **32**, 1077-82

30. Doyle, D. R., McCurely, T. L. and Sergent, J. S. (1983). Fatal polymyositis in D-pencillamine treated rheumatoid arthritis. *Ann Intern. Med.* **98**, 327-30

31. Gronert, G. A. (1980). Malignant hyperthermia. *Anesthesiology*, **53**, 395-423

32. Thompson, D. E. A. and Tallack, J. A. (1973). Co-existent muscle disease and malignant hyperpyrexia. In Gordon, R. A. *et al.* (eds.) *International Symposium on Malignant Hyperthermia.* (Springfield, Ill: Charles C. Thomas), pp. 309-18

33. Leiding, K. G. and Graham, M. D. (1981). Malignant hyperthermia. *Arch. Otolaryngol.*, **107**, 758-60

34. Frank, J. P., Harati, Y., Butler, I. J., Nelson, T. E. and Scott, C. I. (1980). Central core disease and malignant hyperthermia syndrome. *Ann. Neurol.*, **7**, 11-17

35. Brownell, A. K. W., Paasuke, R. T., Elash, R. T., Fowlow, S. B., Seagram, C. G. F., Diewold, R. J. and Friesen, C. (1983). Malignant hyperthermia in Duchenne muscular dystrophy. *Anesthesiology*, **58**, 180-2

36. Rosenberg, H. and Heiman-Patterson, T. (1983). Duchenne's muscular dystrophy and malignant hyperthermia: another warning. *Anesthesiology*, **59**, 362

37. Denborough, M. A., Galloway, G. J. and Hopkinson, K. C. (1982). Malignant hyperpyrexia and sudden infant death. *Lancet*, **2**, 1068-9

38. Kalow, W., Britt, B. A. and Richter, A. (1977). The caffeine test of isolated human muscle in relation to malignant hyperthermia. *Can. Anaesthesiol. Soc. J.*, **24**, 678-94

39. Kalow, W., Butt, B. A. and Peters, P. (1978). Rapid simplified techniques for measuring caffeine contracture for patients with malignant hyperthermia. In Aldrete, J. A. and Britt, B. A. (eds.) *Second International Symposium on Malignant Hyperthermia.* (New York: Grune & Stratton), pp. 339-350

40. Gronert, G. A. (1983). Controversies in malignant hyperthermia. *Anesthesiology*, **59**, 273-4

41. Mambo, N. C., Silver, M. D., McLaughlin, P. R., Huckell, V. F., McEwan, P. M., Britt, B. A. and Morch, J. E. (1980). Malignant hyperthermia susceptibility. *Human Pathol.*, **11**, 381-8

42. Harriman, D. G. F. (1982). The pathology of malignant hyperpyrexia. In Walton, J. and Mastalgia, F. L. (eds.) *Skeletal Muscle Pathology.* (Edinburgh: Churchill Livingstone), pp. 575-91

43. Harriman, D. G. F., Ellis, F. R., Franks, A. J. *et al.* (1978). Malignant hyperthermia: an investigation of 75 families. In Aldrete, J. A. and Britt, B. A. (eds.) *Second International Symposium on Malignant Hyperthermia.* (New York: Grune & Stratton), pp. 67-87

Muscle weakness is a symptom of several endocrine disturbances and is sometimes the presenting feature.

Hyperthyroid Myopathy

Proximal muscle weakness with mild atrophy often develops in patients with thyrotoxicosis. Weakness correlates with the duration and severity of hyperthyroidism and is readily reversed by therapy.

Muscle Biopsy

Changes are usually fairly minor and non-specific (Figures 17.1 and 17.2). There may be atrophy of both fibre types, but notably of type 1 fibres[1,2]. Electron microscopy has revealed increased subsarcolemmal glycogen deposits[1], and other non-specific abnormalities (Figures 17.3 and 17.4). Clinical disability may seem out of proportion to inconspicuous morphological changes, suggesting atrophy is not the only cause of weakness. The metabolic disturbances which impair muscle strength do not necessarily induce obvious histological changes. Atrophy is probably attributable to increased protein degradation[3]. Changes in fibre type composition have been clearly demonstrated in animals, where whole muscles are available. This has been described in man[2], but it is difficult to assess in a small biopsy. In hyperthyroid rats there is an increase in the proportion of fibres which are type 2 with the myosin ATP-ase reaction[4]. Thyroid hormones may effect changes in myosin ATP-ase activity analogous to a switch to a fast motor neuron.

Hypothyroid Myopathy

Mild muscular symptoms are not uncommon in hypothyroidism, but only a minority develop marked muscular weakness. The CPK is usually elevated and the level reflects the severity of hypothyroidism. However, the degree of proximal weakness and histological changes appear to correlate more closely with its duration[5]. The myopathy responds to L-thyroxine and complete recovery can be anticipated, although those with severe clinical symptoms respond slowly. A few patients develop pain and increased weakness on exertion during the initial treatment period. This peculiar phenomenon may be related to a sudden increased metabolic demand that thyroxine imposes upon weakened muscle[5].

Muscle Biopsy

Muscle weakness is characterized by selective type 2 fibre atrophy (Figure 17.5) and sometimes reduction in the proportion of type 2 fibres[2,5]. Although preferentially a type 2 fibre atrophy, atrophic type 1 fibres may be found. There are increased central nuclei, predominantly in type 2 fibres. Abnormal PAS-positive subsarcolemmal deposits have been described in severe cases and also increased perinuclear acid phosphatase activity. Peripheral crescents of acid mucopolysaccharide are often described in early reports, but these observations have not been repeated with newer staining techniques and their validity is questionable. These changes are eventually reversed by therapy, but the CPK may return to normal whilst there is still clinical and morphological evidence of residual myopathy[5,6] The NADH-TR reaction may show slight, patchy myofibrillar disarray in the treatment period.

Electron microscopy has revealed an accumulation of glycogen and numerous abnormal mitochondria with a honeycomb appearance or containing crystalline inclusions. In severe cases membrane-bound collections of lipid and glycogen granules have been described. These probably represent lysosomes and correspond with the increased acid phosphatase activity. Other non-specific fine structural abnormalities, such as concentric laminated bodies, may be found.

Cushing's Disease

The proximal muscle weakness of idiopathic Cushing's disease may be quite severe. The pathogenesis and histological abnormalities are the same in iatrogenic steroid myopathy (Figure 17.6). The dominant change is a selective atrophy of type 2 fibres (Figures 17.7 and 17.8). Muscle wasting is due to decreased protein synthesis and interference with glucose utilization. The susceptibility of fast glycolytic type 2 fibres is related to their dependence on the glycogen substrate and relatively low level of fatty acid metabolism[7].

Osteomalacia

Although this is not primarily an endocrine disturbance it is mentioned here because of the association with secondary hyperparathyroidism. Proximal muscle weakness and sometimes tenderness is not uncommon in patients with osteomalacia[8], but the exact mechanism of weakness is uncertain. It has been attributed to disuse atrophy[9] and certainly bone pain may enforce immobility. In some cases electromyographic and histological findings have suggested a neurogenic

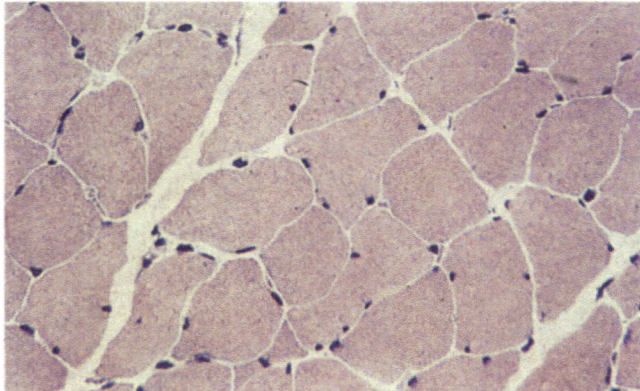

Figure 17.1   Hyperthyroid myopathy. Deltoid biopsy from a 22-year-old man whose symptoms of thyrotoxicosis had been present for several months. On examination he was extremely thin, with proximal muscle weakness and pathologically brisk reflexes. Treatment with carbimazole led to rapid improvement in strength. Despite considerable weakness the biopsy does not show very obvious abnormalities. The fibre diameters are smaller than would be expected in a fit, young man, but there are only scanty severely atrophic fibres. (Same case shown in Figures 17.2–17.4.)   H & E × 180

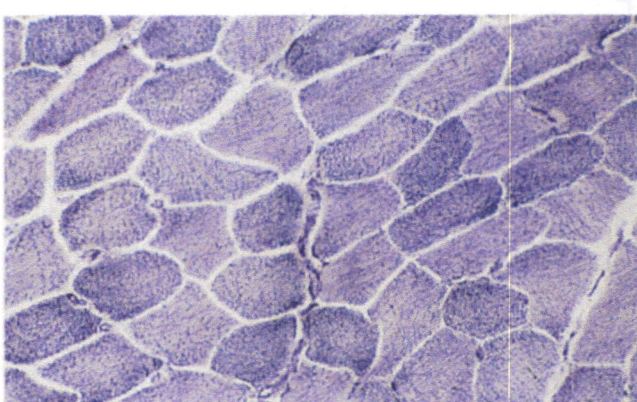

Figure 17.2   Hyperthyroid myopathy. In this biopsy there is normal fibre type distribution and no significant derangement of fibre architecture.   NADH-TR × 180

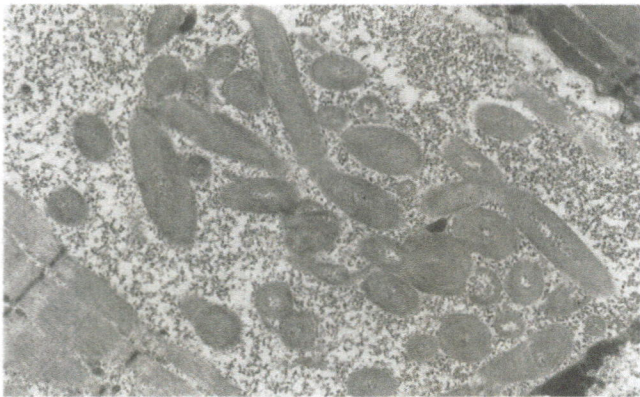

Figure 17.3   Hyperthyroid myopathy. Concentric laminated bodies. The origin of these abnormal cellular constituents is uncertain. They are by no means specific to hyperthyroidism and have been described in a wide variety of myopathies.   EM × 7100

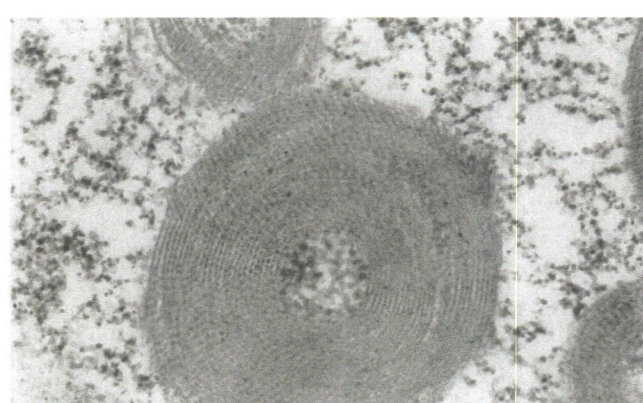

Figure 17.4   Hyperthyroid myopathy. Detail of a concentric laminated body. The regular, concentric bands have a different structure and periodicity from myofilaments and are not thought to be derived from them.   EM × 34 000

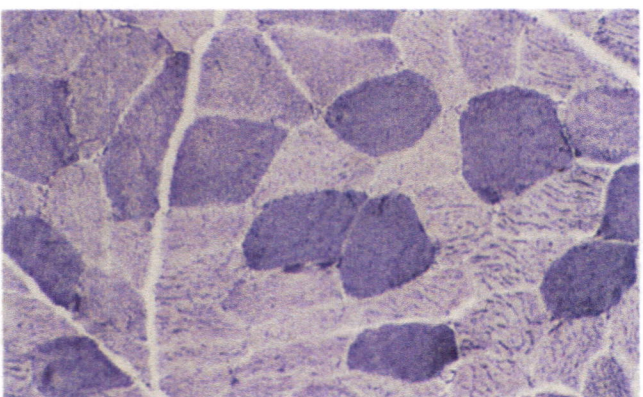

Figure 17.5   Hypothyroid myopathy. Biopsy from a 59-year-old woman with a 4-year history of mild proximal muscle weakness and recently proven hypothyroidism. At the time of the biopsy she had been receiving treatment for hypothyroidism for a few weeks but, although the CPK was normal, muscle weakness persisted. The changes are not very gross. There is mild type 2 fibre atrophy, but no disturbance of cell architecture and normal fibre type composition. This delay in clinical improvement of hypothyroid myopathy is not unusual.   NADH-TR × 180

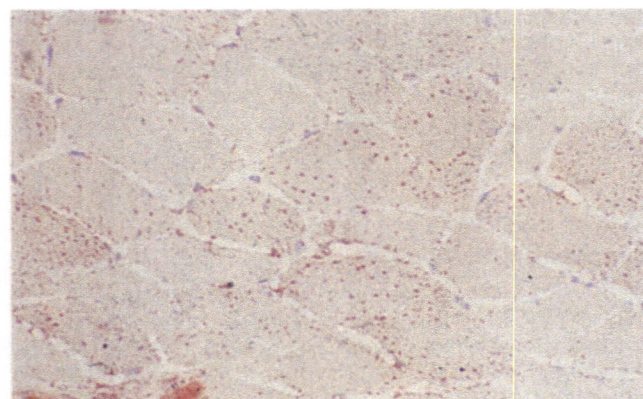

Figure 17.6   Steroid myopathy. An increase in lipid in biopsy from a patient who had been receiving high-dose steroids for only a few weeks. The lipid droplets were present in type 1 fibres. This is an early change in a steroid myopathy.   Oil Red O × 180

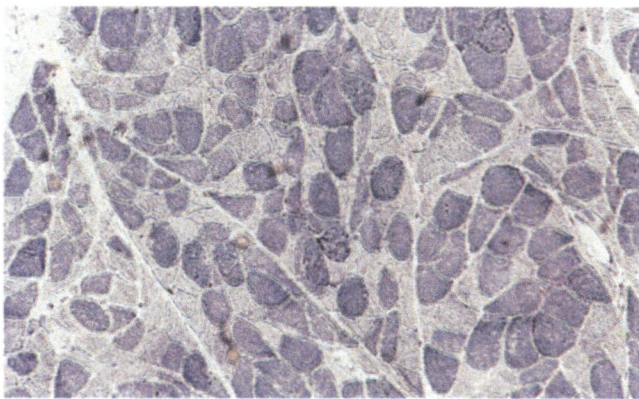

Figure 17.7 Steroid myopathy. Type 2 fibre atrophy in deltoid biopsy of a 71-year-old on long-term steroid therapy for chronic lung disease. (Same case shown in Figure 17.8.) NADH-TR × 75

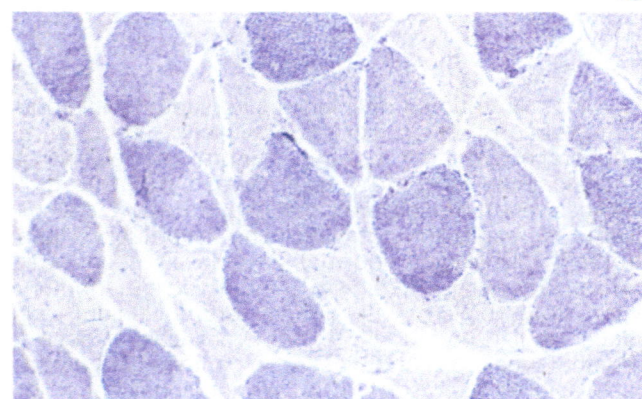

Figure 17.8 Steroid myopathy. Type 2 fibre atrophy. NADH-TR × 180

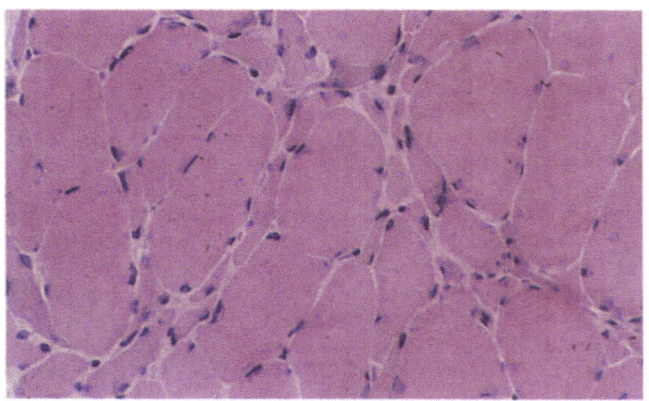

Figure 17.9 Osteomalacic myopathy; 43-year-old man with Crohn's disease who had had extensive small bowel resection. He was hypoprotein-aemic, with ankle oedema and showed considerable generalized loss of muscle bulk and proximal weakness. The CPK was normal. The quadriceps biopsy contains many severely atrophic fibres, with distribution resembling the small group atrophy of denervation. Other investigations showed that he had osteomalacia. When appropriate treatment was begun his muscle weakness was quickly reversed. (Same case shown in Figures 17.10–17.12.) H & E × 180

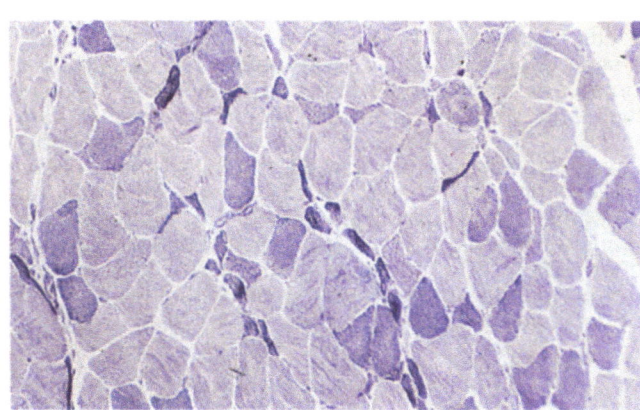

Figure 17.10 Osteomalacic myopathy. Many atrophic angular fibres, of both types, amongst normal-sized fibres. Darkly staining atrophic fibres with the oxidative enzyme reaction increase the similarity with denervation. However, in osteomalacic myopathy there is no compensatory hyper-trophy. NADH-TR × 75

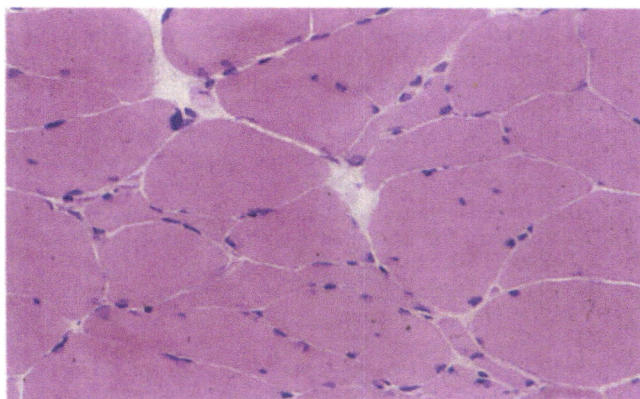

Figure 17.11 Osteomalacic myopathy. There are a few central nuclei. H & E × 180

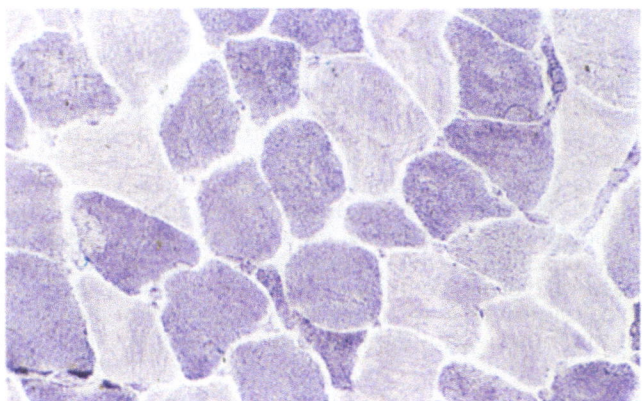

Figure 17.12 Osteomalacic myopathy. Atrophic angulated fibres of both types. Slight patchy staining of type 1 fibres with the oxidative enzyme reaction. NADH-TR × 180

disorder[18]. Nutritional deficiencies in osteomalacia due to malabsorption could conceivably produce a peripheral neuropathy, but this is unproven. The role of hypocalcaemia is controversial. Swash suggests that disturbance of muscle cell calcium transport causes failure of excitation/coupling and eventually fibre atrophy[10]. However, normal muscle is seen with primary hypoparathyroidism[11]. Conversely primary hyperparathyroidism with raised serum calcium can induce similar pathology to osteomalacia[8]. It seems likely that weakness and wasting in patients with osteomalacia is multifactorial. It is an additional cause of weakness in the elderly that is easily overlooked. It has also been described in association with dialysis-induced osteomalacia[12]. Recovery of muscle strength occurs with treatment of osteomalacia, but it may take several months.

Muscle Biopsy

Histological abnormalities are often mild and non-specific. Atrophy of both type 1 and type 2 fibres may be seen (Figure 17.9) or preferential type 2B atrophy. Sometimes the atrophic fibres of both types are very small and may have an angulated contour (Figure 17.10), an appearance that is understandably mistaken for denervation. In the elderly, motor neuron disease may be suspected. However, there is no compensatory hypertrophy. Although necrosis and regeneration are absent, a few central nuclei and minor abnormalities of fibre architecture with the oxidative enzyme reaction may provide additional clues that it is not neurogenic disease (Figures 17.11 and 17.12).

Hypoparathyroidism

Muscle weakness, increased fatiguability and elevated CPK may occur with hypoparathyroidism, but muscle biopsy has been reported as entirely normal by light and electron microscopy[11]. It has been suggested the symptoms are due to functional changes of the muscle cell membrane induced by hypocalcaemia.

Hyperaldosteronism

Primary hyperaldosteronism may present with a rapidly progressive, generalized muscular weakness[13]. The muscles are sometimes tender, but not wasted. Weakness correlates with a very low serum potassium and is quite rapidly reversed when this is corrected. The serum CPK may be very high and myoglobin may appear in the urine[14]. The low serum potassium probably affects the stability of cell membranes. An acute myopathy has also been described with hypokalaemia due to laxative abuse or diuretic therapy. There is clinical and pathological similarity with hypokalaemic periodic paralysis, but the muscle damage in the latter is less severe.

Muscle Biopsy

The biopsy may show fibre necrosis, phagocytosis and regeneration and also vacuolated fibres. Electron microscopy shows that vacuolated fibres contain large membrane-bound vacuoles, sometimes connected with the T tubules[13]. Other fibres without vacuolation may contain dilated sarcoplasmic reticulum and show a honeycomb appearance of the T tubules.

Addison's Disease

Muscle weakness is a recognized symptom of severe adrenocortico-insufficiency. Hyperkalaemia may have a causative role. The muscle weakness is very rapidly reversed by restoration of normal serum ionic concentrations and definite morphological changes have not been described.

References

1. Gruener, R., Stern, L. Z., Payne, C. and Hannapel, L. (1975). Hyperthyroid myopathy: intracellular electrophysiological measurements in biopsied human intercostal muscle. *J. Neurol. Sci.*, **24**, 339–49

2. Wiles, C. M., Young, A., Jones, D. A. and Edwards, R. H. T. (1979). Muscle relaxation rate, fibre type composition and energy turnover in hyper and hypothyroid patients. *Clin. Sci.*, **57**, 375–84

3. De Martino, G. N. and Goldberg, A. L. (1978). Thyroid hormones control lysosomal enzyme activities in liver and skeletal muscle. *Proc. Natl. Acad. Sci. USA*, **75**, 1369–73

4. Ianuzzo, D. *et al.* (1977). Thyroidal trophic influence on skeletal muscle myosin. *Nature*, **270**, 74–6

5. McKeran, R. O., Slavin, G., Andrews, T. M., Ward, P. and Mair, W. G. P. (1975). Muscle fibre changes in hypothyroid myopathy. *J. Clin. Pathol.*, **28**, 659–63

6. Giampetro, O., Boni, C., Carpi, A. and Buzzigoli, G. (1981). Monitoring of the serum levels of muscle enzymes during replacement therapy in hypothyroidism with myopathy. *J. Nucl. Med. Allied Sci.*, **25**, 211–18

7. Livingstone, I., Johnson, M. A. and Mastaglia, F. L. (1981). Effects of dexamethasone on fibre subtypes in rat muscle. *J. Neuropathol. Appl. Neurobiol.*, **7**, 381–98

8. Mallette, L., Patten, B. M. and Engel, W. K. (1975). Neuromuscular disease in secondary hyperparathyroidism. *Ann. Intern. Med.*, **82**, 474–83

9. Dastur, D. K., Gagrat, B. M., Wadia, N. H., Desai, M. M. and Bharucha, E. P. (1975). Nature of muscular change in osteomalacia: light and electron microscope observations. *J. Pathol.* **117**, 211–28

10. Swash, M., Schwartz, M. S. and Sarjeant, M. K. (1979). Osteomalacic myopathy: an experimental approach. *Neuropathol. Appl. Neurobiol.*, **5**, 295–302

11. Kruse, K., Scheunemann, W., Baier, W. and Schaub, J. (1982). Hypocalcaemic myopathy in idiopathic hypoparathryoidism. *Eur. J. Pediatr.*, **138**, 280–2

12. Bautista, J., GilNecija, E., Castilla, J., Chinchon, I. and Rafel, E. (1983). Dialysis myopathy. *Acta Neuropathol. (Berl.)*, **61**, 71–5

13. Atsumi, T., Ishikawa, S., Miyatake, T. and Yoshida, A. (1979). Myopathy and primary aldosteronism: electronmicroscopic study. *Neurology*, **29**, 1348–53

14. Schady, W. and Yuill, G. M. (1981). Myopathy and primary hyperaldosteronism. *Neurology*, **31**, 225–6

Focal Lesions

Primary neoplasms of muscle are beyond the scope of this atlas, but several other causes of localized swelling are briefly described. The histological changes of systemic myopathies to a large extent reflect varying degrees of degeneration or regeneration and repair of skeletal muscle cells. Thus it is not surprising that the same abnormalities often appear in focal reactive lesions and can cause diagnostic difficulty if their fundamental nature is not appreciated.

Mechanical Trauma

Most people have experienced painful, stiff muscles the day after unaccustomed, fairly strenuous exercise; digging the garden, the first game of tennis of the season! We complain for a day or two, but the problem quickly resolves. The symptoms are due to minor focal muscle cell injuries. These are probably initially mechanical, but may be exacerbated by biochemical disturbances in the injured cell. It has been shown that fibre damage is greatest when exercise involves eccentric contractions, i.e. the active muscle is lengthened[1]. The phenomenon of a 'pulled' muscle is merely a more obvious degree of localized muscle damage. However, continued use of the damaged muscle can sometimes produce a localized, chronic swelling, which may be excised because of a suspicion of a neoplasm. The case shown in Figures 18.1 and 18.2 was a firm swelling present for several weeks on the foot of a child, close to a tendinous insertion. Hypercontracted fibres and all stages of necrosis and regeneration can be found alongside hypertrophied fibres, split fibres and interstitial fibrosis; changes compatible with repetitive muscle injury. Segmental necrosis and regeneration will of course follow any wound involving muscle. Surgical specimens that include the site of a recent biopsy may show such changes, e.g. a deep lumpectomy in breast followed by radical mastectomy. Regenerating myoblasts must not be confused with infiltrating carcinoma.

Proliferative Myositis

Proliferative myositis probably represents a vigorous fibroblastic response to local muscle injury. However, there is often no definite history of trauma and the lesion causes concern because it is a rapidly enlarging, painless swelling. It most often occurs in flat muscles of the trunk or shoulder girdle and usually in middle-aged adults[2]. It is less often found in the head and neck[3] region. The swelling may reach 3–4 cm within a week or two of first appearance, but at a later stage it rarely exceeds 6 cm in diameter.

Macroscopically there is poorly circumscribed pale scar-like tissue involving muscle and the muscle sheath. Histology shows a loosely cellular fibroblastic proliferation separating the muscle fibres and widening the fibrous septa between the fascicles (Figures 18.3 and 18.4). Amongst typical spindle cell fibroblasts there are often many giant cells with basophilic cytoplasm, large nuclei and conspicuous nucleoli, somewhat resembling ganglion cells or rhabdomyoblasts (Figures 18.5 and 18.6). These bizarre cells have been responsible for erroneous diagnoses of sarcoma. However, unlike a malignant neoplasm the process does not destroy and replace muscle. The muscle fibres are generally well preserved; occasional necrotic fibres and regenerating myotubes can be found, but they are not a prominent feature. Isolated tiny foci of osteoid are sometimes present in the fibroblastic tissue, but not the broad zone characteristic of myositis ossificans (see below). Electron microscopy shows that the giant cells have abundant rough endoplasmic reticulum and fine actin filaments in the cytoplasm. Despite a resemblance to rhabdomyoblasts, these cells are believed to be modified fibroblasts – myofibroblasts[3]. Identical cells are found in proliferative fasciitis, which is a similar lesion confined to fascia and subcutis and does not involve skeletal muscle. Proliferative myositis is cured by simple excision and it does not recur.

Myositis Ossificans

Focal myositis ossificans is another reactive proliferation of connective tissue in which metaplastic bone formation supervenes. Trauma producing muscle necrosis and haemorrhage is a likely initiating factor. It is usually a well-circumscribed nodule in muscle, but sometimes in tendon or subcutaneous fat[4]. It is most often seen in limb muscles of young active persons. It begins as a tender swelling which gradually becomes firmer and well defined. When it has been present for a few weeks tiny opacities may be visible radiologically. In long-standing lesions this calcification is more distinct.

Histology of the long-standing lesions shows a well-defined partly bony lesion, replacing muscle fascicles (Figures 18.7–18.10). There is definite zonation with an outer shell of mature lamellar bone, which merges on its inner aspect with irregular trabeculae of woven bone, osteoid and sometimes cartilage. In the centre there is cellular fibroblastic tissue. This fully developed lesion does not present diagnostic difficulty, but in the younger lesion mature bone may not have formed and the dense fibroblastic tissue combined with osteoid has been mistaken for soft tissue osteogenic sarcoma. In the benign reactive lesion ossification is always most advanced at the periphery of the lesion, whereas in the

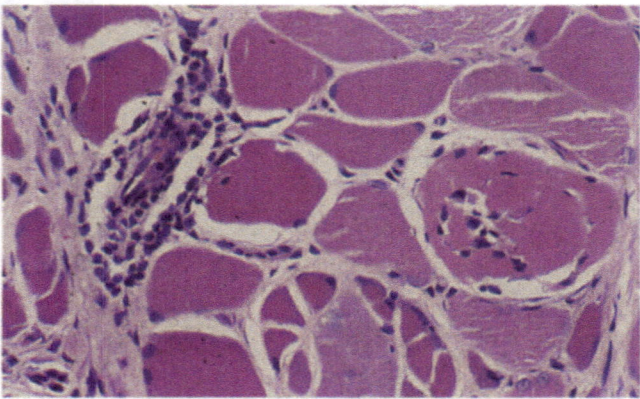

Figure 18.1 Chronic injury – a firm swelling of several weeks' duration on the foot of a young child. The swelling was close to a tendinous insertion. Biopsy shows marked variation in fibre size, with some greatly hypertrophied fibres. There is also focal interstitial chronic inflammation. Mild variation in fibre size and increase in interstitial connective tissue is normal at this site, but the changes here are far in excess of normal and attributable to repetitive injury. The 'pulled' muscle is often damaged near its tendon insertion. (Same case shown in Figure 18.2.) H & E × 180

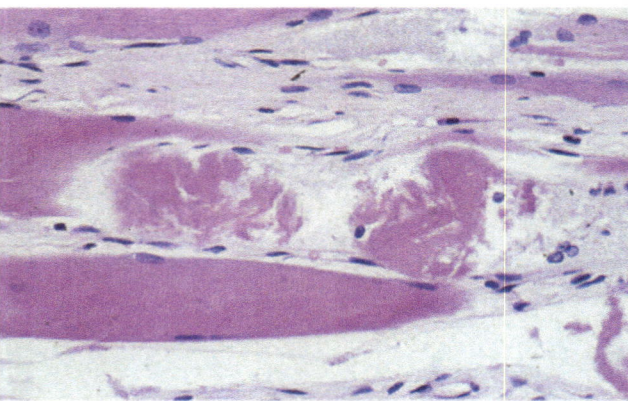

Figure 18.2 Chronic trauma. Hypercontracted fibres were present in this focal muscle swelling indicative of continuing muscle injury. Continued physical activity after initial minor trauma is the likely cause. H & E × 300

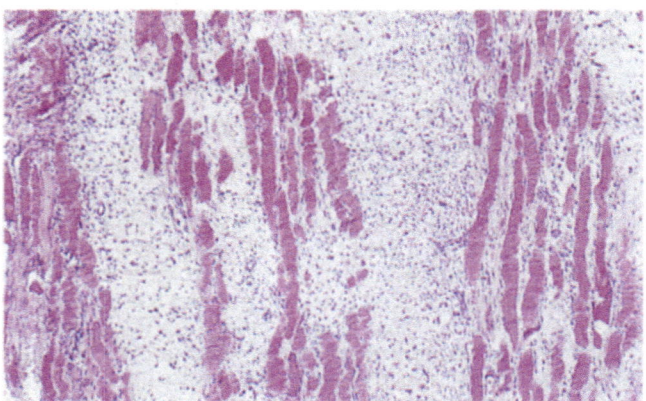

Figure 18.3 Proliferative myositis. Painless swelling in the upper arm of a 69-year-old woman, present for 3 months. On excision a dense white mass 4 cm diameter, surrounded by and involving muscle. Wide separation of the fascicles by loosely cellular fibroblastic tissue. (Same case shown in Figures 18.4–18.6.) H & E × 30

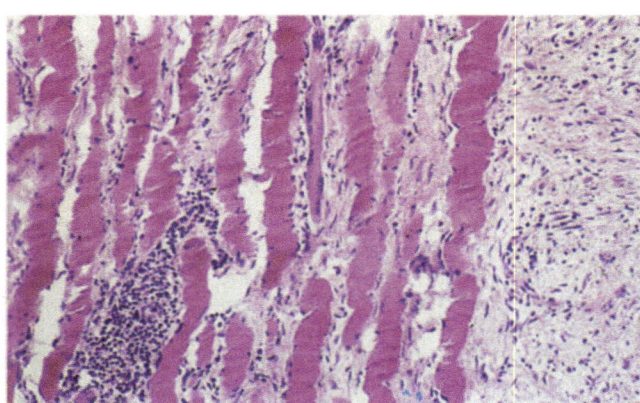

Figure 18.4 Proliferative myositis. Occasional foci of interstitial lymphocytes, necrotic and regenerating fibres may be found, but the majority of muscle fibres are preserved and undamaged. The fibroblastic proliferation does not obliterate muscle fibres. H & E × 75

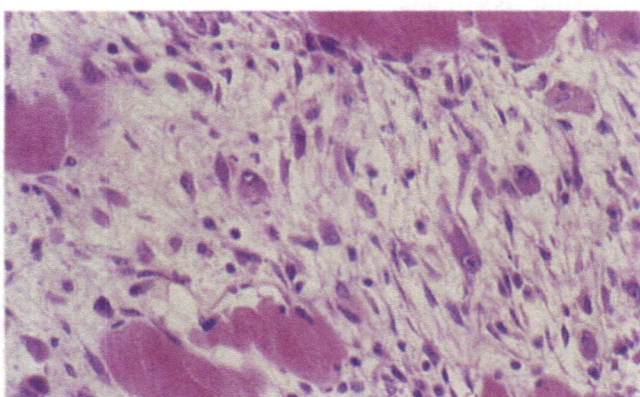

Figure 18.5 Proliferative myositis. The fibroblastic tissue contains typical spindle cell fibroblasts and also larger cells with abundant cytoplasm. H & E × 180

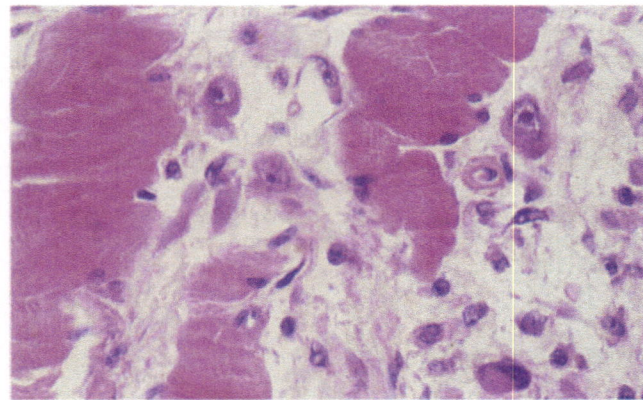

Figure 18.6 Proliferative myositis. The large cells in the interstitium resemble ganglion cells, with abundant cytoplasm, vesicular nuclei and conspicuous nucleoli. These cells are modified fibroblasts – myofibroblasts. H & E × 300

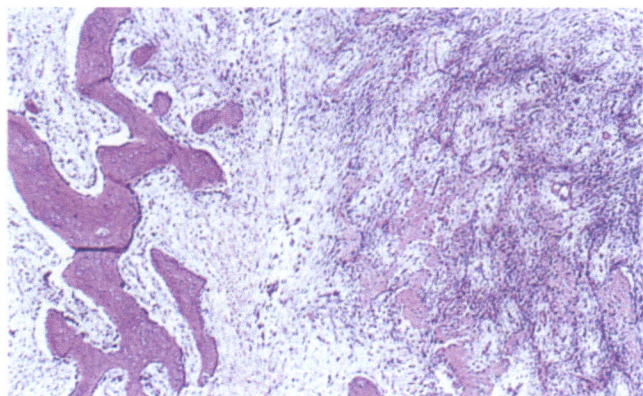

Figure 18.7 Myositis ossificans. Rapidly enlarging mass in the popliteal fossa of a 12-year-old girl, found to be involving the semimembranosus. The focal bony lesion replacing skeletal muscle shows definite zonation. The outer border (left) is formed by trabeculae of mature lamellar bone. Inside this, nearer the centre of the lesion, there is immature woven bone (right). The most central region may contain immature fibroblastic tissue and islands of osteoid, shown in Figures 18.9 and 18.10. (Same case shown in Figures 18.8–18.10.) H & E × 30

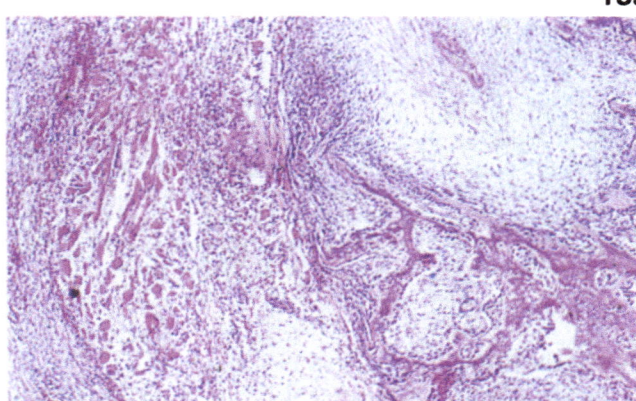

Figure 18.8 Myositis ossificans. Border with skeletal muscle. Trabeculae of woven bone are present at the outer edge of the lesion. When the lesion is developing and before lamellar bone has formed, ossification is always most advanced at the periphery. H & E × 30

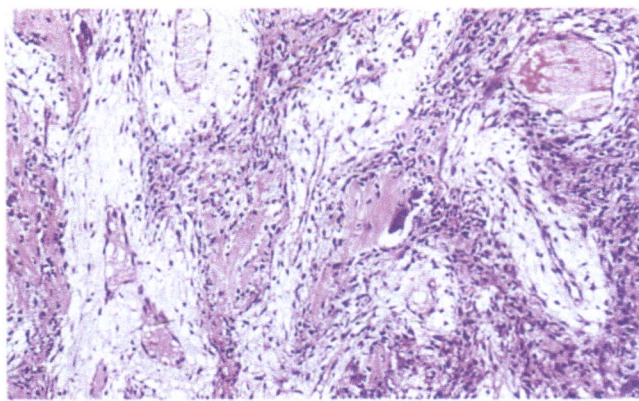

Figure 18.9 Myositis ossificans. Inner zone, beneath lamellar bone, is formed by woven bone which merges in the centre with fibroblastic tissue (right). H & E × 180

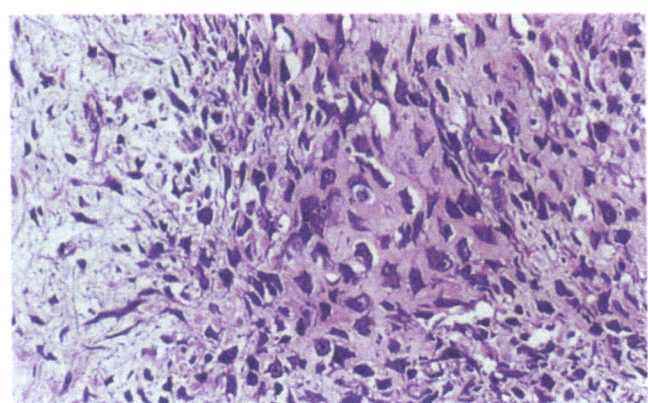

Figure 18.10 Myositis ossificans. Central zone. Fibroblastic proliferation and large cells with hyperchromatic nuclei, surrounded by eosinophilic intercellular material, indicating early osteoid formation. The central region is always the most immature and highly cellular. H & E × 300

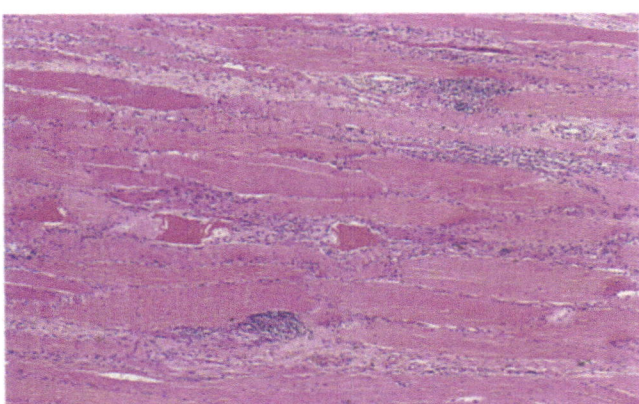

Figure 18.11 Focal myositis. Tender swelling (approximately 6 cm diameter) in the gastrocnemius muscle of a 60-year-old man. No history of injury and no evidence of systemic disease. The excised muscle appeared pale. It shows patchy fibre necrosis and regeneration and interstitial inflammation. No cause was discovered. The patient is in good health with no evidence of recurrence or systemic disease 10 years later. (Same case shown in Figures 18.12 and 18.13.) H & E × 30

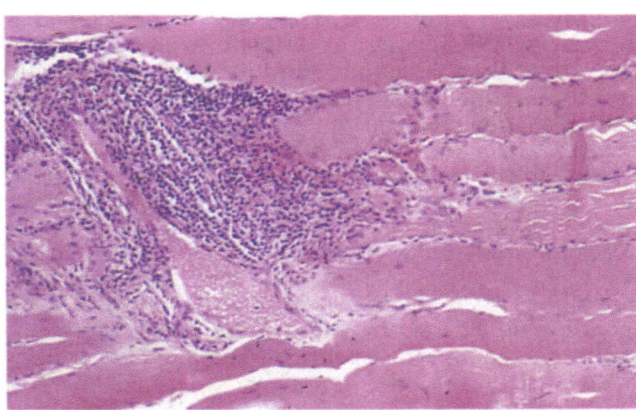

Figure 18.12 Focal myositis. Large perivascular, interstitial aggregate of lymphocytes. H & E × 180

malignant tumour there is an advancing, infiltrative edge of pleomorphic cells.

Fibrodysplasia ossificans progressiva, sometimes referred to as generalized myositis ossificans, is a completely different disorder, characterized by multifocal, soft tissue ossification in childhood and possibly attributable to aberrant periosteal differentiation[5].

Focal Myositis

Focal myositis is another benign, localized swelling of muscle that may be mistaken for a neoplasm. A localized, painful swelling, a few centimetres in diameter, develops over a period of several weeks[6]. It has been described in both adults and children, usually in limb muscles, but also in perioral muscles[7]. Histologically it is obviously a benign inflammatory lesion, with scattered muscle fibre necrosis and regeneration, focal chronic inflammatory cell infiltrates and increased interstitial connective tissue (Figures 18.10–18.15). There may be variation in fibre size with both atrophy and hypertrophy. There is no obvious cause. No organisms can be identified. Eosinophils are on occasion quite numerous, but a search for parasites is unrewarding.

This histology is indistinguishable from polymyositis and furthermore a localized limb swelling is a recognized, albeit rare, mode of presentation of polymyositis[8]. The presence of vasculitis may be a pointer to systemic disease[9]. Other clinical investigations should be performed to exclude this possibility. An EMG may assist in detecting systemic myopathy. The presence of any systemic symptoms, a raised ESR or raised CPK are all very definite indicators of the systemic disorder. When all these other investigations are negative the swelling is probably a genuine focal myositis and there will be no progression[8]. The cause of focal myositis is unknown, but one may speculate that trauma and/or localized infection are involved.

Musculo-Aponeurotic Fibromatoses – Desmoid Tumours

The fibromatoses are a group of proliferative fibroblastic lesions which show infiltrative, local growth, but do not metastasize[10]. This type of lesion can develop at a variety of different sites at different ages[11]. Only the deep musculo-aponeurotic fibromatosis, the desmoid tumour, is mentioned here because it may be confused with other benign focal muscle lesions. Distinction is important because unlike proliferative myositis or focal myositis the fibromatosis tends to recur after incomplete local excision. Clinically the musculo-aponeurotic fibromatosis is usually an insidious painless muscular swelling. It occurs mostly in youngish patients, especially in the second and third decades. The shoulder girdle and lower limb are common sites, but it may develop almost anywhere in the musculature[12]. It frequently reaches 5–10 cm in diameter and can be much larger.

Macroscopically it is an ill-defined, firm pale mass involving muscle and sometimes surrounding fascia and adjacent structures. The lesion is usually only moderately cellular and composed of spindle cell fibroblasts and collagen, frequently orientated in the direction of the muscle fibres. Despite an innocent appearance the fibromatosis engulfs and replaces muscle. At the periphery the advancing infiltrative edge is often more cellular and trapped atrophic muscle

fibres, which have been converted to multinucleate giant cells, can produce a bizarre appearance. Proliferative and focal myositis differ from the fibromatosis in that muscle cells are not obliterated, merely separated by increased, loosely cellular connective tissue. Unlike myositis ossificans, formation of osteoid is exceptional. A fibromatosis must also be distinguished from a low-grade fibrosarcoma. This may be difficult, but greater nuclear pleomorphism, a less orderly arrangement and mitotic activity are the important guides. Any more than scanty mitoses should arouse suspicion of malignancy and hence metastasizing potential.

Metastases in Muscle

Skeletal muscle is often completely spared in disseminated neoplasia. It may be that despite the good blood supply metastases do not take root in muscle because of frequent movement and metabolic changes. However, muscle is by no means exempt from secondary neoplasms. Direct invasion, e.g. involvement of pectoral muscle by breast carcinoma, is well recognized. Less often blood-borne metastases produce focal nodules in muscle and rarely widespread multifocal muscle involvement is responsible for generalized weakness. Two histological patterns of infiltration occur. As in any other tissue a mass of malignant tumour cells may destroy and completely replace skeletal muscle fibres (Figures 18.19 and 18.22). In addition intracellular invasion can occur with preservation of the muscle fibre[13] (Figures 18.23 and 18.24). This unusual metastatic pattern has been described with a variety of neoplasms, including carcinoma of the breast, prostate, urinary bladder, malignant lymphoma and leukaemia[14,15]. Multiple tumour cells are seen within cytoplasmic vacuoles in muscle fibres, which are otherwise intact with normal architecture.

References

1. Newnham, D. J., McPhail, G., Mills, K. R. and Edwards, R. H. T. (1983). Ultrastructural changes after concentric and eccentric contractions of human muscle. *J. Neurol. Sci.*, **61**, 109–22

2. Enzinger, F. M. and Weiss, S. W. (1983). Benign tumours and tumour like lesions of fibrous tissue. In *Soft Tissue Tumours*. (New York: C. V. Mosby), pp. 14–45

3. Orlowski, W., Freedman, P. D. and Lumerman, H. (1983). Proliferative myositis of the masseter muscles. *Cancer*, **52**, 904–8

4. Enzinger, F. M. and Weiss, S. W. (1983). Osseous tumours and tumour like lesions of soft tissue. In *Soft Tissue Tumours*. (New York: C. V. Mosby), pp. 720–44

5. Cramer, S. F., Ruehl, A. and Mandel, M. A. (1981). Fibrodysplasia ossificans progressiva. *Cancer*, **48**, 1016–21

6. Heffner, R. R., Armbrustmacher, V. W. and Earle, K. M. (1977). Focal myositis. *Cancer*, **40**, 301–6

7. Ellis, G. L. and Brannon, R. B. (1979). Focal myositis of the perioral musculature. *Oral Surg.*, **48**, 337–41

8. Heffner, R. R. and Stephen, A. B. (1981). Polymyositis beginning as a focal process. *Arch. Neurol.*, **38**, 439–42

9. Smith, C. A. and Pinals, R. S. (1981). Localised nodular myositis. *J. Rheumatol.*, **8**, 815–19

10. Hajdu, S. I. (1979). Fibromatosis. In *Pathology of Soft Tissue Tumours*. (Philadelphia: Lea & Febiger), pp. 65–77

11. Allen, P. W. (1977). The fibromatoses. A clinicopathologic classification based on 140 cases. *Am. J. Surg. Pathol.*, **1**, 255–69; 305–21

12. Reitamo, J., Hayry, P., Nykyri, E. and Saxen, E. (1982). The desmoid tumour. 1: Incidence, sex, age and anatomical distribution in the Finnish population. *Am. J. Clin. Pathol.*, **77**, 665–73

13. Lasser, A. and Zacks, S. I. (1982). Intraskeletal myofiber metastasis of breast carcinoma. *Human Pathol.*, **13**, 1045–6

14. Rotterdam, H. (1983). Intraskeletal myofiber metastasis of breast carcinoma. *Human Pathol.*, **14**, 828

15. Ioachim, H. L. (1983). Tumour cells within skeletal muscle cells. *Human Pathol.*, **14**, 923–4

Figures 18.13–18.24 may be found overleaf.

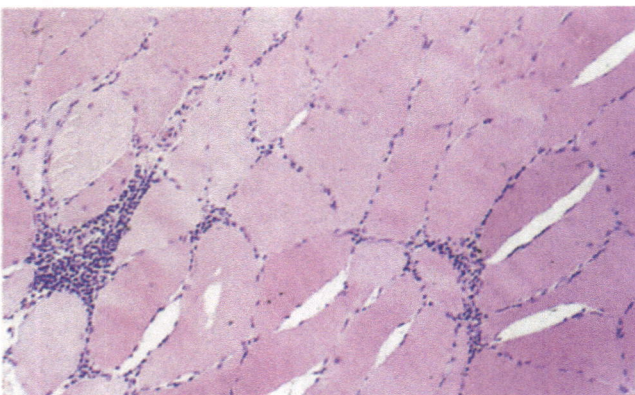

Figure 18.13 Focal myositis. Chronic inflammatory cells, predominantly lymphocytes, also spread between individual muscle fibres in the fascicles. Lymphocytes frequently surround apparently healthy fibres.   H & E × 180

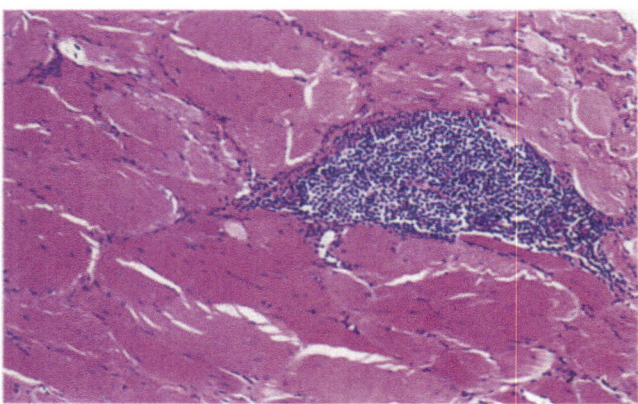

Figure 18.14 Focal myositis in the digastric muscle. Tender swelling in the neck of a middle-aged man. No other symptoms or evidence of systemic disease. The muscle contains scattered aggregates of lymphoid cells. (Same case shown in Figure 18.15.)   H & E × 180

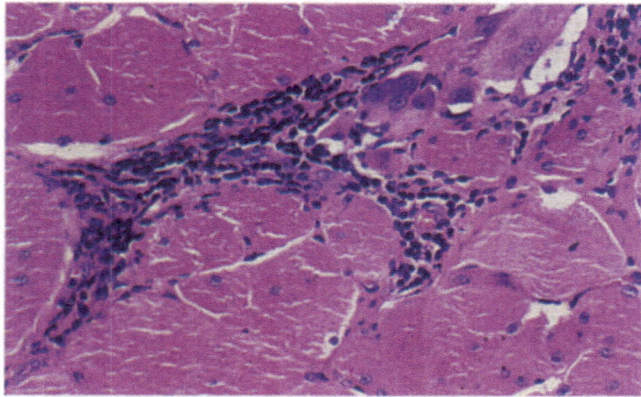

Figure 18.15 Focal myositis. Interstitial lymphocytic infiltrate adjacent to basophilic, regenerating fibres.   H & E × 180

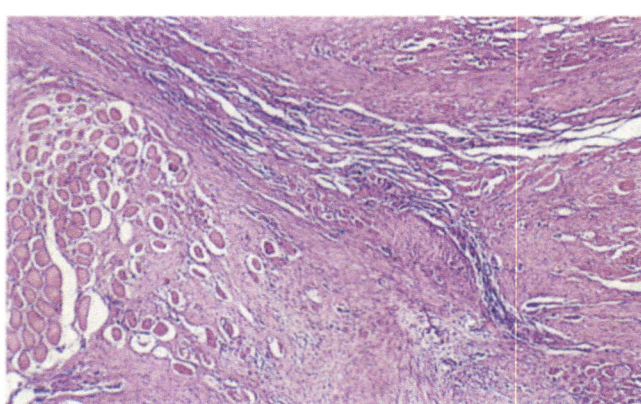

Figure 18.16 Aponeurotic fibromatosis. Recurrent axillary mass involving muscles of the shoulder girdle in a 21-year-old woman. The lesion shows broad bands of fibroblastic tissue infiltrating and replacing skeletal muscle. (Same case shown in Figure 18.17.)   H & E × 30

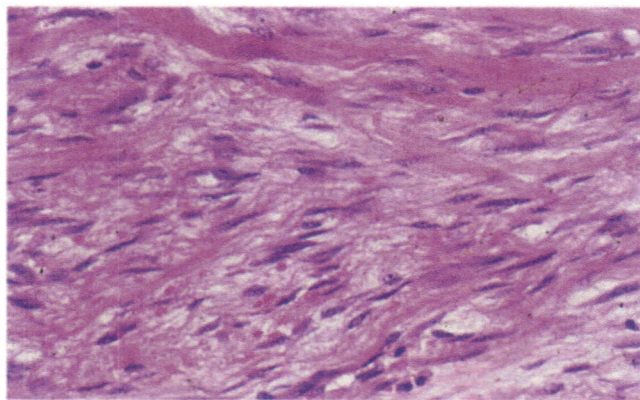

Figure 18.17 Aponeurotic fibromatosis. Mature fibroblasts with roughly parallel arrangement, separated by collagen fibres. The lesion has typically low cellularity and banal appearance. Mitotic figures are absent.   H & E × 180

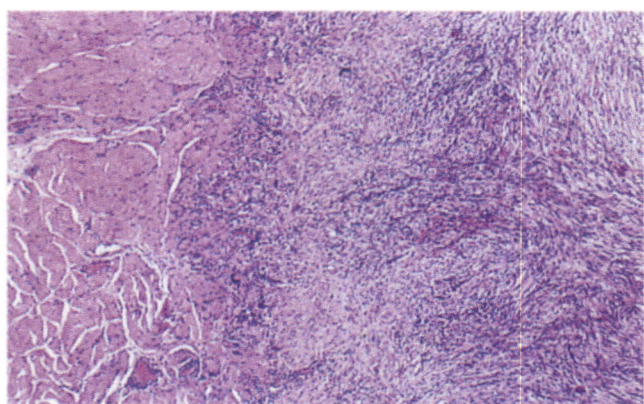

Figure 18.18 Aponeurotic fibromatosis. Painless swelling in the submandibular region of an elderly man. This was a small lesion (2 cm diameter) formed by densely cellular bundles of spindle cell fibroblasts infiltrating and replacing skeletal muscle. (Same lesion shown in Figure 18.19.)   H & E × 30

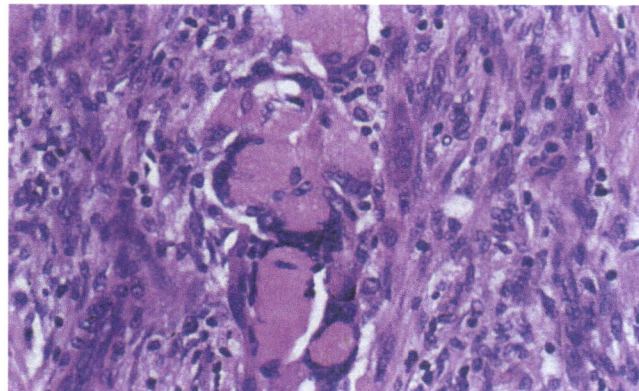

Figure 18.19 Aponeurotic fibromatosis. Skeletal muscle cells at the infiltrating edge, which are being engulfed by the fibroblastic proliferation, may be transformed into bizarre, multinucleate giant cells. The appearance has sometimes been mistaken for a sarcoma. The periphery of this small lesion is more cellular than the central zone. H & E × 180

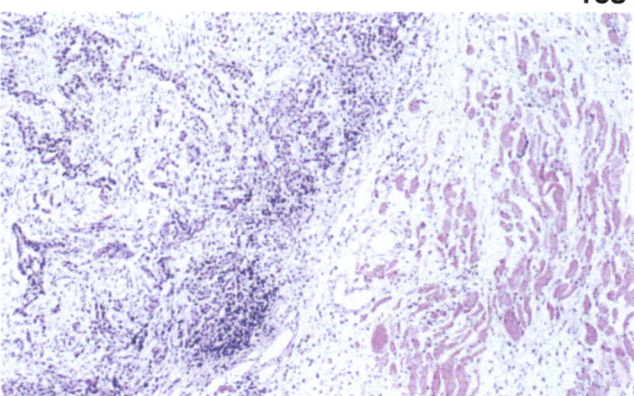

Figure 18.20 Metastatic carcinoma. 80-year-old man with carcinoma of the lung developed proximal muscle weakness a week or two before death. Postmortem examination revealed widely disseminated neoplasm, with multiple tiny nodules (1–2 cm diameter) in skeletal muscles. A nodular deposit of metastatic adenocarcinoma, with a fibrous stromal reaction completely replaces skeletal muscle fibres. (Same case shown in Figures 18.21 and 18.22.) H & E × 30

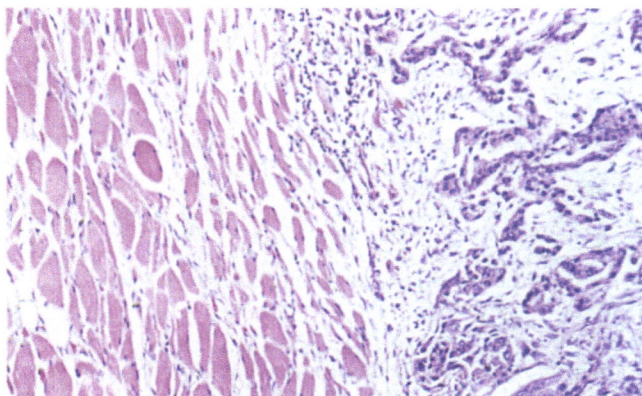

Figure 18.21 Metastatic carcinoma. Nodule in muscle showing boundary with normal tissue. Atrophic muscle fibres adjacent to the expanding tumour. H & E × 75

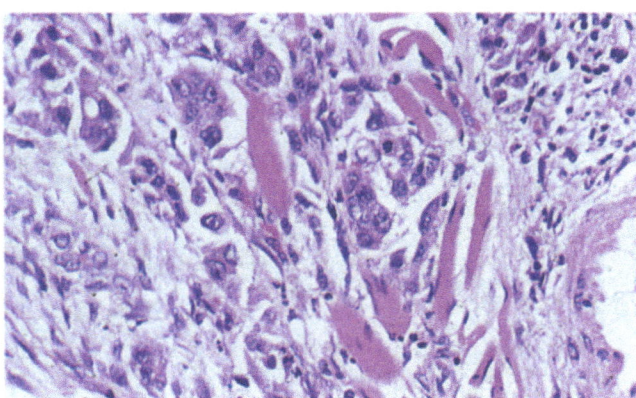

Figure 18.22 Metastatic carcinoma. Adenocarcinoma cells surrounding and obliterating skeletal muscle fibres at the infiltrating edge of the tumour deposit. H & E × 180

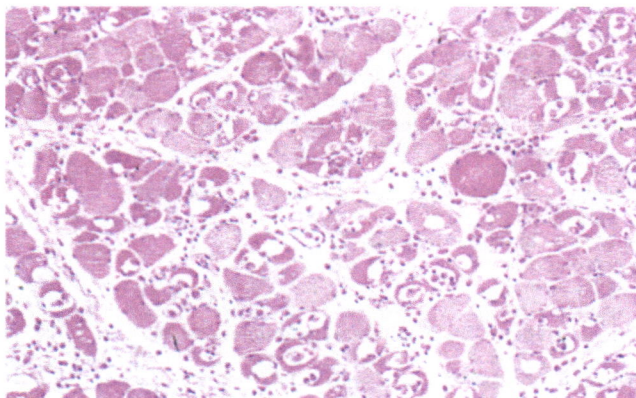

Figure 18.23 Intracellular malignant cells. Muscle obtained at postmortem from intracellular metastases in muscle obtained at postmortem from a patient with disseminated malignant histiocytosis associated with coeliac disease. At low magnification the muscle has the appearance of a vacuolar myopathy. This is due to cytoplasmic vacuoles containing malignant cells. (Same case shown in Figure 18.24.) H & E × 75

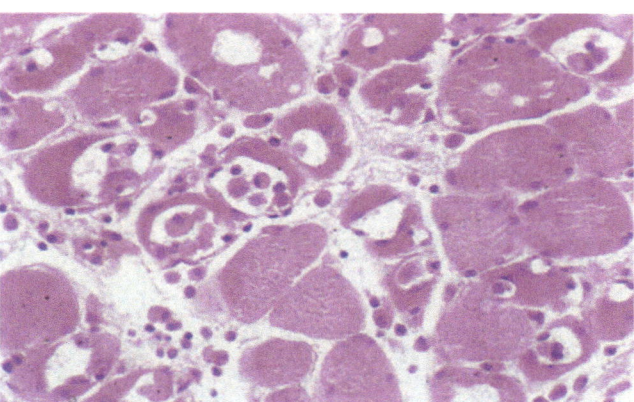

Figure 18.24 Intracellular malignant cells. Cytoplasmic vacuoles contain the malignant histiocytic cells, but the muscle cell membranes appear intact and the rest of the fibres show normal cytoplasm. H & E × 180

Index